CU00943090

Murky waters

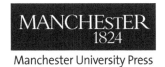

MANCHESTER
1824
Manchester University Press

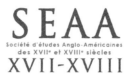

SEVENTEENTH- AND EIGHTEENTH-CENTURY STUDIES

Seventeenth- and Eighteenth-Century Studies promotes interdisciplinary work on the period c.1603–1815, covering all aspects of the literature, culture and history of the British Isles, colonial North America and the early United States, other British colonies and their global connections. The series welcomes academic monographs, as well as collective volumes of essays that combine theoretical and methodological approaches from more than one discipline to further our understanding of the period. It is supported by the Société d'Études Anglo-Américaines des XVIIe et XVIIIe siècles.

General editors
Ladan Niayesh, Université de Paris and Will Slauter, Sorbonne Université

Founding editor
Anne Dunan-Page

Advisory board
Bernadette Andrea, Daniel Carey, Rachel Herrman, Hannah Spahn, Claire Preston and Peter Thompson

To buy or to find out more about the books currently available in this series, please go to:
https://manchesteruniversitypress.co.uk/series/seventeenth-eighteenth-century-studies/
http://1718.fr/

Murky waters

British spas in eighteenth-century medicine and literature

Sophie Vasset

MANCHESTER UNIVERSITY PRESS

Copyright © Sophie Vasset 2022

The right of Sophie Vasset to be identified as the author of this work has been asserted by them in accordance with the Copyright, Designs and Patents Act 1988.

Published by Manchester University Press
Oxford Road, Manchester M13 9PL
www.manchesteruniversitypress.co.uk

British Library Cataloguing-in-Publication Data
A catalogue record for this book is available from the
British Library

ISBN   978 1 5261 5971 7   hardback

First published 2022

The publisher has no responsibility for the persistence or accuracy of URLs for any external or third-party internet websites referred to in this book, and does not guarantee that any content on such websites is, or will remain, accurate or appropriate.

Typeset
by New Best-set Typesetters Ltd

Contents

List of figures   *page* vi
Acknowledgements   viii

Introduction   1
1 Sick bodies   47
2 From bog to jug: a risky remedy?   82
3 Waters of desire: promiscuity, gender and sexuality   120
4 Pump room politics and the murky past of spas   163
5 Pumping and pouring: watering places and the
   money business   212
Conclusion   247
Appendix: Maps of eighteenth-century spas by
   category and by area   256

Bibliography   264
Index   280

Figures

0.1 J. Andrews, 'Map of the mineral waters and bathing places in England', 1797. Coloured etching, 50.5 × 39.5 cm. Private collection.　　　*page* 8

0.2 A map of spas in the British Isles in the long eighteenth century. © Sophie Vasset and Géotéca, Université de Paris.　　　10

0.3 Spas of the Greater London area, by category. © Sophie Vasset and Géotéca, Université de Paris.　　　13

0.4 Benjamin Allen, *The Natural History of the Mineral-Waters of Great-Britain*, London, 1711. © Wellcome Library.　　　16

0.5 'Shower' from Karl Ludwig von Pöllnitz, *Amusemens des eaux d'Aix-la-Chapelle. Ouvrage utile à ceux qui vont y prendre les bains, ou qui sont dans l'usage de ses eaux*, Amsterdam, 1736. © Bibliothèque Nationale de France.　　　22

0.6 'Steam bath' from Karl Ludwig von Pöllnitz, *Amusemens des eaux d'Aix-la-Chapelle. Ouvrage utile à ceux qui vont y prendre les bains, ou qui sont dans l'usage de ses eaux*, Amsterdam, 1736. © Bibliothèque Nationale de France.　　　23

3.1 T. Rowlandson, *Venus Bathing, A fashionable Dip*, c. 1800. Etching with hand colouring, 13.6 × 18.6 cm. © Wellcome Library.　　　125

3.2 T. Rowlandson, *Side Way or Any Way, Venus's Bathing (Margate)*, c. 1800. Etching with hand colouring, 13.6 × 18.6 cm. © Wellcome Library.　　　126

3.3 'The Charms of Dishabille' from *The Musical Entertainer*, 1733. © Trustees of the British Museum. 132

3.4 Frontispiece to 'The Humours of the New Tunbridge Wells at Islington', 1734. 133

3.5 William Faithorne, Frontispiece to Rawlins's play *Tunbridge-Wells*, 1678. Engraving on paper, 19 × 17.1 cm. © Trustees of the British Museum. 145

4.1 'Dickie Dickinson, Governor of Scarborough Spa', 1725. Engraving. © Trustees of the British Museum. 176

4.2 'A Scene at Cheltenham', 1788. Hand-coloured etching, 23 × 34.4 cm. © Trustees of the British Museum. 181

4.3 John Fayram, The Melfort monument in the cross bath, 1739. Engraving. © Bath Reference Library. 183

4.4 Broadside sheet: 'A Description of St. Winefred's at Holy-Well in Flintshire', 1784. 201

A1 Spas by category in the long eighteenth century – Ireland. © Sophie Vasset and Géotéca, Université de Paris. 258

A2 Spas by category in the long eighteenth century – Scotland. © Sophie Vasset and Géotéca, Université de Paris. 259

A3 Spas by category in the long eighteenth century – Wales. © Sophie Vasset and Géotéca, Université de Paris. 260

A4 Spas by category in the long eighteenth century – North England and Yorkshire. © Sophie Vasset and Géotéca, Université de Paris. 261

A5 Spas by category in the long eighteenth century – The Midlands and the East. © Sophie Vasset and Géotéca, Université de Paris. 262

A6 Spas by category in the long eighteenth century – South England. © Sophie Vasset and Géotéca, Université de Paris. 263

Acknowledgements

The first version of this book was presented as part of my *Habilitation à Diriger des Recherches* (Sorbonne-Université, November 2020) and I am grateful to Alexis Tadié, my mentor, for his careful comments on the manuscript and patient revision of the various stages of the work. His support and availability are only matched by the insight of his comments. I am also grateful to the members of the *Habilitation* jury, Daniel Carey, Micheline Louis-Courvoisier, Florence March and Frédéric Ogée, for their precious feedback, which helped me revise and improve the manuscript.

This book would never have been written without the support of the CNRS (Centre National de Recherche Scientifique), which gave me the opportunity to be on research leave (*délégation*) at IHRIM-Clermont. My colleagues Sophie Chiari and Samuel Cuisinier-Delorme's initiative to launch a conference (now a book) on spas in early modern culture provided a wonderful context for my research.

Three research groups at Université de Paris have given me the proper moral, technical and financial support to complete this project: the LARCA (dir. Cécile Roudeau), the 'Person in Medicine Institute' (dir. Céline Lefève) and the Géotéca team of cartographers who worked on all the maps, a two-year-long project led by Violaine Jurie. I am most thankful to my colleagues and friends at Université de Paris, especially Ariane Fennetaux, Ariane Hudelet, François Zanetti and Marine Bellégo for their encouraging feedback throughout.

I would also like to thank the directors of this collection at SEAA17–18: Anne Page, Marie-Jeanne Rossignol, Will Slauter and especially Ladan Niayesh, who supported the project from the beginning and was extremely helpful through the editing process, together with Meredith Carroll.

This book was written in what has been facetiously called by J. Miezkowski the 'long twenty-first century', spanning the years 2020–21. The background setting – numerous lockdowns and constraints, from round-the-clock childcare to online crisis meetings – was far from the quiet retreat and multiple field trips I had envisioned when applying for research leave. In 2020, Bénédicte Miyamoto launched an online writing group which helped us preserve space and time to work efficiently, and I know I won't be the only author in our group to thank her. Antoine Dabrowski, Renaud Boutin and Guillaume Mory generously helped our queer and lively family in so many ways, stepping up for childcare in the midst of serious lockdowns when we most needed it, and I could not have written this book in two years without them. My deepest thanks also go to my parents, and my parents-in-law for their support and care, from a safe sanitary distance to a safe vaccinated proximity. To my children, Irène and Axel, who know more about eighteenth-century spas than any eight- or ten-year-old should, I am grateful for their love and patience. To my wife, Anne Crémieux, I am beyond grateful: she has carefully read, amended and improved my writing with her rhythmical sentences and the occasional pun, and should any clumsy turn of phrase emerge from beneath the clear waters of her revisions, errors remain my own. This book is dedicated to her, and to the amazing collaborator that she has been these past seven years as co-director of the Fondation des États-Unis at Cité internationale universitaire de Paris.

Introduction

It is astonishing to discover how few mineral waters in Britain have survived into the twenty-first century.[1] In France and Germany, many medicinal spas outlived the decline of hydrotherapy in the twentieth century as medical and commercial strategies thrived to promote them, focusing on well-being and chronic diseases.[2] French patients can have their yearly water cure reimbursed by social security if prescribed by a doctor, and one may still bathe in the mineral waters of Vichy, Plombières, Balaruc or Saint-Gervais-les-Bains. By contrast, twenty-first-century English 'spas' tend to refer to luxury services in hotels that do not use mineral waters even when they are located in a spa town like Scarborough, Bristol or Buxton. The Victorian Turkish Baths at Harrogate work with common water. Even better: over the tap that delivers the stinking sulphurous mineral waters outside of the Royal Pump Room stands a sign that reads 'do not drink'. Mineral waters in Cheltenham, Tunbridge and Stoney Middleton in Derbyshire can only be tasted during the summer season as a tourist attraction staged with nostalgic narratives of past grandeur, pump room music and cotillon balls.

The spas of eighteenth-century Britain were numerous, uneven in size, purpose and success, yet all endowed with ambiguous attraction in the publications that celebrated or criticised them. The experience of treatment extended far beyond the pleasant musical walks in between two glasses at the pump room. It was, at best, disagreeable, often an ordeal. The many layers of society shared the experience of a spa town for a season, and sick bodies took centre stage. The very idea of grandeur only concerned the few towns that could invest in architectural developments. Some spa towns were complete failures. Others, like a bubble, rose quickly and disappeared even quicker. For some investors, spas, when properly managed or conveniently located, yielded considerable profits, but others saw their financial dreams gulped down in a sinkhole. From Restoration to Regency, there were up to two hundred locations in Britain, ranging from simple wells to large spa towns, where the waters were generally acknowledged to be medicinal.[3]

The study of the development of spas has been caught in the historical arch-narrative of 'the commercialisation of leisure'. The association of spas with pleasure gardens and early tourism may have resulted in some neglect of the genuine physical distress of spa visitors and the partial relief that the sick seemed to obtain from the water treatment – enough, at least, to go back.[4] Another narrative that recent historians of medicine have been uncomfortable with is the concept of the 'medicalisation' of social and religious practices in the eighteenth century and, in this case, the medicalisation of sacred waters.[5] As I focus the 'murkiness' of spa towns from a literal and figurative point of view, I would like to shift attention away from the polite picture of elite sociability and examine the underpinnings of this elegant social fabric. I started writing this book to challenge the notion that medical treatment was a pretext for visiting watering places in eighteenth-century Britain and to reassert the centrality of sickness and care in spa towns. In doing so, I have launched a larger exploration of eighteenth-century representations of spa visitors and of the people who took care of them, the discourse on the waters, and the medical and social life which unfolded within the great variety of British spas.

Bath and beyond

It is quite impossible to embark on an analysis of spa cultures in eighteenth-century Britain without mentioning Bath. Bath is the first image that comes to mind when eighteenth-century spas are evoked: many fictions are set in Bath and scholarly research abounds, not to mention the exceptional collections at Bath Record Office.[6] The city of Bath has maintained its spa, which siphons the memory of British mineral waters into one exceptional watering place. In Bath, one can bathe in the mineral waters at the New Bath Spa, visit the Roman baths, have breakfast or attend a concert in the pump room, and nibble on Bath buns in a Georgian tea-room while reading about the history of their inventor, Dr William Oliver, one of the famous eighteenth-century 'Bath doctors'.[7] Bath epitomises the experience of the English spa, locating it in the long eighteenth century. The Janeite undertones of a Bath visit make it impossible to escape Austen's portrait in cameo, suggesting that her works define the essence of a spa visit.[8] This book challenges such heritage and centralised views of eighteenth-century British spas by plunging into darker or simply less glamorous representations than those usually associated with Bath, namely well-being, leisure and polite sociability.

The history of other spa towns, wells or early seaside resorts is mostly covered by local or popular history from the 1980s, and few books among these, with the exception of Katherine Denbigh and the nineteenth-century medical doctor A. B. Granville, give a survey of the many spas of Britain.[9] Phyllis Hembry's systematic 1990 investigation into English spas remains the referential scholarly work on the subject. Eighteenth-century printed texts on Bath are copious and diverse, ranging from medical treatises and controversies to songs and satirical poems. By contrast, the publications on the remaining 345 spas, springs and watering places vary greatly in quantity, genre and tone. Some small cold-water spas, like St Mungo's Well in Yorkshire, generated a lot of medical literature, medium-sized spa towns like Scarborough had their own yearly publication of miscellanies, while some highly visited places like Bristol Hotwells are surprisingly largely absent from contemporary writings.

Spa towns are caught in a network of comparisons. Much as any town in Europe with more than three canal ways is likely dubbed the 'Venice' of its region, any spa town with a pump room and a well would call itself 'rival to Bath'. Bath, by contrast, aspired to European fame, and compared itself to other watering places on the continent, looking towards Vichy in France, Baden-Baden in Germany, and Spa in Belgium. John Wood's architectural designs had inscribed Bath's urban aesthetics in the Georgian period, making it an early, self-contained example of urban planning.[10] In medicine, Bath was a centre for medical scholars, the multiple analyses performed on the waters being the object of several controversies, while the General Infirmary stood as a model for the monitoring of the sick poor.[11] Bath was also known for its cultural life, attracting the best performers of the time. The figure of its master of ceremonies, Beau Nash, stands out. He presided over social gatherings, balls, concerts and games for fifty-seven seasons, from 1704 to 1761.[12] Bath, therefore, cannot be excluded from this book, but will be taken for what it was: an exception that should be acknowledged as such; a model and a counter-model for the spas that developed in the long eighteenth century, not an example like any other, and certainly not a representative example of the wider phenomenon of eighteenth-century British spas.

In the first part of this introduction, I would like to give an overview of spas other than Bath. Beyond Hembry's remarkable inventory of English spas published in 1990, little work has been done to categorise the remaining 346 spas and wells of eighteenth-century Britain. In fact, they are regularly represented as a single, undifferentiated phenomenon generating a bulk of indistinct medical and literary writings, mostly spurred by commercial interest. In her introduction to the study of the Scottish spa town of Moffat, Katharine Glover confirms and deplores the lack of proper analytical tools that such categories would provide: 'Although Moffat was perhaps distinctive in its status as a "national institution" for the Scottish elite', she writes, 'there were many such smaller spas across Britain, yet remarkably little scholarly interest has been paid to their social function, particularly in comparison with that lavished on their more glamorous counterparts, most notably Bath'.[13] The reason for such a lack might lie in a tendency to reduce the proliferation of spas to a fashionable phenomenon.[14] Recent scholarly work has shown that fashion is neither despicable nor self-explanatory, and I will come back to these notions when dealing with the question of medical publicity in the second chapter.[15]

For now, I would like to establish a few elements of classification in this introduction to explain where spas were located, what services were provided there, and what kind of treatment was to be found.[16] Eighteenth-century British spas can be organised in four main categories, along the following criteria: architectural size, medical repute, cultural life and attractivity. The various terms of 'spa', 'spa town', 'watering place', 'springs' and 'wells' overlap in their use and meaning, and such categorisation is meant to disentangle the multiple realities of the places in which one could find therapeutic waters.[17] The development of spa towns has too often been presented as one unfathomable and ever-evolving group of minor spas that attempted – and often failed – to mimic Bath, which is a category of its own, since it entertained unequalled fame and outreach on the continent. Some spa towns, in fact, grew quite independently of the image of Bath, and were sometimes preferred by royal visitors, while others attracted pilgrims and sick people from the lower classes, and others still built their reputation on a specific treatment.

A first category consists of national spa towns, attracting visitors from all over the country and occasionally beyond the national borders. Their reputation grew through the protection and financial support of royal and noble patronage. As a result, they could invest in urban developments, provide public spaces for gathering, gardens and walks, build lodgings for their visitors, and erect premises for a variety of entertainments. The social life of their visitors was monitored and centralised during a specific season and some spas were careful to keep their seasons apart.[18] Entertainments were often overseen by a master of ceremonies according to a schedule published in the town, and in guidebooks. This category includes the main spa towns, in chronological order of their development and success: Buxton (1620s), Tunbridge Wells (1660s), Epsom (1670s), Harrogate (1710s), Bristol Hotwells (1720s), Cheltenham (1750s) and Malvern (1760s).[19] The sick would take the waters in various ways, drinking or bathing, and sometimes from various springs within the same spa town which conveniently offered diverse chemical components. Buxton had one chalybeate and eight saline springs; Harrogate boasted five different wells in the mid-eighteenth century; while in the early nineteenth century, the Cheltenham waters could be tasted in four different wells.[20]

A second category comprises local spas which enjoyed a good reputation in their surroundings – and sometimes beyond – and were often supported by noble patronage. They were the object of one or several treatises and could easily become the subject of a poem or a play. They invested in their housing capacity for new visitors, as well as in facilities to provide additional entertainment such as balls, plays or concerts. Dulwich in Lewisham (London area), Matlock in Derbyshire and Llandrindod Wells in Wales were all reasonably attractive and depended on the will of a few local people for their maintenance rather than on organised corporations as in larger spa towns. They were therefore more fragile and less sustainable. Occasional distinguished visitors were recorded and celebrated, improving the reputation of the spa, or undoing it if the visit were unsatisfactory. Most of them kept a 'season' during which concerts and entertainments were provided, and the life of visitors could be monitored by a schedule which started with early morning drinking and ended with early evening balls or games.

A third category of mineral waters – the largest by far – consisted in local wells or springs that would occasionally include extra installations to access the waters: a shed to protect visitors from the rain, a rail or a stone wall around the well. Some of these were located in the close environment of a more established spa town, while others could be lost in the woods or in the hills of a mining area, such as the multiple wells of Yorkshire inventoried by Thomas Short in 1734.[21] Many a London spa, like St Govor's Well in Kensington Gardens or the chalybeate well of Notting Hill House, enjoyed a neighbourhood reputation and could be the subject of a medical or a local pamphlet.[22] The reputation of some of these wells could extend beyond the local clientele when their waters were thought to have specific medicinal properties. St Mungo's Well in Yorkshire, for example, reputed to cure children's diseases, was regularly mentioned in early eighteenth-century treatises on cold water.[23]

A fourth, and perhaps more surprising, category includes early seaside resorts and mixed mineral water and sea water spa towns like Scarborough, Brighton and Weymouth. Although seaside resorts are often seen as a phenomenon that emerged in the late eighteenth century, and heralded a major shift in early tourism, I argue that a survey of the discourse on watering places in the long eighteenth century cannot exclude seaside villages, let alone the therapeutic use of sea water. First, the presence of both mineral and sea water in the same place justifies it. When George III visited Weymouth in 1789, he enjoyed both sea-bathing and drinking the sulphurous waters of Nottington Well.[24] Secondly, the idea of a 'watering place' by the 1750s would be inclusive of Margate and Ramsgate, which had no mineral water but offered medical treatment, as Richard Russell explains in his treatise on the use of sea water first published in 1753.[25] Of course, the presence of the sea, and the proximity of harbours and seaside market towns, gave these spas a specific character that would later evolve into another type of resort, but this is a retrospective take on their history. As I hope to show with several examples throughout the book, eighteenth-century seaside watering places should be considered as a sub-category of spa towns.

Further scholarly work is needed to refine these categories and understand the social and economic dynamics of each.[26] Undoubtedly, the proliferation of watering places entailed strategies of competition and rivalry in the writings meant to promote them. Most famously, the racy satirical poem published at the end of the seventeenth century, *An Exclamation from Tunbridge and Epsom against the Newfound Wells at Islington*, stages the two older spas in a mock attack of their newly created rival, denoting fierce competition:

> Behold the fickleness of *Fortunes* Wheel! The instability of things under the *changeable* Moon! So shall you find it foretold in *Mother Shipton Manuscript Prophecies* (never yet printed) p. 409:
>
> Tunbridge was, Epsom is, Islington shall be
>
> The greatest Bog-house of the squittering three.[27]

The scatological imagery evoking the purging effects of the waters is only matched by the disparaging view of fashionable places, where spa towns compete for attention. Such gendered representation of spas and their fashion victims ready to kill each other for a beauty prize may have influenced later representations of spa towns as run by the fickle tides of fashion. Yet, the urban historian Peter Borsay gives a more nuanced account of this competition, asserting that 'The relationships between towns could also be of a non-competitive, supportive nature. Malvern benefited from the expansion of Cheltenham in the early nineteenth century, acting as an overflow for it. Small watering places might profit from the proximity of larger ones.'[28] The ambivalent relationship between spa towns and local spas of a competitive, supportive, and complementary nature can be seen as a form of 'coopetition', a term used by sociologists to describe twenty-first-century spa towns.[29]

Putting spas on the map, over- and underground

Location was a main factor in the emergence of a spa town, from their mineral origins underground to their accessibility over ground. Although many synopses and lists of mineral waters by type, region and country were available, very few maps of British mineral waters were published in the eighteenth century. I was only acquainted with one map of English spas, established in John Andrews's 1797 *Historical Atlas of England*.[30] Andrews's beautiful map (Figure 0.1) is most probably based on medical publications such as Rutty and Short's.[31] Just like them, Andrews considers mineral waters in their

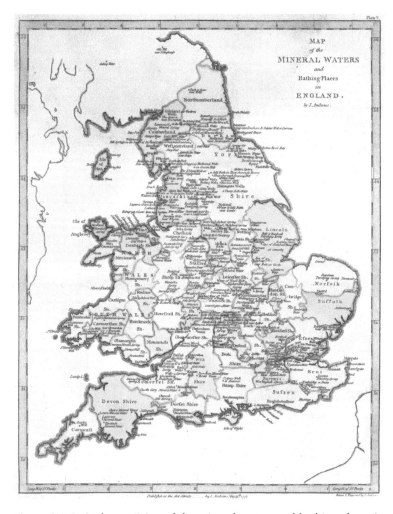

Figure 0.1 J. Andrews, 'Map of the mineral waters and bathing places in England', 1797, private collection.

great variety, from the 'medicine water near Brancepeth' in County Durham to the multiple petrifying wells and springs, both a visitor's attraction and an opportunity to try calcareous waters. The map thus charts all watering places, including seaside resorts, wells, springs and even some lakes of Cumberland and Derbyshire. Although the map is hard to read in a regular book format, it clearly shows that spa towns were not evenly distributed in eighteenth-century England, and that their density is greater inland than on the coastal regions.

In the twentieth century, Phyllis Hembry's map published in *The English Spa*, which lists 152 English spas, reveals the density of spa towns between 1560 and 1815. Yet, like Andrews's map, it fails to acknowledge the size and period of each spa. A more specific overview of British spas in the long eighteenth century by period and by category can be found in the various maps at the end of this book. Based on a collaboration between historians and geographers, the map pictured in Figure 0.2 shows both density and size. It clearly appears that most English people were within reasonable distance of a middle-sized spa, and smaller spas were even more accessible, both in rural and urban areas.

The density of spas exceeded other regions in four main areas: Yorkshire, Derbyshire, the London area, and the Somerset region with the neighbouring country of Gloucestershire. These sites were perceived in the collective imagination of the country with cultural ramifications which extended far beyond the mere facts of topography, as some regions had rural, mining, coastal or urban identities.

Such was the case for Yorkshire, famous for the sulphurous waters of Harrogate and saline and chalybeate waters of Scarborough. The entire region was roamed by Thomas Short, a Sheffield-based water doctor of the mid-eighteenth century, who was eagerly searching for any kind of spring or well to measure the presence of minerals.[32] Yorkshire had started to develop its mining industry in the middle ages: collieries flourished in the western part and lead-mining in the Dales. In his books, Short draws on regional knowledge about digging for coal and finding water or identifying different kinds of gas. He also collected local histories and anecdotes from miners, which gave him information about the geological components of the underground, the lines of metal and mineral seams. Just south of Yorkshire, the abundance of spas in Derbyshire and Leicestershire in the East Midlands could also be explained by the rich and varied composition

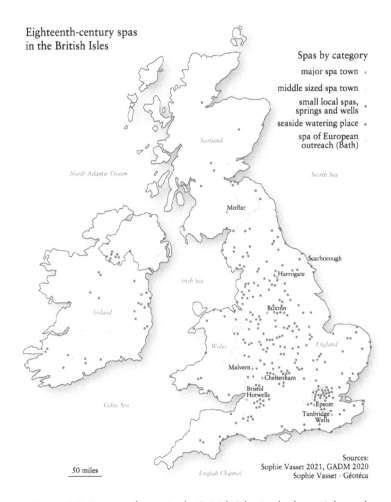

Eighteenth-century spas
in the British Isles

Spas by category

major spa town .

middle sized spa town

small local spas,
springs and wells

seaside watering place .

spa of European
outreach (Bath)

North Atlantic Ocean

Scotland

North Sea

Moffat

Scarborough

Harrogate

Irish Sea

Buxton

Ireland

Wales

England

Malvern

Cheltenham

Bristol
Hotwells

Celtic Sea

Epsom
Tunbridge
Wells

50 miles

English Channel

Sources:
Sophie Vasset 2021, GADM 2020
Sophie Vasset - Géotéca

Figure 0.2 A map of spas in the British Isles in the long eighteenth
century

of the soil. At the turn of the nineteenth century, for example, the
Moira waters in north Leicestershire were found within a coal mine
and attracted visitors directly to the pit.

The early success of Buxton in the Peak District, in north-west
Derbyshire, probably spurred surrounding towns to look for their
own mineral springs. The town of Matlock, for example, was yet
another spring discovered by miners, where investors successfully

improved the premises as the reputation of the spa steadily grew to become an important centre for hydropathy in the nineteenth century. Similar logic must have prompted the cities of Somerset and Gloucestershire in the south-west to invest in the spas and springs they found in the hilly and fertile grounds of the Cotswolds and wetlands of north Somerset. Bath, Bristol, Cheltenham and Malvern were close to each other, and sick patients could travel from one spa to another within a day. Contrary to Yorkshire, however, the Somerset and Gloucestershire area saw its larger spa towns prosper more than small wells or local springs. Finally, the attraction for coastal spas and warmer weather were certainly instrumental in the development of the spas of the south, in Sussex and Kent. Brighton and Southampton both offered mineral water-drinking and sea water-bathing, which was an advantage over the towns of Margate and Ramsgate that relied only on the medicinal properties of sea water promoted in 1753 by Richard Russell.[33]

Many spa towns were seen as distinct from other provincial market towns as they provided a rural experience imbued with elaborate pastoral aesthetics. According to Barbara Benedict, the idealised countryside of provincial spa towns was emphasised by architects, editors of miscellanies and promoters of early tourism in discourses which turned nature into a commodity.[34] The organised consumption of nature was encouraged by a larger medical environment, influenced by the Hippocratic revival of the previous century, and especially by the treatise *Air, Water, Situation*.[35] Provincial spas, with their wholesome air, carefully crafted natural environment and healing waters, could be seen as an early form of environmental medicine which counteracted the growing anxiety about the toxicity of urban environments.[36] Towns and cities were perceived as unwholesome for several reasons: not only did urban crowds and narrow streets create a sense of suffocation in some metropolitan centres, but, more broadly, the urban atmosphere was thought to be toxic because of a medical belief in the quality of air and airborne particles bringing diseases.[37]

Paradoxically, watering places stood on the continuum between town and country, especially in the Georgian era, after the major improvement of roads and turnpikes made them more accessible.[38] Revising the spatial categories that tended to oppose country house and cottage to city buildings, Borsay explains: 'From early on, watering-places had been constructed and projected to reflect the ideal of *rus in urbe*'.[39] The urban design of spa towns celebrated nature with its multiple gardens, cascades, vistas, walks and promenades. Borsay even notes that 'the spas in close vicinity to the metropolis, such as Epsom and Tunbridge Wells, were particularly prone to this treatment, clearly intended to satisfy the Londoners' appetite for the pastoral myth'.[40] Spas in and around London have often been neglected in historical studies of spas as they do not fit the countryside vision of spa towns as a resort out of the city, and yet a quick look at a map of early modern spa towns shows their pre-eminence (Figure 0.3). The density of spas is striking for the London area and its neighbouring counties, Surrey, Hertfordshire and Essex.

The proliferation of London spas in the eighteenth century was the product of both contextual and geological causes. First, the growing success of spas in other regions attracting the citizens of London out of town inspired several investors in the metropolis to seek profit from such interest in mineral waters.[41] Medieval holy wells no longer in use since the Reformation reappeared, such as St Chad's in north London. Some were 'rediscovered' in forgotten cellars, most famously Sadler's Wells in Islington, which rose to fame during the Restoration as 'The New Tunbridge Wells'.[42] Secondly, the underlying geology of the British capital and its surrounding counties was exceptionally fertile for water sources (whether mineral or common), as is the case for most European capitals. Again, the development of turnpikes, roads and coaches made it possible to take a day trip and escape to a semi-rural environment just outside of London. As Mrs Rubrick explains to her sister in the 1779 comedy by George Colman, *The spleen, or, Islington Spa*: 'Come! Don't be uneasy though the family are at such a *distance*! There's above forty coaches pass within a hundred yards of the place every day, and you may hear of us every quarter of an hour'.[43] According to Elizabeth McKellar, the relationship between centre and periphery in eighteenth-century London should be redefined by focusing on the example of Richmond and Islington:

> [T]he spas adjacent to London marketed themselves as a more convenient alternative to those further afield, particularly Epsom and Tunbridge Wells. To emphasize the purity of their product, the spa owners sought to perpetuate a rustic environment redolent of healthiness

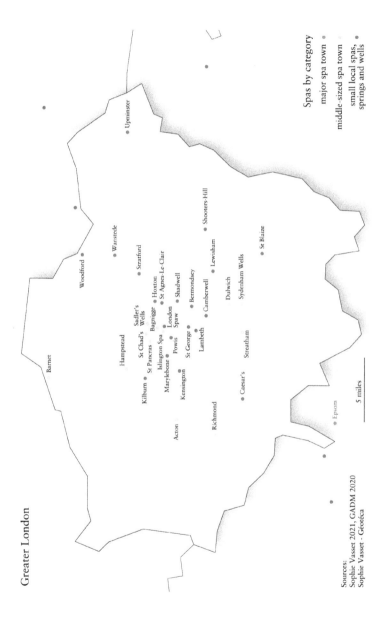

Figure 0.3 Spas of the Greater London area, by category

and tranquillity, even paradoxically, as this was being undermined by the large number of townspeople who flocked to them.[44]

Outside of the city, any town that could boast of a spa would have an interest in developing its facilities and offering easy access, which explains the emergence of a 'ring of spas' in the counties surrounding London.[45]

London was also in dialogue with other spas, much farther afield, in the countries colonised by the British. In the non-European contexts of colonised territories overseas, mineral waters could stir up local political and religious debates between the colonised and colonisers. Spa towns flourished in Jamaica, as the mountains were abundant with hot springs, and the south east colonies of North America. The springs of Virginia, called Bath and White Suphur were thoroughly analysed by the physician Benjamin Rush, and as Charlene Lewis and Vaughn Scribner explain, became a place of cure and sociability for planters.[46] Closer to the English capital, Scotland, Wales and Ireland had their own spas, which generated representations in dialogue with renowned English spas, yet remained specific to each culture. Scottish spas and seaside resorts, as Alastair Durie explains, were promoted and closely investigated by the great number of Scottish doctors disseminated in all the territories of eighteenth-century Britain.[47] Donald Monro and William Buchan wrote about them, and the centrality of Moffat, the genteel source of the Lowlands studied by Katharine Glover,[48] did not prevent other spa towns like Peterhead, Pannanich and Pitkeathly from flourishing in the second half of the eighteenth century. Even more than in Scotland, numerous waters in Wales and Ireland were pivotal points of a Catholic culture of thaumaturgic waters inherited from medieval holy wells.[49] The aggressive discourse of English and recently converted Irish Protestant crusaders against these spas did not prevent other Protestant users from taking the waters.

Stone, salt and metal: the minerals in mineral waters

Beyond size and place, geology mattered. Spa waters were called 'mineral waters', whether they were bottled and drunk or applied externally, which emphasised the presence of the mineral components of the water rather than its warmth as was the case with thermal waters. Mineral waters thus crossed the path of the natural history of minerals celebrated in Pope's grotto, and the development of the mining industry.[50] A lot of treatises gave a thorough account of the exploration, measurement and analysis of mineral content as a key to evaluate healing potential. The emphasis on the minerality of waters was partly inherited from earlier medicine and natural history, such as Georgius Agricola's treatise, *De Re Metallica* (1556), in which water is seen as the mobilising factor for all minerals, as suggested by Tiffany Werth.[51] In William Baily's late sixteenth-century *Discourse on certain Bathes*, Werth retrieved a remarkable oxymoron expressing the minerality of spa waters. 'There is in these waters some stone juice', Baily writes, observing how the deposits of the evaporated waters on objects form a crust.[52]

To make these microscopic mineral particles visible to his readers, Benjamin Allen inserts a plate at the beginning of his *Natural History of Mineral-Waters* published in 1711 (Figure 0.4).[53] It displays the various forms of salts present in the water, and their specific appearance. Just like the expression 'stone juice', this plate shifts the attention from the liquid tangibility of water to its invisible solid elements, especially as salts were recognisable by their shape.[54] In fact, drinkers and bathers could well perceive the presence of solids as many waters were literally murky: a glass of mineral waters was likely to be thick and cloudy, leaving red iron stains or a beige crust on the taps that delivered them or at the bottom of a basin.

The Yorkshire physician Thomas Short still defined the waters along these lines in 1765: 'By Mineral Waters are intended such as contain, or bring along with them, in their Interstices or Pores, Particles of Minerals of one or more Kinds, in greater or lesser Quantities or Proportions'.[55] Short is adamant to draw a clear distinction between common and mineral waters, adding that the latter 'derive to the simple Vehicle some notable Properties beyond common Water, or additional Improvements, or natural Assistants to it, to the great Benefit of the Sick'.[56] Many of the mineral elements found in spa waters could be identified through several processes such as distillation, evaporation, cooking, microscope observation and dyeing by dipping oak galls in the water.[57] A few British doctors launched systematic studies of waters and established detailed comparative classification tables for the waters they collected.[58] The aim was to

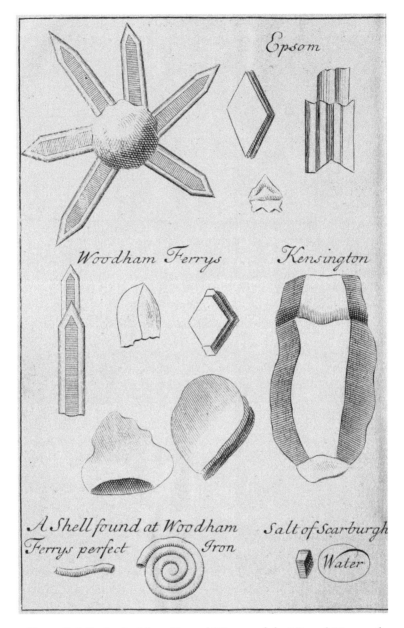

Figure 0.4 Benjamin Allen, *Natural History of the Mineral-Waters of Great-Britain*, 1711

understand their composition in minerals and gas, which the physicians called 'apporhea', or 'volatile parts'. Mineral waters were thus perceived as the powerful reunion of three of the four elements – earth, air and water. Upon the examination of the Malvern waters, for example, John Wall concludes that 'there is also a fine, subtle, penetrating Spirit conceal'd in these Waters'.[59] Water doctors tried to make their readers measure the action of invisible elements in the water through notions of subtlety, volatility and permeability.

Although many tools were available for the analysis of mineral waters, the place of early chemistry within the larger range of early medicine and science practice was ambivalent. Christopher Hamlin explains that 'promoters of springs were usually willing to seek out good news where it could be found'[60] and turned to the analyses of contents to attest to the presence of active minerals. He observes an evolution in the status of chemistry throughout the century, which gradually served as a discourse of legitimisation for the medical use of waters, even though physicians and apothecaries did not rely solely on chemical analyses and complemented them with numerous case studies and other principles of mechanical medicine. As Noel Coley argues, the methods of analysis fluctuated, the composition of the minerals contained in the water were similar to each other, and the density of the elements in a specific water was unstable as it depended on the season, the climate and the hour of extraction.[61] This, together with the competitive context of spa medicine in eighteenth-century Britain, resulted in several controversies, most famously the sulphur controversy over the Bath waters. Other controversies focused either on particular spas such as the waters of Scarborough just after the Restoration, or on the solvability of a particular element in water such as 'fixed air' (carbon dioxide).[62]

The status of eighteenth-century chemistry has sometimes been simplified in a linear narrative of Enlightenment science, in which it would have gradually been disentangled from alchemy and improved in status to become a leading discipline in the nineteenth century. And yet, the differentiation between chemistry and alchemy was not clear-cut in early modern science, as William Newman and Lawrence Principe have made clear.[63] Alchemy, they argue, cannot be reduced to the mere study of metallic transmutations: some of Newton's works, for example, are largely indebted to alchemy.[64]

The complex status of chemistry was thus reflected in the controversies on the components of water and methods of analysis. Clearly, several physicians writing on mineral waters wanted to differentiate themselves from those who, like Thomas Short or his rival Peter Shaw, were committed to taking down the results of their experiments on waters at various times of the day and night, in various climates and various seasons.[65] These chemical disputes remained hard to decipher for other physicians and laymen. The extended chemical analyses of waters tended to be distilled into more digestible notions of water types that could easily be identified by potential visitors and their medical advisors.

What were, then, the main mineral components of the waters? In their analyses, physicians and apothecaries found metal (iron and copper), sulphur, limestone and 'salts' (nitre, magnesia, sodium, vitriol, aluminium).[66] In the fashion of eighteenth-century natural historians, I will need to enter into another few principles of categorisation based on the early attempts of eighteenth-century water doctors to delineate the six main types of water. The most convincing and helpful summary is undoubtedly to be found in William Buchan's pedagogical appendix to his 1786 edition of *Domestic Medicine*. Buchan saw that the practice of taking the waters had been increasing and he found it necessary to deliver 'a few hints or cautions to persons who bathe, or drink the mineral waters, without being able to put themselves under the care of a physician'.[67] In his *Cautions Concerning Cold Bathing, and Drinking the Mineral Waters* he identified four main categories of mineral waters:

> [M]ineral waters are classed as hot and cold, and as Chalybeate, Saline, Sulphureous, and Calcareous, as they are impregnated with iron, salts, sulphur, or lime. Chalybeates may be distinguished as simple chalybeates, having no prominent impregnation but iron; and saline or purgative chalybeates, having a strong mixture of purging salts, which are very different from the others, both in taste and effect. Tunbridge is at the head of the former, and Cheltenham of the latter class.[68]

Most water doctors agreed with the first three categories, but on the last there was less consensus and it was often divided into sub-categories. Other eighteenth-century water doctors, namely Linden, Rutty, Short and Allen, usually classified the waters in the following categories: chalybeate waters, containing iron, with their unmistakable reddish taint; saline or purging waters containing salts such as nitre, magnesium or alum; a compound of saline and iron commonly called 'chalybeate purging'; sulphurous waters easily identifiable by a smell of rotten eggs; and, finally, calcareous waters, also called 'steamy' because they were thought to be extremely volatile, with a component of limestone. Among these, sea water, prescribed and drunk like the others, was often included as a sub-category of the saline.[69] And yet, strict categorisation would be too reductive of the multiple attempts and methods of mineral water analysis: the identification of chemical components often led to the conclusion that the waters under study were unique in their combination of minerals. The analysers also gauged other aspects of the waters, such as warmth, thickness or unctuosity, and the presence of gas. These categories were thus made to make the variety of spas readable to a wider public and helped identify certain elements and improve or reproduce them, but they were unstable and some of the water doctors disregarded them. The subtlety and complexity of waters' composition, which was an easy object of controversy, might explain the reluctance to use simpler categories.

Mineral waters could also be amended in their composition, as we will see in the first chapter, and physicians often prescribed them with additional drugs, either mixed with the waters, or administered before and after taking them. Several waters from the continent were bottled and exported to Britain, the most popular being the Spa, Pyrmont and Seltzer waters, but the mineral waters trade in Britain was alive and well.[70] What's more, with the technical developments of chemistry, some waters could be reproduced artificially.[71] Throughout the eighteenth century, artificial waters were being tested in various European capitals, and England acquired an artificial spa in Brighton in the early nineteenth century. Set up by German doctor Friedrich Struve, it brought a specific variety of reconstituted German spa waters to English patients.[72]

Water every way, and many drops to drink

As explained above, the medical approach to mineral waters was not limited to chemistry. Drinking and bathing were thought to put

the fibres and inner fluids in motion, which was highly encouraged
by early modern mechanical and humoral medical thought. In the
hundreds of treatises on mineral waters published in the eighteenth
century,[73] case histories almost always systematically accompanied
the results of analyses and provided their authors with a rhetoric
of proof which expertly navigated between miracle cure and clinical
observation.[74] They put forward specific ailments that would be
cured by the waters, and sometimes provided explanations for such
cures. I will enter into more detail on the various medical accounts
given for the healing processes of mineral waters in the first chapter
of this book. For now, suffice it to say that the main medical principles
invoked to account for the action of mineral waters were porosity,
nourishment, evacuation and fortification. As the skin was considered
porous, the minerals were thought to impregnate the body and
nourish the blood, juices and internal organs.[75] Conversely, after a
bath many patients were wrapped in blankets for an hour, which
increased sudation, promoting the evacuation of 'crudities' and other
unwanted fluids in the body. Finally, water temperature was thought
to have an effect on bodily fibres – muscles, nerves and the membranes
of the organs – relaxing them when hot, strengthening them if cold.
The solvent contained in the saline and calcareous waters was thought
to dissolve potential tumours, excrescences or anything that could
clog the circulating fluids. The 'drying' properties of sulphur were
considered helpful in skin diseases. The properties of each type of
water were not fixed, however, and varied according to the opinion
of doctors and patients.

The healing properties of mineral waters were nothing new for
eighteenth-century doctors and patients, as water treatment was
inherited from Antiquity and medieval medicine. Even 'modern'
doctors, who claimed to trust experiment more than early medical
works, mentioned the ancient use of Roman baths and thermae when
they wrote about Bath and Buxton,[76] establishing a connection with
the medical principles of Antiquity.[77] Naturally hot waters such as
in Bath were highly prized, as they did not require 'hypocausts',
the expensive installation of a furnace system underneath the *tepidarium* (hot baths), originally maintained by enslaved people, which
Antiquarians had recently discovered in various Roman thermae
and villas.[78] It would be tempting to see the revival of Roman
practices as part of a larger revival of Antiquity which pervaded the

neoclassical poetic and architectural revival of the times, but there is little evidence in literature confirming such representations. Later uses of water were equally influential on eighteenth-century water doctors, who inherited many principles from medieval medicine and early modern water treatises. Marylin Nicoud's analyses of European medieval treatises on mineral waters follows the development of several infrastructures in Poretta and Acqui Terme in the north of Italy, for example. She also shows how balneotherapy gained more ground in Germany between the fourteenth and sixteenth centuries. In parallel, she explains, medical dissertations on mineral waters became a recognisable genre of medical treatises in the fourteenth century.[79] Medicinal bathing was gradually distinguished from the recreational steam baths of medieval towns, which tended to be associated with brothels.[80] A continuity can therefore be established between the regulations dictated by fifteenth-century doctors and the cautionary prescriptions of eighteenth-century physicians. As David Harley recalls, a wrong prescription of mineral waters was seen as 'a sword in a madman's hand'.[81]

Early modern accounts of bathing practices seem to challenge the assumption that early modern bodies were not in regular contact with water, supported by historians of the body like George Vigarello.[82] In *Concepts of Cleanliness*, for example, Vigarello depicted the methods of 'dry cleaning' performed, with linen absorbing the sebum and sweat of the body, and the gradual defiance of public baths that developed throughout the sixteenth century. Bathing, Vigarello explains, was considered dangerous because the skin was believed to be porous to air and water. He describes the feeling of increased vulnerability as fears of contamination grew with the multiple plague epidemics of the sixteenth century:

> [A] frightful image of the body emerges from the first coordinated fights against the plague from the sixteenth century onwards: the body is thought to be composed of permeable envelopes. Its surface may be penetrated by water or by air, making its borders ever more uncertain against a disease whose materiality is invisible, and corporeal borders become even more indeterminate as the material aspects of contamination are invisible.[83]

For this very reason, however, doctors and patients strongly believed in the medicinal virtues of mineral waters: 'water that penetrates

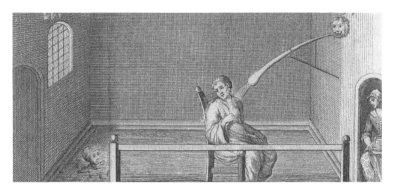

Figure 0.5 'Shower' from Karl Ludwig von Pöllnitz, *Amusemens des eaux d'Aix-la-Chapelle*, 1736

the skin implies specific manipulations. In some cases (at least for hydrotherapy), this mechanism is therapeutic.'[84]

In the eighteenth century, water treatment came in various ways. The method of treatment prescribed was as important – if not more so – than the composition of the waters taken. Doctors determined how, when and how much water should be drunk by their patients. 'Bathing' covered a variety of immersions, from walking or swimming in large pools to dipping one's body in a tank brought along to the wells and filled on the spot. The time spent in the water mattered, and so did the time spent sweating afterwards. In some bathing facilities, showers were available to modify the force of application onto the skin (Figure 0.5). There were also several forms of local applications, such as foot baths or covering one's limb with a wet cloth.[85] Steam baths revisited the medieval steam rooms: bathers took steam baths in individual wooden steam cabins or were exposed to steam spurting out of nozzles at the end of heating pipes (Figure 0.6). Finally, the waters could be drunk at the pump room, where glasses were distributed by water women, and passed from one person to the next, or at the wells where drinkers often had to bring their own tankard. The quantity ingested was usually gradually increased, accompanied by other drug treatments, based on how well the patient reacted to the cure.

Taking the waters was monitored, advised and prescribed by many 'water doctors' in the eighteenth century. By this I mean primarily the authors of medical treatises who claimed some degree of

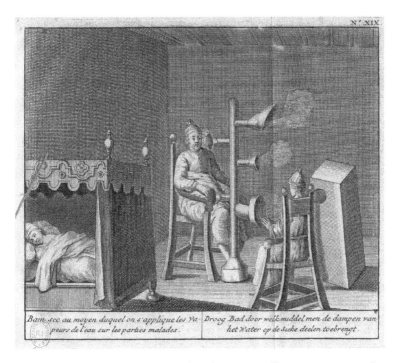

Figure 0.6 'Steam bath' from Karl Ludwig von Pöllnitz, *Amusemens des eaux d'Aix-la-Chapelle*, 1736

expertise in their accounts of mineral waters. Others had established a practice in a spa town where they would welcome patients sent by their local doctors to try the waters, follow them during the season and possibly correspond with them afterwards. Medical treatises on waters keep pointing out the risk taken by many patients who drink the waters with no prescription at all, an object of vexation and anxiety for the water doctors, as will be discussed in the second chapter. This category of self-prescribing patients is the target of William Buchan's cautionary advice which he contrasts with other water treatises: 'We have indeed many books on the mineral waters, and some of them are written with much ingenuity; but they are chiefly employed in ascertaining the contents of the waters by chymical analysis'.[86] While water treatises have often been perceived as a group of indeterminate writings engrossed in the promotion of a particular spa, some clarity can be brought to sort out the bulk of the production of writing doctors. In fact, Buchan's *Cautions Concerning Cold Bathing* itself belonged to a particular subgenre of mineral water treatises.

Water writings, from medicine to literature

In 1990, Christopher Hamlin criticised the recurrent trend among his fellow historians to disparage publications on mineral waters. Commenting on the historian William Addison's work on English spas in the 1950s, he wrote: 'like most later historians, Addison chose to see the spa mainly as a phenomenon of social history, of changes in manners, morals, and amusements. Yet our neglect of those thousands of often lengthy and passionate medical and chemical treatises and pamphlets is surely unwise.'[87] One step towards a clearer epistemological approach to water medicine is to determine the main trends in which these passionate debates were channelled. In medical treatises, as in other types of literature, each genre provides readers with a frame of expectations that helps them navigate through the text. Water doctors and authors writing on the medical properties of mineral waters generally chose to write in a particular pre-existing genre, be it a comparative treatise on several spas or on several types of bathing, a spa analysis, observations and case histories, a preventative treatise or a list of extraordinary cures. Books on mineral waters were often a mix of several genres, each of them requiring specific codes and conventions.

Among the medical treatises on waters published in the long eighteenth century, several subgenres can thus be identified: comparative treatises analysing the mineral composition of waters;[88] treatises focusing on the types of bathing, especially between cold and hot water such as John Floyer's *Psychrolousia*, and others focusing on the chemical analysis of one particular spa; compilations of observations written in the tradition of 'consilia' such as Pierce's 1697 treatise on Bath waters; preventative treatises extolling the long-term benefits of bathing and drinking; and, finally, lists of extraordinary cures verging on the style of quack pamphlets. Medical advice and accounts also appeared in travel guides, periodicals and encyclopaedias, which were instrumental in the circulation of knowledge, and acted as an interface between medical and public opinion on the waters.

The other source of information available on mineral waters came from popular literature, poetry and songs. Spa waters and spa visitors were written about in guidebooks, periodicals, novels, satire in all its forms – pamphlets, libels and lampoons; often bound together and sold as miscellanies. Miscellanies are emblematic of the seasonal culture of spas. In one of the rare articles on this neglected minor genre, Jennifer Batt draws attention to their relationship to time and space, singling out the 'resort-based miscellanies'[89] as a subgenre, and insisting on the role of the printers and editors of these collections, and their agency in shaping the literary world. She refers to Michael Suarez's account of the relationship that this specific genre entertains with time: 'The Miscellany, then, typically celebrates – and indeed constructs – taste, novelty, and contemporaneity in assembling a synchronous body of material'.[90] They sometimes feel like a bric-a-brac of disconnected genres, ranging from satirical poems *à clef* to neoclassical descriptions of pastoral scenes. They were published in the major spas of the first category and reflect the dialogue between popular and elite cultures.

Such 'water poetry' is the target of *The Guardian*, Richard Steele's short-lived periodical in 1713:

> The *Water Poets* are an innocent Tribe and deserve all Encouragement I can give them. It would be barbarous to treat those Authors with Bitterness, who never write out of the *Season*, and whose Works are useful with the Waters. I made it my Care therefore to sweeten some sour Critics, who were sharp upon a few Sonnets, which, to speak in the Language of the *Bath*, were the *Alkalies*. I took particular Notice of a *Lenitive Electuary*, which was wrapt up in some of these gentle Compositions, and am persuaded, that the pretty one who took it, was as much relieved by the Cover as the Medicine. There are hundred general Topicks put into Metre every Year, *viz. The Lover is inflamed in the Water*; or, *he finds his Death where he sought his Cure*; or, *the Nymph feels her own Pain, without regarding her Lover's Torment*. These being for ever repeated, have at present a very good Effect; and a Physician assures me, that *Laudanum* is almost out of Doors at the *Bath*.[91]

Such jubilant satire of literature as therapy is a precious source for the interdisciplinary study of medicine and literature, and this particular issue will be a recurrent reference throughout the book. In a long run-on metaphor on spa treatment, Nestor 'Ironside', whose name is already minerally impressed, mocks the chemical discourse and quack rhetoric on spas, and the pompousness of seasonal poetry, as well as the boredom of repetitive life in spa towns mirrored by the exploitation of hackneyed and old-fashioned courtship verse.[92] 'Water poetry' quickly became associated with bad literature. These types of collections, together with songs, pamphlets, broadside sheets and satirical poems, contributed to creating a sense of community among their targeted readers. I will investigate the ways in which spa visitors thus represented themselves and created a common imaginary space of pastoral nostalgia, satirical therapy, political and social transgression, and pleasure pervaded by the shared concern for sickness, and recovered health.

Other literary genres came to be associated with spas. A word must be said on 'spa comedies', a small subgenre that overlaps Restoration comedies and comedies of manners. The action is set in a spa town, as the title usually indicates, such as Colman's *The spleen, or, Islington Spa*, which starts with Mrs Rubrick's exclamation: 'No, give me fresh air, and Islington! – All the world shut up their houses in London at this time of the year, and resort to the watering places.'[93] Spa comedies have a particular way of weaving the plot, integrating sick characters, ball scenes or water-drinking scenes into the conventional love triangles and comedy-of-errors motifs. I hope to show that they revealed a general culture of performance in spa towns, and a reflection on the theatricality of sociability, with carnivalesque undertones.

As one would expect, spas were abundantly described in various forms of travel literature – guidebooks, letters, gazetteers and journey narratives. One of the most well-known journey narratives for the study of eighteenth-century spas was written by Celia Fiennes, who travelled through England in the early eighteenth century in pursuit of health. Her travel accounts were not published until 1811, however, and would not have been available to the reading public at the time. They remain a rich source to examine the expectations, surprises and disappointments she encountered when she tried a new spa: twenty-three in total.[94] Guidebooks, which, unlike Fiennes's journal, were available to contemporaries, compiled useful information on the cultural life of spas and their environment. They also provided historical and medical background, as well as social advice on protocol, dress and behaviour. This served as a model for satirical literature which reprocessed travel-writing into satirical letters, memoirs and guides. The most famous example of mock-travel accounts is Christopher Anstey's popular *New Bath Guide, or, memoirs of the B-n-r-d family*, which inspired many a sequel and copies in other contexts such as *The Cheltenham guide; or, Memoirs of the B-n-r-d family continued*, another example of the ongoing cultural dialogue between Bath and other spas.[95]

The canonical eighteenth-century novels dealing with British spas in the second part of the eighteenth century should be placed in this wider context of spa literature. Smollett's *Humphry Clinker*, Austen's *Persuasion* and *Northanger Abbey*, and Burney's *Evelina* stem out of a wider culture of playful and creative spa writings that were available in spas and in London and reproduced in periodicals.[96] *Humphry Clinker* stages a grumpy, gouty man who travels from one spa to another in search of a satisfying therapy. Because it tends to blur the frontier between fiction and documentary accounts, it is sometimes used by historians to justify their analysis of a spa culture.[97] Yet Smollett's novels, no matter how documented they were by his own knowledge of medicine, are built on the satirical criticism of the vain pursuits of a corrupt elite, and should be understood as such. Burney's *Evelina* uses the space of Bristol Hotwells and Bath to create encounters outside of the parental control of the heroine's guardian, allowing Evelina to explore other forms of sociability. Austen's novels *Persuasion* and *Northanger Abbey* portray the sociable circles of Bath but in two different manners: *Persuasion* focuses mostly on private parties and their elitist rhetoric of exclusion, while *Northanger Abbey* deals with the more socially mixed assembly rooms, pump rooms and bath. The list of canonical novels would not be complete without Jane Austen's unfinished novel *Sanditon*, which engages in satirical depictions of manners and greed, representing the hubris of a man who is committed to the development of a seaside resort and looks everywhere for a surgeon to attract respectable visitors.[98]

Eighteenth-century spas: theoretical watermarks

As self-contained bubbles of health, nature and leisure, spa towns constituted fertile grounds for fiction and satire, as well as theoretical systems of interpretation. Towards the end of his life, Michel Foucault gave several talks on the notion of 'heterotopia' – or 'other spaces' in which alternative behaviours are made possible. He defines 'heterotopia' as 'the sites of temporary relaxation such as cafes, cinemas, beaches'.[99] Their inherently fleeting nature and seasonal organisation opened up many possibilities of exploring other forms of social interaction, dress, schedule and deportment, as they 'suspend, neutralize, or reverse the set of relations that they happen to designate, mirror, reflect'.[100] As I hope to show in the third chapter of this book, the way spas may correspond to Foucault's notion of a *topos* for otherness is confirmed by the many examples of transgressive behaviour, scandal and carnivalesque aesthetics in the literary representations of large and medium spa towns. Yet Foucault, who was particularly attentive to various large-scale enterprises of health, did not mention spa towns in his examples. As I will argue in the first chapter, spas revolved around the care of the sick and were represented as such. They cannot be reduced to the entertaining and liberating qualities of a holiday resort, nor can their baths – and even sea baths – be seen as a mere place of relaxation, especially as most water treatments were anything but relaxing.

Parallel to Foucault's heterotopias, it would be tempting to see spa towns as pockets of Habermasian ideals.[101] The numerous meeting places, from the pump room to the promenades, offered possibilities of alternative sociability similar to the role of the coffeehouse in a metropolitan context. The political stakes of spa societies require further investigation that may show how some of the Habermasian notions on the political force of public space and on the construction of public opinion outside of central power could apply, in part, to certain spas, especially those attracting enough visits. Yet the political perception of the role of spas should not leave aside other forms of political interactions, such as the strategies developed to monitor the visitors' bodies, the relationship between medicine, town council and commerce, and the religious inheritance of the healing waters.

Another tempting interpretational frame is based on fashion. A recurrent criticism in contemporary writings condemned spa visitors as fashion victims, mocking their hairstyles, their affectations and even doubting the sincerity of their 'fashionable diseases'. The term has been critically studied in recent years to reveal the modes of co-construction by medical and literary cultures covering many forms of vulnerability among the eighteenth-century sick.[102] Anita O'Connell, Annick Cossic, Rose McCormack and Rachael Johnson have all contributed to the reflection on eighteenth-century coverage of spa and seaside resort-visiting as a fashionable trend, focusing mainly on female visitors and their independence, their relationships and their diseases. Their work illustrates how spa culture promoted female correspondence and fostered some models of independence. O'Connell and Cossic in particular show the difficult negotiations that the idea of 'fashionable diseases' brought to the experience of those suffering from the experience of sickness.[103]

Groundwork investigation into the history of English spas is extensive. Even though we greatly differ in our scope and methodology, I am much indebted to Phyllis Hembry's social history of English spa towns, published in 1990, *The English Spa, 1560–1815*. Hembry, who incidentally was based in Cheltenham, achieved a major survey of the development of spas in early modern Britain, documented thoroughly with a table of promoters, a chronology of the development of spas and detailed accounts of famous visitors. Medical and literary issues are peripheral to her analysis, as her work focuses mostly on urban development and patronage. Since 1990, however, no other book has approached English spas in their entirety. John Eglin's book on Beau Nash, the master of ceremonies of Bath and Tunbridge Wells, focuses on gaming and sociability, and remains within the bounds of those two major English spas.[104] Peter Borsay's book, which extends beyond the eighteenth century, is a useful entry into urban spaces and Georgian architecture and the memory of spa towns, but is still very much focused on Bath.[105] Annick Cossic and Patrick Gaillou's volume on eighteenth- and nineteenth-century spas brings interesting comparative information on French and English spas, beyond the scope of this book.[106]

Historians of medicine have devoted some attention to British watering places before the nineteenth century, although rather less so than their continental counterparts.[107] Roy Porter's view of spa medicine, like Hembry's, was rather economical, and probably influenced by his approach of the London medical market fostering aggressive competition and opportunistic publications. He edited a special issue of the *Bulletin of the History of Medicine* in which Noel Coley and Christopher Hamlin discussed the chemical analyses of spas in the seventeenth and eighteenth centuries.[108] Similarly,

Anne Borsay's excellent study of the General Infirmary, *Medicine and Charity in Georgian Bath* (1999), is helpful to account for the ways in which the poor were integrated in spas, and how they were treated and monitored in town. It remains specific to Bath, however, and does not cover other spa towns and their attempts to monitor the movements of the poor, as I explain in my last chapter.

Scholars of cultural history and literature have delved into the ambivalent representations of spas, as I do here. Since the publication of Daniel Cottom's seminal cultural study of spas in literature, 'In the bowels of the novel: the exchange of fluids in the Beau Monde', several other articles have been published on the inner contradictions of eighteenth-century spa towns, all of which call for further research on spas, which I hope this book will provide. According to Cottom, mineral waters are 'a phantasm invested with the life of contemporary anxieties and desires'.[109] For all its stimulating entries into the role of spas in the collective imagination of eighteenth-century Britain, Cottom's focus on the *Beau Monde*, and his partial adherence to the belief that diseases were a pretext to visit spas, are debatable. Nonetheless, his ideas about the 'fluidity of social exchanges' in watering places are thought-provoking: spas, Cottom argues, were attractive to the *Beau Monde* precisely because they were so repulsive. Ten years after Cottom's publication, scholarly interest in eighteenth-century mineral waters has grown through the publication of several stimulating articles on secondary watering places such as Tunbridge Wells, Margate, Scarborough and Moffat, yet each article is limited to one particular spa, calling for a broader perspective on the scope of the phenomenon at national level.[110]

One of the most stimulating areas for research on eighteenth-century spa towns has been women studies. The groundbreaking work of Elaine Chalus and Amanda Herbert on female sociability in health resorts and spa towns shows the renewed scholarly interest in watering places in the field of gender history. Chalus looks at the political role of eighteenth-century elite women and their influence in creating social circles that engaged in political debates, in London as well as in several watering places across the country.[111] Amanda Herbert's book, *Female Alliances*, an innovative study of female relationships within public and private space and their role in the construction of early modern social and cultural practices, has an entire chapter dedicated to spa towns as meeting places for women who notably gathered around confectionary-making, as sweets and lozenges were offered to counteract the bitter, rotten or salty taste of waters.[112]

The cultural history of mineral waters is necessarily connected to the history of water in general, and recent developments of eco-criticism have renewed the interest in the history of the relationship between humankind and water. Cohen and Duckert's reflexion on elemental eco-criticism, for example, which suggests thinking *with* the elements rather than *about* them, takes a fresh look at the materiality of air, water, earth and fire, and fosters new heuristic modes that could certainly be applied to the history of mineral waters.[113] Set beyond the scope of this book, it will certainly trigger further research on the history of healing waters, their materiality and their role in structuring communities before the Anthropocene. French studies on the cultural history of waters and its connection to the four elements precede Cohen and Duckert's *Elemental Ecocriticism*, such as Alain Corbin's book on climatology, fresh water and sea water, *Le ciel et la mer*, which draws heavily on Gaston Bachelard's seminal study at the crossroads of epistemology, psychoanalysis and literature: *Water and Dreams: An Essay on the Imagination of Matter*.[114] Corbin follows Bachelard, elaborating a distinction between fresh waters, violent waters and deep waters: 'The healthy, clear waters from the spring; the tempestuous, violent waters running down to submerge and drown; the deep, sometimes thick and swarming, sometimes dead waters'.[115] This book hopes to show how the discourse on mineral waters in eighteenth-century Britain combined all three properties: as spring waters (for spa towns), they were healing and beneficial, yet their therapeutic powers made them potentially dangerous if not taken properly, and finally, their provenance from 'the bowels of the earth' connected them to waters deep underground, charged with minerals and invisible gas.

The course of the book

The notion of 'murky waters' constitutes a closely followed thread in the five chapters that evolve in concentric circles, from sick bodies to financial structures. I use 'murkiness' as an invitation to consider the material and metaphorical aspect of mineral waters, in contrast with ideas of cleanliness, transparency, well-being and refinement that twenty-first-century readers spontaneously associate with spas.

The first two chapters of the book are focused on the medical use of mineral waters. In the first chapter, 'Sick bodies', I reassert the importance of illness and medicine in watering places. Sick bodies, I argue, took centre stage, and spa towns were first and foremost places of cure and care rather than the clean and sparkling Georgian places of leisure to which they have sometimes been reduced. The chapter explores the cultural forms of trust in the therapeutic powers of mineral waters, and explains the medical principles that accounted for those powers. I take a look at the representation of chronic diseases and their connection to spa treatment. The second chapter, 'From bog to jug: a risky remedy?', explores the multiple representations of the dangers of the water cure. It challenges the idea that mineral waters were yet another cure-all in the quack pharmacopoeia of the eighteenth-century commercialised and competitive medical world. I come back to the notion of 'pharmakon' to investigate medical representations of water treatment as a corrosive and potentially dangerous remedy. Waters themselves showed worrying signs of literal murkiness: some drinking wells gave out stinking smells and cloudy waters, and their origins could easily be traced back to the muddy ponds of nearby swamps. Some contemporary descriptions of baths and bathing facilities are frankly revolting. Many a watering place was satirised as a house of office, and the results of constant purging were exposed to the reader in rich scatological imagery.

Moving on from scatology to sexuality, the third chapter shows how spa towns were a favourite setting for narratives of transgression. Watering places were an imaginary space opening up possibilities of otherness in the self-fashioning strategies of spa visitors and in their seasonal relationships. The chapter centres on bodily behaviours and cultural constructions of the body. It starts on 'Nudity', from the desirable neoclassical nudity of bathing women to the farcical nakedness of men trapped on the beach with no clothes. The unusual proximity of bodies, or the 'dishabille' or 'riding dress' of women portrayed in songs and satire, created a suitable setting to explore the dynamics of the marriage market, and its natural derivation, adultery. A spa visit, in comedies and novels, triggered many possibilities of dangerous meetings and secret relationships. Spa comedies revolved around the idea that the multiple public spaces of spa towns fostered performance in all manners of relationships. Finally, I look at gender roles and gender fluidity to investigate excessive performative behaviours and the gender-bending possibilities they opened up in the imaginary spaces associated with spa towns, the pump room, the promenade, the ballroom, and the baths or wells.

The fourth chapter, 'Pump room politics and the murky past of spas', takes a look at the political impact of spa societies on temporary visitors who gathered for a season before returning to their homes, bearing new ideas and new information. The chapter starts with an obsession in contemporary writings on spas: gossip. At the interface of private and public spheres, gossip is shown as a dangerous political weapon within the close world of watering places. Such cultures of secret and uncontrollable circulation of information reflected national anxieties, where spas could easily become places of political and religious dissent. By contrast, other discourses on British spas celebrated them as waters that could heal the nation, specifically through the bodies of kings and queens, but also by nurturing international relationships with continental visitors. Colonial spas were also seen as instrumental in 'curing the colonisers', to paraphrase E. T. Jennings's work on nineteenth-century France.[116] Quite specific to Britain, one lurking political and religious issue was characteristic of early modern spas: the feared resurgence of Catholicism. This unfortunate history was negotiated in the discourse of medical doctors, visitors and literary authors. Relying on the work of A. Walsham on the reformation of holy waters, and their disappearance yet persistence in early modern culture, I investigate eighteenth-century sites of Roman Catholicism in mineral waters' original holiness.

In the fifth and final chapter, 'Pumping and pouring: watering places and the money business', I look at the representation of investment, speculation and the circulation of money at private and public level. As early as the eighteenth century, watering places were associated with gambling or 'gaming'. The metaphor of gambling extended to the ambitious investors in the development of spas. Their hubris was exposed in narratives of failure or corruption such as Austen's *Sanditon*. At the other end of the spectrum, lack of money was a lurking phenomenon in spa literature. In the major spas, medical doctors published propositions for monitoring the poor by both regulating and financing their access to the baths or the wells. In medium-sized spas, the discrepancy between advertising tracts and the poor quality (and quantity) of lodgings was often pointed at. In all of them, social promiscuity was an object of constant worry, and fortune-hunting was represented as a favourite sport.

Rather than claiming any kind of exhaustivity – too many spas for too small a book – I have probed into the stories, treatises, songs, satires and poems on spas to embrace the ambivalence of diverse discourses on watering places, the inherent tensions between sickness and leisure, isolation and sociability, disgust and desire, policy and plotting, greed and charity. From the dangers of treatment to the reminiscence of healing miracles, the literature on spa visits represents them as potentially fraught with danger as much as – and perhaps because they could also be – restorative and transformative.

Notes

1 In the eighteenth century, 'mineral waters' were not restricted to bottled waters. They referred to waters with a high mineral content, by contrast with common water. A 'spring' was the place where the water naturally surged from the ground (or dripped, depending on the intensity of the flow). In this book, the term 'spa' encompasses all other terms, as it did in the eighteenth century. A 'spa' could refer to a spring of mineral waters or, by extension, to the facilities built around it, or even to the whole city, more often called 'spa town'. A 'well' (often plural) could either be a simple well from which mineral waters were extracted and distributed for drinking, or it could be equipped with a basin. A 'pump room' was usually more elaborate than a well and furnished with taps that were directly connected to the spring; the water was distributed to drinkers by water women according to doctors' prescriptions. A 'bathing house' would have one or several baths, collective or individual, and could be private or owned by the corporation. A 'watering place' is a village or town organised around the therapeutic use of water, be it mineral or sea water.

2 France has seven hundred springs officially acknowledged as thermal springs ('La médecine thermale aujourd'hui: le thermalisme en Chiffres', www.medecinethermale.fr/curistes/la-medecine-thermale-aujourdhui/le-thermalisme-en-chiffres.html (last consulted 30 May 2020)). On the new uses of spas in France, see A. Sonnet, L. Lestrelin and M.

Honta, 'La fabrique des territoires du "bien vieillir": recompositions du thermalisme et gouvernement municipal en France', *Lien social et Politiques*, 79 (2017), 53–72.

3 In her inventory of early modern spa towns in England, *The English Spa, 1560–1815: A Social History* (London: Athlone Press, 1990), Phyllis Hembry counts 135 spas over the whole period: she argues that 44 new spas were created in England between 1660 and 1710, reaching a total of 65 in 1710. I have expanded this inventory to the spas of eighteenth-century Britain (not just England) and added a few spas, springs and wells that Hembry had not registered, which resulted in a total of 346 spas (appendix). My investigation was mostly run through the comparative lists of two British water doctors, J. Rutty and T. Short. Further work is needed to update Hembry's referential history of spas with systematic inventories relying on twenty-first-century online catalogues and databases of printed texts, periodicals and correspondences. Such research goes beyond the immediate purpose of this present work, which aims at opening up new ways of looking at spas and will hopefully trigger further interdisciplinary study of the phenomenon.

4 Several critics have pointed out that the history of spa towns has been too centralised and too focused on the elite. Jon Stobart, for example, in his article comparing the cultural life in spa towns and other provincial market towns, argues: 'From the Restoration to the Regency, spa towns were the ultimate product and symbol of specialised and commercialised leisure, but are too often seen as either individually or collectively isolated in this role'. J. Stobart, 'In search of a leisure hierarchy: English spa towns and their place in the eighteenth-century urban system', in P. Borsay, G. Hirschfelder and R. E. Mohrmann (eds), *New Directions in Urban History: Aspects of European Art, Health Tourism and Leisure since the Enlightenment* (Munich: Waxmann, 2000), p. 19.

5 As David M. Turner argued, 'medicalisation' tends to present disease, treatment and health as the sole province of medical doctors, leaving little agency to the sick, their families and other agents of care within the wide range of medical professions. D. M. Turner, *Disability in Eighteenth-Century England: Imagining Physical Impairment* (New York: Routledge, 2012), p. 6.

6 In 2014, Bath Record Office obtained a grant to catalogue the exceptional collections of the Bath City Council Archives from the twelfth to the twenty-first century (www.batharchives.co.uk/sites/bath_record_office/files/heritage/BathCityRecords.pdf (last consulted 10 August 2020)).

 7 There are, in fact, two doctors with the same name. William Oliver
    (1658–1716) wrote *A Practical Dissertation on Bath Waters* (Bath:
    James Leake, 1737) but did not reside in Bath while William Oliver
    (1695–1764), the alleged inventor of the 'Oliver', or bath bun, was
    involved in the governing body of the General Infirmary of which
    he became the main physician (A. Borsay, 'William Oliver', *Oxford
    Dictionary of National Bibliography*, 2004).

 8 In his introduction to a *Medical History Supplement* dedicated to the
    history of spas in 1990, Roy Porter noted that 'the culture of spa – so
    vital even in the gilded age of Edward VII – has fossilized into a
    fact of "heritage"' (R. Porter, 'Introduction: the medical history of
    waters and spas', *Medical History Supplement* (1990), p. vii). Further
    reflection on the nostalgic culture of spas and their initial association
    with eighteenth-century Jacobitism, as well as the persistence of Roman
    Catholicism, will be discussed in chapter 4.

 9 K. Denbigh, *A Hundred British Spas: A Pictorial History* (London:
    Spa, 1981); A. B. Granville, *Spas of England and Principal Sea-Bathing
    Places* (Bath: Adams & Dart, 1971). Single-authored books on specific
    spas like Cheltenham, Scarborough, Tunbridge and Harrogate are
    listed in the bibliography.

10 This model of urban planning influenced other European spa towns
    in the nineteenth century, as Jérôme Penez explains in his article on
    watering places as ideal cities in nineteenth-century France. J. Penez,
    'Les stations thermales françaises: des villes idéales?', in A. Cossic
    and P. Galliou (eds), *Spas in Britain and in France in the Eighteenth
    and Nineteenth Centuries* (Newcastle: Cambridge Scholars Publishing,
    2006), p. 97. On the Georgian heritage of Bath, see P. Borsay, *The
    Image of Georgian Bath, 1700–2000: Towns, Heritage, and History*
    (Cambridge: Cambridge University Press, 2000).

11 See A. Borsay, *Medicine and Charity in Georgian Bath: A Social
    History of the General Infirmary, c. 1739–1830* (Aldershot: Ashgate,
    1999).

12 See O. Goldsmith, *The life of Richard Nash, of Bath* (London: J.
    Newbury, 1762); J. Eglin, *The Imaginary Autocrat: Beau Nash and
    the Invention of Bath* (London: Profile Books, 2005).

13 K. Glover, 'Polite society and the rural resort: the meanings of Moffat
    Spa in the eighteenth century', *Journal for Eighteenth-Century Studies*,
    34:1 (2011), p. 65.

14 See chapter 2, 'A cure-all?', p. 92.

15 See, for example, A. O'Connell and C. Lawlor, 'Fashioning illness in
    the long eighteenth century', *Journal for Eighteenth-Century Studies*,
    40:4 (2017), 491–501.

16 These categories are heavily indebted to Hembry's inventorial work, which is the basis for my own inventory (see appendix). I have deliberately used slightly different approaches for each category because I focus on the ways in which spas were perceived. Our perception shifts categories as it embraces new objects, and sea water is relevant to the fourth category, while specific treatment is more important for small wells than it is for larger spa towns which could have various springs with various therapeutic indications.

17 See n. 1.

18 According to A. Kerhervé, 'It is commonly admitted that the Bristol waters attracted more visitors from the end of April until September, the Tunbridge waters from May till October, the Scarborough waters in July': A. Kerhervé, 'Writing letters from Georgian spas: the impression of a few English ladies', in Cossic and Galliou (eds), *Spas in Britain and in France*, p. 115. 'Early rivalry between Bath, Epsom, and Tunbridge Wells may have led the Somerset spa to adopt a spring and autumn season, leaving the summer open to its competitors'; P. Borsay, 'Health and leisure resorts', in *The Cambridge Urban History of Britain* (Cambridge: Cambridge University Press, 2000), p. 783.

19 The dates given here are rough indications of periods of development in the long eighteenth century, they do not mean that the spas did not exist before. Buxton, for example, had been known since Roman times.

20 In Harrogate, visitors could drink the waters at the Tewit Well, Johns Wells and the Starbeck Well in High Harrogate and the Sulphur spa of Low Harrogate. There were also three mineral springs in the neighbouring village of Knaresborough, two sulphurs and one chalybeate (Hembry, *The English Spa*, p. 96). In Cheltenham, rival spas developed after the visit of George III in 1788: the Old Well (the original spa), the King's Well (in honour of George III), the Montpellier Wells (opened in 1809) and the Sherborne Well (Hembry, *The English Spa*, pp. 255–6).

21 T. Short, *The Natural, Experimental and Medicinal History of the Mineral waters of Derbyshire, Lincolnshire, and Yorkshire* (London: F. Gyles, 1734).

22 S. Sunderland, *Old London's Spas, Baths, and Wells* (London: Bales, 1915) is still a useful resource on London spas.

23 J. Floyer, *Psychrolousia: Or, the History of Cold Bathing: Both Ancient and Modern* (London: Smith and Walford, 1706), p. 133.

24 Hembry, *The English Spa*, p. 285.

25 R. Russell, *A Dissertation Concerning the Use of Sea Water in Diseases of the Glands* (Oxford: J. Fletcher, 1753).

26 Further social historical investigation is necessary to confirm the
    relevance of these categories. As Jon Stobart explains, for example,
    the size of a spa town can be measured through the register of arrivals
    that was kept by the town council. Stobart, 'In search of a leisure
    hierarchy', pp. 19–21.
27 *An Exclamation from Tunbridge and Epsom against the Newfound
    Wells at Islington* (London: J. How, 1684), p. 1.
28 Borsay, 'Health and leisure resorts', p. 784.
29 Adrien Sonnet accounts for the solidarity and competition of spa
    actors with this notion, which comes from game theory. Sonnet, *Des
    villes en quête de capacité politique: permanences et recompositions
    du gouvernement municipal du thermalisme: une analyse comparée
    Dax (Nouvelle-Aquitaine) – Bagnoles de l'Orne (Normandie)* (PhD
    Thesis, Bordeaux, 2020).
30 J. Andrews, *Historical Atlas of England: Physical, Political, Astronomi-
    cal, Civil and Ecclesiastical, Biographical, Naval, Parliamentary, and
    Geographical; Ancient and Modern; from the Deluge to the Present
    Time in Which Are Described Its Minerals, Curiosities, Inland Fisheries
    and Navigation, Commerce, Peerages, Noblemen and Gentlemen's
    Seats* (London: Smeeton, 1797). I am grateful to Aude de Mezerac
    and François Zanetti, who gave me this map and made me discover
    new spas and springs of which I was unaware.
31 J. Rutty, *A Methodical Synopsis of Mineral Waters, Comprehending
    the Most Celebrated Medicinal Waters, Both Cold and Hot, of Great-
    Britain, Ireland, France, Germany, and Italy, and Several Other Parts
    of the World* (London: W. Johnston, 1757).
32 T. Short, *A General Treatise on Various Cold Mineral Waters in
    England, but more Particularly on those at Harrogate, Thorp-Arch,
    Dorst-Hill, Wigglesworth, Nevill-Holt, and Others of the like Nature.
    With Their Principles, Virtues and Uses* (London: A. Millar, 1765).
33 Russell, *A Dissertation Concerning the Use of Sea Water*.
34 'The use of natural imagery in spa verse, including satire, serves to
    naturalize, and so legitimize, the pleasure spas sell; this discourse
    collapses the distinction between the natural and the artificial so
    that nature becomes a commodity'. B. M. Benedict, 'Consumptive
    communities: commodifying nature in spa society', *The Eighteenth
    Century*, 36:3 (1995), p. 208.
35 Hippocrates, *Upon Air, Water, and Situation*, ed. F. Clifton (London:
    J. Watts, 1734). On the consumption of Nature, see Borsay, 'Health
    and leisure resorts'.
36 Environmental medicine is a late twentieth-century discipline which
    focuses on the relationship between toxic environments and health.

37 See, for example, J. C. Riley and S. Smala, 'Medical geography and medical climatology', in J. C. Riley and S. Smala, *The Eighteenth-Century Campaign to Avoid Disease* (London: Springer, 1987), pp. 31–54.

38 B. Albert, *The Turnpike Road System in England: 1663–1840* (Cambridge: Cambridge University Press, 1972); D. Bogart, 'Turnpike trusts, infrastructure investment, and the road transportation revolution in eighteenth-century England', *Journal of Economic History*, 65:2 (2005), 540–43.

39 Borsay, 'Health and leisure resorts', p. 800.

40 Borsay, 'Health and leisure resorts', p. 799.

41 A more detailed inventory of the spas of London can be found in J. S. Curl, *Spas, Wells, and Pleasure-Gardens of London* (London: Historical, 2010) and the early twentieth-century account by Sunderland, *Old London's Spas*.

42 The question of ancient holy wells, which is both political and religious, is still a subject of controversy today. It will be discussed in chapter 4. Alexandra Walsham's referential work on the question has brought the debate out of the linear narrative of 'desacralisation of the world' in which the destruction of holy wells has often been caught. A. Walsham, 'Reforming the waters: holy wells and healing springs in Protestant England', *Studies in Church History Subsidia*, 12 (1999), 227–55.

43 G. Colman, *The spleen, or, Islington Spa: a Comick Piece* (London: T. Becket, 1776), p. 9.

44 E. McKellar, 'Peripheral visions: alternative aspects and rural presences in mid-eighteenth-century London', *Art History*, 22:4 (1999), p. 504.

45 The expression 'ring of spas' comes from Denbigh, *A Hundred British Spas*, pp. 75–101.

46 C. M. B. Lewis, *Ladies and Gentlemen on Display: Planter Society at the Virginia Springs, 1790–1860* (Charlottesville, VA: University of Virginia Press, 2001); V. Scribner, '"The happy effects of these waters": colonial American mineral spas and the British civilizing mission', *Early American Studies: An Interdisciplinary Journal*, 14:3 (2016), 409–49.

47 A. Durie, 'Medicine, health and economic development: promoting spa and seaside resorts in Scotland c. 1750–1830', *Medical History*, 47:2 (2003), 195–216.

48 Glover, 'Polite society and the rural resort'.

49 See J. Kelly '"Drinking the waters": balneotherapeutic medicine in Ireland, 1660–1850', *Studia Hibernica*, 35 (2008), 99–146.

50 A. B. Willson, 'Alexander Pope's grotto in Twickenham', *Garden History*, 26:1 (1998), 31–59.

51 T. J. Werth, 'Taking the cure, mineral waters and love's folly in Lady Mary Worth's *Urania*', in S. Chiari and S. Cuisinier-Delorme (eds), *Spa Culture and Literature in England, 1500–1800* (Basingstoke: Palgrave Macmillan, 2021).

52 W. Baley, *A Briefe Discours of Certain Bathes or Medicinall Waters in the Countie of Warwicke Neere Vnto a Village Called Newnam Regis* (London, 1587), p. 11.

53 B. Allen, *The Natural History of the Mineral-Waters of Great-Britain* (London: W. Innys, 1711).

54 N. G. Coley, '"Cures without care": "chymical physicians" and mineral waters in seventeenth-century English medicine', *Medical History*, 23:2 (1979), p. 211.

55 Short, *A General Treatise on Various Cold Mineral Waters in England*, p. 12.

56 Short, *A General Treatise on Various Cold Mineral Waters in England*, p. 12.

57 Oak galls – a parasite of the oak and apple tree – were used to determine the presence of iron in the water. Galls were dipped in the water, which turned black when iron was present.

58 Most of the publications on mineral waters concern only one or two spas, or the spas of a particular region. The following works by Allen, Short, Rutty, Lucas and Linden are the most extensive comparative studies of British mineral waters in the eighteenth century: Allen, *Natural History of the Mineral-Waters*; T. Short, *An Essay towards a Natural, Experimental, and Medicinal History of the Principle Mineral Waters of Cumberland, Northumberland, Westmoreland, Bishop-prick of Durham, Lancashire, Cheshire, Staffordshire, Shropshire, Worcestershire, Glocestershire, Warwickshire, Northamptonshire, Leicestershire, and Nottinghamshire* (Sheffield: J. Garnet, 1740); Rutty, *A Methodical Synopsis of Mineral Waters* ; C. Lucas, *An Essay on Waters: In three parts. Treating, I. Of simple waters. II. Of cold, Medicated Waters. III. Of Natural Baths* (London: A. Millar, 1756); D. W. Linden, *A Treatise on the Origin, Nature, and Virtues of Chalybeat Waters: and Natural Hot Baths. with a Description of Several Mineral Waters in England and in Germany* (London: T. Osborne, 1752).

59 J. Wall, *Experiments and Observations on the Malvern Waters* (1756; Worcester: R. Lewis, 1763), p. 24.

60 C. Hamlin, 'Chemistry, medicine, and the legitimization of English spas, 1740–1840', *Medical History Supplement*, 10 (1990), pp. 67–81.

61 N. G. Coley, 'Physicians and the chemical analysis of mineral waters in eighteenth-century England', *Medical History*, 26:2 (1982), pp. 123–44.

62 On the sulphur controversy see G. S. Rousseau, 'Matt Bramble and the Sulphur Controversy in the XVIIIth century: medical background of *Humphry Clinker*', *Journal of the History of Ideas*, 28:4 (1967), 577–89; on the dispute between Wittie and Simpson on the Scarborough waters in the 1660s see A. Brodie, 'Scarborough in the 1730s – spa, sea and sex', *Journal of Tourism History*, 4:2 (August 2012), p. 131; on the question of fixed air see Coley, 'Physicians and the chemical analysis of mineral waters'.

63 W. R. Newman and L. M. Principe, 'Alchemy vs. chemistry: the etymological origins of a historiographic mistake', *Early Science and Medicine*, 3:1 (1998), 32–65.

64 L. M. Principe, 'Reflections on Newton's alchemy in light of the new historiography of alchemy', in J. E. Force and S. Hutton (eds), *Newton and Newtonianism: New Studies* (Dordrecht: Springer Netherlands, 2004), pp. 205–19.

65 See Smollett's harangue against chemistry in chapter 2, 'A cure-all?'. Peter Shaw questions Thomas Short's methods and results on the analysis of the Scarborough waters: P. Shaw, *An Enquiry into the Contents: Virtues, and Uses, of the Scarborough Spaw-Waters: with The Method of examining any other Mineral-Water* (London: F. Gyles, 1734).

66 Coley warns against rash attempts at retrospective classification: 'The term "salt" and "alum" often indicated no more than a salty or bitter taste, whilst "vitriol" and "nitre" each referred to a variety of ill-defined substances'. Coley, 'Physicians and the chemical analysis of mineral waters', p. 124.

67 W. Buchan, *Cautions Concerning Cold Bathing, and Drinking the Mineral Waters. Being an Additional Chapter to the Ninth Edition of His Domestic Medicine* (London: A. Strahan, 1786), p. 5.

68 Buchan, *Cautions Concerning Cold Bathing*, p. 5.

69 S. Mcintyre, 'The mineral water trade in the eighteenth century', *Journal of Transport History*, 1 (1973), p. 6.

70 See Mcintyre, 'The mineral water trade'.

71 See N. G. Coley, 'The preparation and uses of artificial mineral waters (ca. 1680–1825)', *Ambix*, 31:1 (1984), 32–48.

72 P. Hembry, M. Cowie and E. E. Cowie, *British Spas from 1815 to the Present: A Social History* (London: Athlone Press, 1997), p. 113.

73 Around three hundred treatises were published on British mineral waters between 1680 and 1820, if we include subsequent editions. A bibliography of British medical sources on mineral waters can be found at https://thermal1719.hypotheses.org/a-propos (last consulted 31 October 2021).

74 I will come back to case histories and the rhetoric of proof in chapter 1, drawing on G. Pomata's work on case histories. G. Pomata, 'Sharing cases: the *Observationes* in early modern medicine', *Early Science and Medicine*, 15:3 (2010), 193–236.

75 In 1765 Thomas Short concluded from his experiments on bathing that 'in tepid bathing there is both an ingress of some water, and egress of some water through the skin at the same time in the bath'. Short, *A General Treatise on Various Cold Mineral Waters in England*, p. 99.

76 '['T]is certain, that as to priority of Writings, the *Bath* in *Somersetshire*, and *Buxton* in *Derbyshire*, challenge without all dispute having been as well known to the *Romans* as the former; which is evident, first from the Remains of the ancient *Roman* Brickwall about St. *Anne's* Well, which, together with its Bason, was totally razed in 1709 when Thomas Deives of Cheshire erected the present beautiful Arch over that noble tepid Fountain'. Short, *Natural, Experimental, and Medicinal History of the Principle Mineral Waters*, p. 67.

77 Recent scholarly work has shed doubt on the medical value of ancient balneology. See J. Scheid et al. (eds), *Le thermalisme: approches historiques et archéologiques d'un phénomène culturel et médical* (Paris: CNRS Éditions, 2019). Evelyne Semama, Henry Broise and Philippe Mudry discuss the relative absence of medical thought related to bathing, which seemed more associated with religious sanctuaries than actual medical prescriptions. Eighteenth-century medical doctors, on the contrary, tend to invoke the memory of ancient balneology they associated with several discoveries of hypocausts and other ruins of Roman baths (see G. Savani, 'The lure of the past: ancient balneology at the turn of the eighteenth century', *Journal for Eighteenth-Century Studies*, 43:4 (2020), 433–45).

78 See Savani, 'The lure of the past'.

79 M. Nicoud, 'Les médecins italiens et le bain thermal à la fin du Moyen Âge', *Médiévales*, 21:43 (2002), 13–40.

80 This is not the case for all steam baths or public baths, as some were provided by monasteries, which tended to separate men and women bathing. M. Nicoud, 'Le thermalisme médiéval et le gouvernement des corps ' in Scheid et al. (eds), *Le thermalisme*, pp. 79–104.

81 D. Harley, 'A sword in a madman's hand: professional opposition to popular consumption in the waters literature of southern England and the Midlands, 1570–1870', *Medical History Supplement*, 10 (1990), 48–55.

82 G. Vigarello, *Concepts of Cleanliness* (Cambridge: Cambridge University Press, 1988); G. Vigarello, *Le Propre et le Sale* (Paris: Seuil, 1985).

83 Vigarello, *Concepts of Cleanliness*, p. 32.

84 Vigarello, *Concepts of Cleanliness*, p. 34.

85 John Wall asks one patient to 'cover the parts with Cloths dipt in the same water and moistened from time to time'. Wall, *Experiments, and Observations*, p. 37.

86 Buchan, *Cautions Concerning Cold Bathing*, p. 6.

87 C. Hamlin, 'Chemistry, medicine', p. 67.

88 Benjamin Allen in the 1710s, Thomas Short in the 1740s and John Rutty in the 1750s compared many spas of Britain. By contrast, Diederick Wessel Linden, still in the 1750s, and Charles Lucas in the 1760s included some examples from the continent while Benjamin Rush focused on early American colonies in the 1770s.

89 J. Batt, 'Eighteenth-century verse miscellanies', *Literature Compass*, 9:6 (2012), p. 396.

90 M. F. Suarez, 'The production and consumption of the eighteenth-century poetic miscellany', in I. Rivers (ed.), *Books and Their Readers in Eighteenth-Century England: New Essays* (Leicester: Leicester University Press, 2001), pp. 217–51. In her article on spas and bluestockings, Alison Hurley argues that 'The format had peaked and disappeared by mid-century'. A. E. Hurley, 'A conversation of their own: watering-place correspondence among the Bluestockings', *Eighteenth-Century Studies*, 40:1 (2006), p. 20, n. 41. Although the term 'Miscellany' tends to disappear from titles after the 1750s, anthologies of poetry on watering places – less satirical, perhaps – continued to be published, such as *Water poetry: A collection of verses written at several public places, most of them never before printed* (London: G. Pearch, 1771). See also C. Watson, *Miscellanies, Poetry, and Authorship, 1680–1800* (Basingstoke: Palgrave Macmillan, 2021).

91 *The Guardian*, 174 (September 1713), p. 504. This letter was originally published in an earlier miscellany entitled *A Packet from Will's* (London, S. Briscoe, 1705). See n.89 p. 80.

92 On the long-lasting association of water poetry with bad literature, see for example P. Hembry's derogatory description of the water poets: 'Many spas inspired more literary efforts and their virtues were often celebrated in poetry by the so-called water-poets, patrons with leisure to spare between bouts of drinking and bathing. At Tunbridge Wells such verse offerings for public perusal were inscribed in a book kept at the bookseller's on the Walks. The occasional poem or doggerel verse often revealed the quality of local life.' Hembry, *The English Spa*, p. 169.

93 Colman, *The spleen, or, Islington Spa*, p. 8.

94 Excerpts from Fiennes's writings were made public in 1811 by the romantic poet Robert Southey, and published in 1811 under the title

Through England on a Side Saddle. The referential edition for this study is C. Morris (ed.), *The Illustrated Journeys of Celia Fiennes 1685–c1712* (London: McDonald, 1982). See also B. Osborne and C. Weaver, *Aquae Britannia: Rediscovering 17th Century Springs and Spas: In the Footsteps of Celia Fiennes* (Malvern: Cora Weaver, 1996).

95 C. Anstey, *The New Bath Guide or Memoirs of the B—R—D Family*, ed. A. Cossic (1766; London: Peter Lang, 2010); W. Fordyce Mavor, *The Cheltenham guide; or, Memoirs of the B-n-r-d family continued: In a series of poetical epistles* (London: Harrison, 1781).

96 T. Smollett, *The Expedition of Humphry Clinker* (1771; Oxford: Oxford World's Classics, 1998); J. Austen, *Persuasion* (1817; Oxford: Oxford University Press, 2004); J. Austen, *Northanger Abbey* (1817, New York: Norton, 2004), F. Burney, *Evelina, or the History of a Young Lady's Entrance into the World* (1778; Oxford: Oxford World's Classics, 2002).

97 See for example John Stobart's article 'In search of a leisure hierarchy', in which he insists that the primary goal of spa towns was health holidays, yet concludes by saying that, by the second part of the eighteenth century, visitors sought recreation more than restoration, quoting *Humphry Clinker* to illustrate his statement.

98 J. Austen, *Sanditon* (Oxford: Oxford University Press, 2019).

99 M. Foucault, 'Des espaces autres', *Empan*, 54:2 (2004), p. 14; M. Foucault, trans. J. Miskowiec, 'Of other spaces', *Diacritics*, 16:1 (1986), p. 24.

100 Foucault, trans. Miskowiec, 'Of other spaces', p. 24.

101 J. Habermas, *The Structural Transformation of the Public Sphere: An Inquiry into a Category of Bourgeois Society* (1963; Cambridge, MA: MIT Press, 1989).

102 See for example J. Andrews and C. Lawlor, '"An exclusive privilege … to complain": framing fashionable diseases in the long eighteenth century', *Literature and Medicine*, 35:2 (2017), 239–69; O'Connell and Lawlor, 'Fashioning illness'.

103 R. Johnson, 'The Venus of Margate: fashion and disease at the seaside', *Journal for Eighteenth-Century Studies*, 40:4 (2017), 587–602. R. A. McCormack, '"An assembly of disorders": exploring illness as a motive for female spa-visiting at Bath and Tunbridge Wells throughout the long eighteenth century', *Journal for Eighteenth-Century Studies*, 40:4 (2017), 555–69. A. O'Connell, 'Fashionable discourse of disease at the watering-places of literature, 1770–1820', *Journal for Eighteenth-Century Studies*, 40:4 (2017), 571–86. A. Cossic, 'Fashionable diseases in Georgian Bath: fiction and the emergence of a British model of

spa sociability', *Journal for Eighteenth-Century Studies*, 40 (2017), 537–53.

104 Eglin, *The Imaginary Autocrat*.

105 Borsay, *The Image of Georgian Bath*.

106 Cossic and Galliou (eds), *Spas in Britain and in France*.

107 In France, for example, Marylin Nicoud and Didier Boisseuil have published a volume on the history of European spa towns from the middle ages to early modern times: D. Boisseuil and M. Nicoud (eds), *Séjourner au bain: le thermalisme entre médecine et société, XIVe–XVIe siècle* (Lyon: Presses universitaires de Lyon, 2010). Another volume by the same group of scholars is dedicated to mineral waters on the *longue durée*: Scheid et al. (eds), *Le thermalisme*.

108 Porter, 'Introduction', pp. xvii–xii.

109 D. Cottom, 'In the bowels of the novel: the exchange of fluids in the Beau Monde', *NOVEL: A Forum on Fiction*, 32:2 (1999), 157–86, 179.

110 Chiari and Cuisinier-Delorme (eds), *Spa Culture and Literature in England*; R. W. Cooley, '"Sexy in a 'Tunbridge Wells' sort of way": a study in the literary iconography of place', *Journal for Early Modern Cultural Studies*, 15:1 (2015), 90–118; Glover, 'Polite society and the rural resort'; Johnson, 'The Venus of Margate'; Brodie, 'Scarborough in the 1730s. Rachael Johnson's PhD thesis on watering places in Kent must be mentioned, especially her work on masters of ceremonies (R. M. Johnson, 'Spas and seaside resorts in Kent, 1660–1820' (PhD Thesis, University of Leeds, 2013), http://etheses.whiterose.ac.uk/5857/ (last consulted 15 June 2020)).

111 E. Chalus, 'Elite women, social politics, and the political world of late eighteenth-century England', *Historical Journal*, 43:3 (2000), 669–97; E. Chalus, *Spaces of Sociability in Fashionable Society* (New York: Routledge, 2019).

112 A. E. Herbert, *Female Alliances: Gender, Identity, and Friendship in Early Modern Britain* (New Haven, CT: Yale University Press, 2014). This study elaborates on an earlier article on early modern spas in which Herbert gives a detailed account of the various functions of women in sixteenth- and seventeenth-century spas, from cleaners to bath women, who stayed in the waters for hours, accompanying bathers and selling sweets. A. E. Herbert, 'Gender and the spa: space, sociability and self at British health spas, 1640–1714', *Journal of Social History*, 43:2 (2009), 361–83.

113 J. J. Cohen and L. Duckert, *Elemental Ecocriticism: Thinking with Earth, Air, Water, and Fire* (Minneapolis, MN: University of Minnesota Press, 2015).

114 The scope of Corbin's book extends beyond what is announced in his title, as he tackles the question of the history of watering places, spas and seaside resorts: A. Corbin, *Le ciel et la mer* (Paris: Bayard, 2005); G. Bachelard, *Water and Dreams: An Essay on the Imagination of Matter* (Dallas, TX: Pegasus Foundation, 1983); G. Bachelard, *L'eau et les rêves: essai sur l'imagination de la matière* (Paris: J. Corti, 1947).

115 Corbin, *Le ciel et la mer*, pp. 66–67. My translation.

116 E. T. Jennings, *Curing the Colonizers: Hydrotherapy, Climatology, and French Colonial Spas* (Durham, NC: Duke University Press, 2006).

1

Sick bodies

In 1776, in response to David Hume's request to publish his auto-biographical account *My Own Life* after his death,[1] Adam Smith encourages his ailing friend to follow his physician Sir John Pringle's advice for a course of mineral waters: 'A mineral water is as much a drug as any that comes out of the Apothecaries Shop',[2] he argues. Smith, however, questions Pringle's prescription of yet another course of the Bath waters:

> I reckon it probable that the Bath Waters had never agreed with you, but that the good effects of your journey not being spent when you began to use them, you continued for some time to recover, not by means of them, but in spite of them. Is it probable that the Buxton waters will do you more good?[3]

Hume's sickness was well advanced in June 1776, and he had only two more months to live. Yet Smith, whose theory of moral sentiments shows his interest in the workings of the body, agrees with Hume's physician in promoting the use of mineral waters when nothing else seems to work. Smith even adds that, should the waters of Buxton fail to work, 'the journey to Buxton, however, may be of great service',[4] suggesting that the whole process of taking the waters started with the departure from home on a therapeutic trip.

That mineral waters were valid drugs is the starting point of this chapter. Spa towns, big or small, attracted ailing persons, whose sick bodies had often tried another drug, or, like Hume, another mineral water. Starting with the most widespread spa narratives of eighteenth-century Britain, Austen, Smollett and Burney, this chapter revisits the representation of spa towns in literature and medicine to investigate the ways in which sick bodies inhabited them. It

therefore starts with a few Bath examples, only to establish that
even in Bath sickness was central, and not necessarily feigned as a
pretext to go to the spa. After shifting the focus onto secondary spa
towns, I intend to show how Adam Smith's advice to his ailing
friend was far from isolated. Mineral waters were prescribed for a
variety of diseases, which I will endeavour to arrange in four main
categories around which medical prescription was organised. In
each group, medical theories accounting for the physiological effects
of mineral waters on the body will be invoked, even though these
theories regularly overlapped in the same treatise. In most cases,
however, long-term afflictions were the object of water treatment,
and the study of mineral waters opens a window on the nature of
these complex diseases which affected bodies in multiple ways and
spurred the sick to look for relief.

Places of cure and care

Eighteenth-century spas have their classic portrayals, in which they
are depicted as commercial and social hotspots: Jane Austen's
Northanger Abbey (1817) and *Persuasion* (1817), Fanny Burney's
Evelina (1778) and Smollett's *Humphry Clinker* (1771). Most of
them, as mentioned previously, have been instrumental in building
a Bath-centred image of spas revolving around leisure and tourism.
And yet, in each of these narratives – even when Bath is the setting
– illness ranks as a primary motive among the many reasons that
bring each protagonist to visit a spa town. Sickness can affect a
secondary character, a plot device often interpreted as a pretext for
a spa visit: Mr Allen's 'gouty constitution'[5] in Jane Austen's *Northanger Abbey* is a reason to go to Bath which leads the heroine,
Catherine Morland, to meet with Isabella and John Thorpe and the
delightful Mr Tilney. In spite of its obvious service to the plot, the
character's sickness remains quite tangible in the narrative. Allen's
gout, which is certainly peripheral, does not escape Austen's unfailing
capacity to debunk a few cultural clichés. John Thorpe, who entertains
no critical distance with the world, exclaims: 'Does he drink his
bottle a-day now?',[6] only to have his aphorism swept away by
Catherine's swift response: 'His bottle a-day! – No. Why should
you think of such a thing? He is a very temperate man.'[7] Rather

than being the sour consequence of intemperance and fashionable excesses,[8] gout is evoked as a chronic disease that affects temperate and intemperate people alike: no other sign of Allen's intemperance is given anywhere in the novel, confirming the heroine's indignation. What we know of Allen is that he joins others after the dance, doesn't move much, dabbles in meteorological science and dislikes too much company. His illness, at the margin of the plot, is a mark of old age. The gout gives him a grumpy temper and makes of him a sobering presence for his household.

In *Persuasion*, as a counterpoint to the threatening rules of sociability, the heroine, Anne Elliot, is in search of reliable networks of care. Austen enters into more detail on the pains and difficulties of life with a long-term disease. Mrs Smith, Anne's friend, driven to dire circumstances by widowhood and illness, tells her story to Anne: 'There had been a time, Mrs Smith told her, when her spirits had nearly failed. She could not call herself an invalid now, compared with her state on first reaching Bath.'[9] This contrasts with glorious Janeite images of Georgian Bath, encouraged by the private and public marketing strategies of the town. Austen clearly presents Bath as a destination for invalids, including the poor and incapacitated. Mrs Smith's physical and financial pains are further exposed:

> Then, she had indeed been a pitiable object – for she had caught cold on the journey, and had hardly taken possession of her lodgings, before she was again confined to her bed, and suffering under severe and constant pain; and all this among strangers – with the absolute necessity of having a regular nurse, and finances at that moment particularly unfit to meet any extraordinary expense.[10]

The signs of a severe chronic illness requiring constant treatment bring to the fore the dangers of solitude for those who were not supported by friends or family. Mrs Smith, like so many isolated women in Jane Austen, depended on the goodness of strangers. Her care was undertaken by the sister of her landlady, a nurse who was living at her house when unemployed, and tended her 'most admirably'.[11]

This furtive example of women's networks of solidarity weaving the social fabric of everyday care is a significant entry into the social life of Bath. Far from the social pomp usually associated with the town or with the professional circles of medical men, the scene is a tableau of the nursing role of women, and their involvement in curing and caring beyond mere medical acts. Nurse Rooke holds a function in the plot that I would describe, in Mary Fissell's words, as a form of healing that took place 'outside of the economic exchange'.[12] In addition to everyday care, Nurse Rooke helps Mrs Smith to feel useful and to socialise: she teaches her how to knit, and to make 'little thread-cases, pincushions and card-racks', finding the means of 'doing a little good to one or two very poor families in this neighbourhood'.[13] Mrs Smith's cure is thus both physical, moral and social: Nurse Rooke understands the multiple aspects of care.[14] This dialogue acts as a counterpoint to the pump room scenes, reminding the reader of the intrinsic nature of spa towns, that is, a town swarming with sick bodies and vulnerable characters. It sheds light on the possibilities of care offered by the multiple private lodgings and their small domestic sociability, quite distinct from the hotels and palaces of the nineteenth and twentieth centuries.

In Frances Burney's epistolary novel *Evelina* (1778), the eponymous heroine visits a watering place of second rank: Bristol Hotwells. This was located beneath the sublime prospect of St Vincent's Rock, close to the river Avon, and the warm, mildly saline water was much threatened by the overflow of the muddy river. It was developed into an 'established spa' only after being rescued in the late seventeenth century by a group of 'Merchant Venturers' who invested in the pump room and helped the development of the town.[15] By choosing this spa town as a destination over Bath, Burney reinforces the provincial aspect of the narrative in *Evelina*:

> Bristol Hotwell, August 28.
>
> You will be again surprised, my dear Maria, at seeing whence I date my letter: but I have been very ill, and Mr. Villars was so much alarmed, that he not only insisted upon my accompanying Mrs. Selwyn hither, but earnestly desired she would hasten her intended journey.
>
> We travelled very slowly, and I did not find myself so much fatigued as I expected. We are situated upon a most delightful spot; the prospect is beautiful, the air pure, and the weather very favourable to invalids. I am already better, and I doubt not but I shall soon be well; as well, in regard to mere health, as I wish to be.[16]

Reverend Villars, Evelina's tutor, insists on his ward's going along with the witty and unconventional Mrs Selwyn (whom he genuinely dislikes) and specifically advises her to drink the waters: 'his anxiety that I should try the effect of the Bristol waters, overcame his dislike to committing me to her care'.[17] Readers of *Evelina*, measuring Villars's protectiveness of his ward, will thus understand that the Bristol waters are expected to be an efficient treatment, potentially active in case of an emergency. Evelina's letter corroborates her guardian's trust in the Hotwells waters, as her condition improves rapidly. She perceives the bettering of her health in accordance with contemporary medical ideas on the effect of waters on the body. Just as the waters purge her melancholy and act upon the organs and fluids internally, the external effects of the climate, the exercise provided by the journey and the pure air around their nearby lodgings at Clifton Heights, combine to restore her health. This effect, which a twenty-first-century reader would be tempted to see as psychological, was in fact perceived as a physical, soft action of the local environment that affected the patient's mind and body alike.

More details on water treatment are given in another epistolary novel published seven years before *Evelina*, Tobias Smollett's *Humphry Clinker* (1771). The novel has been the basis for many investigations into the history of spas, their representation in literature and their medical functions, and remains a major influence on representations of eighteenth-century spas.[18] Matthew Bramble, the main character, regularly writes to his medical doctor and friend, Dr Lewis. He is pained by gout, a splenetic constitution and multiple ailments he jokingly calls 'old age'. Following his doctor's orders, he travels through England and visits several watering places, including Bristol Hotwells, Bath and Harrogate, in pursuit of better health. He describes them in the most critical and disparaging manner, except for the town of Scarborough, where he finally admits having 'benefited, both from the chalybeate and the sea', as Scarborough offered the opportunity for sea-bathing as well as mineral water-drinking.[19] Tobias Smollett, who was trained as a surgeon and was awarded the degree of Medical Doctor from the University of Aberdeen, had also written a medical pamphlet entitled *An Essay on the External Use of Water*, twenty years earlier in 1752, which might explain why the character Matthew Bramble's accounts on water treatments have regularly been considered, sometimes a little too quickly, as almost documentary.

One of Bramble's comments on Scarborough echoes contemporary reflections on the opportunism of spa-builders and water doctors, and may have influenced historical ideas about spas. 'There are fifty spas in England as efficacious and salutary, as that of Scarborough, though they have not yet risen to fame', Bramble writes to Dr Lewis, before adding sarcastically: 'and, perhaps, never will, unless some medical encomiasts should find an interest in displaying their virtues to the public view'.[20] Bramble scornfully compares water doctors to the Grubstreet opportunistic encomium writers. His rebuke was familiar to eighteenth-century readers, as hinted by the discomfort of the well-known water doctor, Diederick Wessel Linden, the author of a pamphlet on the Shadwell waters had expressed in his preface. His printers made no effort to avoid any conflict of interest as it is 'printed for the proprietor; and to be had at the Shadwell-Spaw, in Sun-Tavern-Fields, Shadwell; and F. Jones, Mineral Water Purveyor to His Royal Highness the Duke of Cumberland, in Tavistock-Street, Covent-Garden'.[21] Yet, Linden refutes any particular interest at the beginning of his treatise: 'It may perhaps be suggested, by some haughty and supercilious Critics, that the signing of my Name to such Bills and Directions, is by no means suitable to the State and Decorum of the Faculty; or that is it far beneath the Dignity of a regular and graduate Physician to extend and familiarize his prescriptions in such a manner', he writes, objecting that he has 'nothing so much at heart, as the Wellfare of mankind'.[22] Linden's mention of his diploma echoes Bramble's implication that the authors of water treatises are not always licensed doctors. This might explain why Linden is one of the targets of Smollett's satire; the Westphalian doctor is, in fact, a recognisable caricature in *Humphry Clinker*.[23] Their praise of the spa virtues may be proportional to their financial interests in the business of the spa town. If we follow Bramble's cynical remark, unintentionally supported by Linden's defensive comments, the hundreds of medical treatises dedicated to specific spas in the eighteenth century would only have been written as a means of promotion rather than as an impartial investigation into the medicinal effects of the waters.

Both Phyllis Hembry and Roy Porter, in their seminal studies of eighteenth-century spas published in the 1990s, seem to agree with Doctor Smollett's unveiled accusation in *Humphry Clinker* of the commercial interests of his peers.[24] Such a view has tended to narrow the role of doctors in the publication of mineral water treatises as instrumental to the development of the credentials of a particular spa and to the construction of the author's reputation as its expert. In her chapter on minor spas in *The English Spa*, Hembry expands this notion to other health professionals whom she sees as agents in the development of the spa – 'the local apothecary could join the physician in giving credibility to the virtues of neighbouring mineral waters'.[25] Porter expressed similar ideas on eighteenth-century British medical publications on waters: 'in Britain at least, rival claims over the efficacy of special waters, and rival techniques for utilizing them, became the focus of disputes between doctors far more murky and sulphurous than the waters whose virtues they were touting'.[26] Porter thus catches the controversial nature of medical exchange, which Anita Guerrini, Margaret Pelling and Frances White have mapped out for the medical networks of early modern and eighteenth-century London.[27] If we follow Porter's argument, medical controversy on waters is primarily a marketing strategy, an eighteenth-century version of buzz-making created by the competitive context of the rapid ascension and proliferation of spa towns in England. Such views were corroborated by Daniel Cottom's study of spas in literature. He addresses the medical authors' economic motive in a rash statement attacking retrospectively the hundreds of medical authors as 'writers more concerned to puff the medicinal virtues of the waters'.[28]

A closer look at the multitude of published medical treatises and pamphlets dedicated to mineral waters in the eighteenth century both confirms and invalidates this view: many medical authors engaged in the blatant promotion of a particular spa and vigorously doubted the medical reasoning of their opponents, creating major or minor controversies around the nature of the mineral waters, the directions for their use and the account of their effects. At the same time, several eighteenth-century doctors launched themselves into systematic comparative studies of British and European spas. Such was the case of Benjamin Allen, Thomas Short, John Rutty, Charles Lucas, Diederick Wessel Linden and Donald Monro.[29] Some of these doctors fought against each other, such as John Rutty and Charles Lucas, but their controversies cannot be traced to the potential financial benefits they might have received from promoting one particular spa. Although we can hardly investigate the motivation behind their research, at the crossroads of natural history and case-based medicine, these publications do testify to a wider curiosity about the nature and effects of mineral waters than the self-serving interest pointed at by Porter and Hembry, in line with Bramble's criticism of 'medical encomiasts'. Promotion and competition are too obvious in all these treatises to be ignored, but were not the only reasons for their publication: promotional discourse was often woven in a larger interest in therapeutics, puzzling cases and natural history. Water treatises were a lively medical genre with a long history rooted in the late medieval period in Italy.[30] In water treatises, authors ingeniously combine various medical theories, chemical analysis and medical observations, not to mention the numerous anecdotes illustrating cases and discoveries.

The efforts and ideas of the publishing medical world do not, however, represent all that is medical in the eighteenth century, as social, cultural and feminist historians of medicine have persistently reminded us since the 1990s. This is also true of watering places. Reasserting the centrality of health in watering places implies that wider initiatives of care should not be neglected. The building of a hospital, the development of new therapies, the management of the poor, the monitoring of public and private spaces for the transportation of the sick, the multitude of small jobs related to the management of the sick, the development of parks and pathways, the regulation of time within the city, and the small actions of everyday care provided by nurses, companions and family, were all part of the therapeutic experience of watering places. Following Anne Borsay's seminal study on Bath General Infirmary which shed light on the institutional management of the sick and the poor, several social historians have also investigated the development of medical and social institutions and their pivotal role in the social fabric of spa towns.[31] Such a shift of focus, from the fashionable to the care of the sick, is also to be encouraged in literary studies in which multiple examples of sickness, medical concerns and care have been displayed. Even in Austen, Burney and Smollett, whose novels abound in scenes of eighteenth-century fashionable spa sociability, sickness lurks in the background, remaining the initial motive for a visit to the spa. In this perspective, Amanda Herbert's investigation of female sociability in spa towns and Rose McCormack's analysis of illness as motive for visiting spas agree that early modern and eighteenth-century spas remained places for health, and refute the idea that health, more often than not, would have been used as a pretext to visit the spa. As McCormack argues, 'Scholarly attention has been given to the spas as health resorts, but there is a recurring argument in spa historiography that illness was often feigned and that it declined as a genuine motive for spa-visiting throughout the eighteenth century'.[32] In the same vein, Herbert insists on the visitors' genuine hope for treatment: 'Women and men stayed for weeks or even months at a time in spa cities in order to seek cures', adding that 'women and men of both high and low status went to the spa'.[33]

The non-fictional writings of the *salonnière* and Blue Stockings Society leader Elizabeth Robinson Montagu corroborate the idea that spa-visiting was driven by the direct and indirect experience of sickness. She regularly visited Bath and Tunbridge, and some of her lively descriptions have recurrently been quoted in scholarly articles, as they capture the mood of the place.[34] Montagu's letters on Tunbridge Wells differ from those of Bath, as she genuinely recommended the use of Tunbridge waters when she wrote to Anne Donnellan, who belonged to the circle of friends around the Duchess of Portland:

> I flattered myself they came to inform me of your recovery, and I was sorry immediately to learn your relapse. I hope Tunbridge will be of great service to you, I think nothing gives such great spirits as those waters, and the air of the place is excellent. I was there two seasons for my health, and I found vast benefit by the waters.[35]

By 'spirits' she refers to a more internal healing process beyond a general state of mind: the regeneration of the 'animal spirits', an ethereal fluid often invoked in early modern medicine, and still present in the eighteenth century, which was part of the medical representation of the effects of the waters on the internal organs.[36] Montagu's immediate association of waters and air also reflects how water cures were always more than water. In the minds of patients and doctors alike, the whole environment took part in the healing process. She jokingly adds, 'I wish I had any excuse, but illness, to go this year; I should enjoy your company extremely', implying that illness was indeed the main motive for such a visit, and that she was in pain when she last visited Tunbridge.[37] She spells out the appeal: 'for the wildness of the country, and romantic air of everything, gives great pleasure to those who are fond of the beauties of nature; and I think the variety of such a mixture of retirement and lonely solitude, with the resort of company at other hours, very agreeable.'[38] The natural environment, seen through the eyes of a spa-goer, is entirely serviceable to the cure, as is sociability and the relaxed atmosphere of countryside relationships, potentially less pressurised than those of the metropolis, driven by urban protocol.

Montagu's dramatic conclusion to this laudatory description contrasts with the peaceful and inspiring tableau she has just drawn: 'If you recover your health by the help of the waters, I shall still love them better; and I think I have some obligation to them already, for I believe I owe my life to their assistance.'[39] Her style is usually marked by excess and playfulness, and her disease is not specified so that one can hardly measure whether her life was truly endangered, and yet this dramatic contrast between the bucolic scene and the intensity of her conclusion can be explained by the sense of care that she experienced from the Tunbridge cure. She doesn't reduce the experience of healing to the sole medicinal virtues of the waters, even though she fully asserts her confidence in their efficiency, but places the restorative process in the wider natural and social environment of the spa. In other words, through the eyes of the young Elizabeth Robinson (as she was not then married), a visit to Tunbridge Wells has a curative effect for two reasons: it gives access to an efficient medicine, and it provides other ways of improving one's health by breathing pure air, contemplating nature, exercising, socialising moderately and resting. This is the kind of care to which she 'owes her life' and that she wishes for her friend: it is not a doctor/patient prescription, and ranges among the many examples of medical advice one obtained, and regularly followed, through friends and family. A few months later, she congratulates her friend on following her guidance: 'she [Miss Scott] wrote me you went from Tunbridge in good health',[40] which confirms the impact that such advice could have. We do not know, however, what kind of 'illness' Elizabeth Robinson and Anne Donnellan were suffering. Propriety might have spurred these young women to self-censorship where sick bodies were mentioned. The advice they provided for each other did not seem to focus on diagnosis.[41] In the same vein, Alain Kerhervé notes that the famous letter-writers, when visiting spas, mostly wrote 'ordinary' letters attesting to the prevalence of sickness and cure during their stay, such as Hester Lynch Piozzi's complaint in 1798: 'I promise your Ladyship a pretty letter from Bath, but how shall I keep my word? I see nobody and nothing but the Doctors.'[42]

Should we then disregard the narrative of fashion, sociability and leisure as biased and exaggerated? Such a conclusion would not be any less biased and is surely unnecessary: the whole interest of the study of eighteenth-century spas lies in the tension between pleasure and sickness. Such tension even pervaded the economic organisation of spas: the conflicts between doctors, who were trying to keep control over the urban organisation of the spa, and other actors such as mayors, merchants and service providers who were trying to shape the spa into an attractive place to visit.[43] As we will see in subsequent chapters, pleasure calls for leisure, and sickness for care. Alexandra Walsham captures this ambivalence: 'An uneasy alliance of contradictory impulses – sickness and sociability, compassion and commercialization, religion and profit – was central to the identity of the celebrated wells and spas of the seventeenth and eighteenth centuries'.[44]

Leisure and care sometimes meet, sometimes remain at odds. They are not mutually exclusive because they represent crucial elements of the experience of spas, making spa scenes in novels ambiguous and interesting, usually a turning point in the plot. This is also why spas were an easy target for satire: to the happily healthy, sickness and sociability did not belong together. Sickness should not be regarded as a false motive, and spa treatment should be considered as it was then: a real treatment in the pharmacopoeia of the time, often prescribed for chronic diseases and complex symptoms, and sometimes for desperate cases. Taking the medical aspect of spas at face value is essential to understand the complexity of watering places, their development and their role in the culture of the times. Otherwise, the easy and rather monolithic narrative of 'the commercialisation of leisure' takes over, and the long and difficult history of sick bodies, water-drinking, bathing and creative modes of care gets swallowed into a blurred vision of what is too often reduced to inefficient treatments and false sickness, when mineral waters frequently relieved and were, in any case, very much sought after.

A catalogue of diseases

'Spas are invalid-friendly', writes Annick Cossic in a note to her article on female invalids and spa therapy:

> those affected by gout or by venereal diseases could exhibit their grotesque bodies or their stained faces, sometimes disfigured, unashamedly in the spa environment, like Queen Anne at the turn of the century. This involved a changing attitude to the deformed body, which had previously 'elicited not only suspicion of moral character but also ridicule'.[45]

The term 'invalid-friendly', reminiscent of what twenty-first-century readers would call 'accessible', is worth exploring. Spa towns were organised, culturally and physically, around sick bodies. They were structured in time and space to facilitate access to the wells, the pump room or the baths. The flow of visitors had to be monitored, and their circulation was eased around town. In literature, in the shadows of the scenes of sociability, the overwhelming presence of sick bodies in spa towns is depicted in a variety of sources, from letters to medical treatises. Visual satire staged deformed bodies, gouty patients and poxed women at the centre of the crowd.[46] Rowlandson's 'Comforts of Bath' series of eight coloured prints, for example, abounds in recumbent bodies carried by servants, crutches, and wheelchairs or 'Merlin chairs'. The overwhelming presence of sick bodies at the bath, at the pump room, and in the town lodgings, weighed on the experience of the water cure. The sickly crowd acted as a constant mirror to one's own physical condition.

What kind of sickness did they suffer from, and what were the water treatments prescribed for? Although the list could be long, as I will explain in the next chapter, four main groups of diseases emerge from the perusal of medical treatises and literary representations of spa treatment. These 'complaints' – the eighteenth-century term aptly focused on patient experience – were rarely isolated and often belonged to a larger symptomatic tableau. Their evolution was long term, uncertain and recorded as such: some complaints, relieved by taking the waters, would reappear a few months or a few years later. Sometimes, it made them worse. The first group revolves around rheumatic diseases, including partial or complete paralysis, gout and palsy. A second group consists of nervous diseases – the term is to be understood broadly, from the highly gendered hysteria and green sickness to stomach and bowel complaints related to melancholy or hypochondria.[47] Thirdly, sex-related complaints, from 'the whites' and irregular courses to venereal disease and barrenness, attracted the most tragic and comic representations in the medical and satirical literature of the times. Finally, diseases of the skin and eyes – including ulcers, sarcomas and cancers – were the subject of hundreds of successful cases in medical literature.

Gout and other rheumatic complaints are worth looking at first because they are deeply entangled with visual and literary representations of eighteenth-century sick bodies in spa towns. Rheumatic complaints, palsy, paralyses and gout, were some of the best represented diseases in the visual and literary culture of spas. In such cases, bathing was recommended, and sulphurous and chalybeate waters preferred. The historian of chemistry Noel Coley confirms that sulphurous waters such as Bath or Buxton were usually prescribed for the gout, which was commonly considered the 'disease of the affluent'.[48] Literary representations of gouty characters looking for spa treatment abound in eighteenth-century novels: Matthew Bramble in Smollett's *Humphry Clinker*, Admiral Croft in Austen's *Persuasion*, Mr Allan in Austen's *Northanger Abbey*, to name but a few, are all grumpy and wealthy men who seem to resent their treatment even more than their disease. The history of gout has been largely determined by Roy Porter and George Rousseau's seminal study, which investigated the cultural and medical heritage of the representations of the disease since Antiquity.[49] They surveyed the major debates on the supposed benefits and inheritance of the disease, pinpointing the publication of William Cadogan's 1771 treatise, *A Dissertation on the Gout and all Chronic Diseases*, as a turning point in the explanatory frame of the disease.

Cadogan, a renowned physician who was also the Governor of the Foundling Hospital, argued that gout was not beneficial in any way, that it should – and could – be treated, and that it was not, as was believed, hereditary.[50] Cadogan's treatise is based on three moral principles: indolence, intemperance and vexation. His proposed treatment relies on diet and exercise, and he rarely mentions the use of mineral water, except to contrast it with wine: 'Water is the only liquor nature knows or has provided for animals', he writes, in line with the natural approach of treatment promoted two decades earlier by John Wesley,[51] 'and whatever Nature gives us, we may depend upon it, it is safest and best for us'.[52] Cadogan's perception is representative of the mechanical approach of the use of water: his explanation of the effects of mineral water on gout is both moral and physiological, and no credit is given to the early chemical analysis of the mineral elements within the water:

> when we have committed any excesses or mistakes of any kind, and suffer from them, it is water that relieves ... it is the element that dilutes and carries off the crudities and indigestion, the mineral virtues they contain makes them tolerable to the stomach in their passage but do, as I believe, little more in the body: it is the water that cures.[53]

By their relaxing effect on rigid fibres, and their action on the concretions of the skin, sulphurous mineral waters such as Bath, Buxton, Harrogate and Moffat waters were preferred for the treatment of the gout, which, in eighteenth-century medical thought, could affect the body beyond the hands, feet and knees. Porter and Rousseau throw light on a lesser-known form of that same disease in eighteenth-century medical thought: the internal or 'repelled' gout.[54] Internal gout meant that the 'crudities', unable to be purged out of the body through painful and salutary crises in the joints, turned back against the organs. Queen Anne, for example, was diagnosed with internal gout – hence her multiple visits to the royal spas of Tunbridge Wells and Bath, aimed at both treating her gout and promoting her fertility.[55] Once this fatal stage had been reached, spas were prescribed for pain relief, since they channelled the course of the 'gouty matter' out of the organs, through the joints and out of the skin. Warm baths were recommended, as were early means of 'packing', that is to say, wrapping in wet blankets to make the patient sweat. Through the purgative process of sudation, like purging, bleeding or salivating, gout was expected to be driven out of the body.[56]

Readers can follow the course of such treatment in Smollett's novel *Humphry Clinker* as Matthew Bramble narrates his bathing experience in the sulphurous waters of Harrogate with medical gothic undertones: 'At night, I was conducted into a dark hole on the ground floor, where the tub smoked and stunk like the pot of Acheron, in one corner, and in another stood a dirty bed provided with thick blankets, in which I was to sweat after coming out of the bath.'[57] Bramble stresses the ambivalence of the treatment by evoking the underground river Acheron: in Ovid, the river was a branch of the Styx and a way into hell, while other texts saw it as a place of healing and cleansing. His vision of the water cure closely intertwines physical ordeal and medical treatment: 'My heart seemed to die within me when I entered this dismal bagnio, and found my brain assaulted by such insufferable effluvia',[58] he continues, putting himself in the submissive role of an objectified patient whose refusal of treatment would be seen as a lack of courage: 'ashamed to recoil upon the threshold, I submitted to the process'.[59] In Bramble's words, the violence of a disembodied cure predominates over care – no bather, no nurse is presented in this scene. The patient's subjectivity is strongly asserted by his satirical voice, in contrast with the passivity of his gouty body, packed in blankets, nauseated by the smell of sulphur, almost imprisoned in what sounds more like a vault than a place for caring for the sick. The treatment does not prove successful and yet Bramble wanders off to other spas, looking for temporary relief, which he will only find in Scarborough. After such a description, the character's persistence in his pursuit of a spa treatment is quite stunning, considering his overall resistance to medical prescriptions. And yet, pain spurs him, and what proves inefficient in one spa town might work in another context, with other mineral content. Such an attitude reflects a common trait of spa patients found in the medical cases published by doctors as well as in the correspondence of the times: each spa was specific, and what didn't work in Bath could well work in Scarborough.

The second group of diseases, which revolves around nervous complaints, from hysteria to 'windy melancholy', was addressed in various ways, but would generally be cured by drinking purging waters to fortify the patient's 'laxed fibres'. This was a condition that applied to organs, muscles and nerves alike, and was often seen as the cause of hysteria, hypochondria, the vapours and green sickness.[60] Diederick Wessel Linden, the Westphalian doctor who had come to settle in England with the Hanoverian regime,[61] based much of his investigation into the chalybeate waters of England on a comparison with German waters.[62] Linden describes 'two sorts of baths prepared of the Chalybeat Waters'. One method, which consists in the use of a 'wooden machine' and of iron pipes to avoid any attraction of the particles of the iron already contained in the water

by any other metal, is deemed more efficient for nervous complaints.
The water is heated, and patients are placed in a bath covered with
'canvas, or any other matter of an open texture, sufficient to admit
air to prevent suffocation, which is let down when the patient is
bathing'.[63] It is thus carefully prepared 'to preserve of the volatile
spirits as is possible'.[64] Linden's promises are hopeful:

> the Bath, so prepared, is then made use of when these spirits are in
> action, for being then capable of penetrating through the *Skin*, Sinews,
> Nerves and Muscles, it irritates the same, and by this means elevates
> the laxed and Weak Vessels, and restores them to their natural strength
> and substance, when the Nervous system by this method receives its
> natural strength again.[65]

The rationale behind water treatment is not the relaxation of the
body – more of a twenty-first-century concept – but the strengthening
of the fibres and the rehabilitation of weakened nerves.

The nervous spectrum was large, and the symptoms associated
with nervous diseases, as Micheline Louis-Courvoisier explains, often
connected melancholia with painful digestion, connecting the bowels
and the brain.[66] In his *Methodical Synopsis of Mineral Waters*, the
Irish water doctor John Rutty depicts the symptoms of a lady who,
'after a nervous fever, fell into great pains of the head and back,
with privation of heat and motion of the limbs, with the *fluor albus*,
loss of flesh and appetite, and her stomach retained nothing that she
took'.[67] The case appears in the account of the purging waters of
the small Irish spa of Mont Pallas (County Cavan), thirty-nine miles
from Dublin, near the house of 'Ignatius Pallas, Esq.', who, on top
of giving his name to the spa, invited the Dublin doctor to analyse
his waters on the spot. Because of this mind–bowel connection,
purging waters were a powerful treatment for nervous complaints:

> In this languid state she betook herself to the use of this water on
> the spot, drinking three pints a day. It first vomited, then purged her
> prodigiously, her excrement sharp and excoriating; it also proved
> diuretic and her urine was highly foetid, like smiths forge water, but
> more intolerable: in six days she found sensible benefit, and in process
> of time was entirely restored in all respects.[68]

The graphic description of the bodily fluids justifies the violence of
the purge. The violence of the cleansing waters delivers the body
from intoxicating and stagnating internal matter, which weighed on

the nerves, muscles and stomach. The cure is a highly trying method that shakes the insides of the woman, restoring her to her senses. Nervous complaints, which were highly gendered illnesses, were thus both a genuine medical concern and the target of satire.[69] The gendering of diseases like hysteria and green sickness, or 'the hyp' – hypochondria was the masculine counterpart of hysteria – were part of the gender paradigm on display in the satirical literature on spa towns, as we will see in chapter 3.

In the same vein, sex-related diseases, ranging from the much represented venereal diseases to the more complex forms of male and female barrenness, were an ongoing subject of spa satire.[70] Venereal disease occupies a major place in eighteenth-century medical cultures, especially as the underlying social and physical issues they contained made them a handy metaphor for the ills of society, as Noelle Gallagher convincingly argues in *Itch, Clap, Pox*. Venereal diseases also allow good observation of the social processes at work around the advent of illness. Regarding the matter of mineral waters as medicine, however, venereal diseases are treated within a wider array of afflictions, and medical discourse seemed concerned with proper ways of implementing a cure for these diseases rather than vilifying their cause. Chalybeate waters, more than other types of mineral waters, were recurrently advised to fight venereal disease.

The idea that mineral waters were a good treatment for venereal diseases came from the previous century. In the first edition (1632) of his treatise on Tunbridge Wells, the doctor Lodwick Rowzee had drawn a distinction between 'Gonorrhea simplex', an irritation of the genitalia that occurs spontaneously, and 'Gonorrhea Venerea', the consequences of sexual intercourse:

> It [the water] helpeth also the running of the reines, whether it be *Gonorrhea simplex* or *Venerea*, and the distemper of the *Parastatae* arising from thence, as likewise a certain carnositie, which groweth sometimes in the conduite of the urine, nay and the Poxe also, the water having an notable potentiall drying facultie.[71]

Rowzee considers Tunbridge chalybeate waters as a medicine like a syrup or a balm. The 1725 edition does not mention venereal disease and leaves out Rowzee's remark. Were Tunbridge doctors afraid that such information would attract a crowd of patients with light morals, as suggested by the popular literature of the time? The circulation

of the Earl of Rochester's lewd poem 'Tunbridge Wells' certainly
didn't help lift such reputation.[72] In fact, at the other end of the long
eighteenth century, the waters of Tunbridge Wells were still identified
as efficient for sex-related diseases. In his *Medical Guide for the
Invalid to the Principal Watering Places of Great Britain* published
in 1804, the prolific and practical writer physician William Nisbet
advises that the Tunbridge waters be taken for 'irregular courses
or amenorrhoea'; 'flooding at the passive stage', the 'whites' and
'constitutional weakness as a result of venereal disease'.[73]

   Tunbridge Wells was far from being the only spa recommended for
venereal diseases, but chalybeate waters such as those of Tunbridge
seemed to have been preferred in many cases. The great advocate
of chalybeate waters was the above-mentioned Westphalian doctor
Diederick Wessel Linden, whose survey of the *Origins, Nature and
Virtues of the Chalybeate Waters* was published four times in five
years. Like Rowzee and later Nisbet, Linden recommended the use
of these waters for venereal distempers, for which he was careful
to assign other potential causes than sexual intemperance: 'for
Ulcers in the kidneys in consequences of the *Venereal Distemper*
(or otherwise contracted), these Waters [Tunbridge] are of sovereign
use'.[74] He also gives a case of *Gonorrhoea simplex* that is worth
quoting at length:

> A Young Man, 20 years of age, was afflicted with Gonorrhoea simplex;
> not contracted from a venereal infection: and therefore, more difficult
> to cure. He was so bad, that a consumption was visibly coming upon
> him; there was nothing omitted by his friends; but as soon as they
> came to the knowledge of it, caused proper means to be made use
> of for his recovery; and when the Materia Medica would yield no
> relief, he was sent to *Bristol*, and from thence to *Bath*, and for a
> considerable time used these Waters, under proper advice; and when
> these failed, the *Lyncomb* Chalybeate-waters, near Bath, were also
> fruitlessly tried. Some months after, he had made use of these waters,
> he became my Patient, and was completely cured, by an equal mixture
> of Chalybeate, and Saline, Purging-water.
>
> N.B. It must be observed, that he constantly had taken a small quantity
> of Glauber Salts, with the *Lyncomb* Spa-waters; a method, frequently
> recommended, where the Chalybeate-waters, as those of Lyncomb,
> are without salt, but I never could, from Experience, find any greatly
> salutary effects from it.[75]

The complexity of this medical history is also found in similar cases that will be presented throughout this study, and several elements are worth commenting upon here. On the social background of disease, the young man's 'friends' – a general term to describe friends and family supporting him – are eager to help him and invest in his cure. As a patient, he is not disconnected from his social support system, which is part of the caring process, and recorded as such from the doctor's point of view. The experience of disease is thus lived within a social network that is altered by the sickness of one individual. On the therapeutic context, the term 'Materia Medica' is juxtaposed here with mineral waters, prescribed once other drugs have been deemed inefficient.[76] Hence mineral waters are integrated in the *materia medica* with other medicinal treatments, and at the same time they stand apart as a prescription given in particularly complex and resistant cases. Were mineral waters thus considered a last-chance therapy? It certainly was a regular strategy of medical rhetoric to present a treatment in this way, and should therefore be interpreted with caution. The mention of Glauber salts and what appears to be Linden's own mixture of various waters is an example of their status within the *materia medica* of the time. He blends several types of waters and adds other components, as one would prepare a medicine with various doses of active principles. In fact, mineral waters were often mixed with other elements, if not other waters. Finally, Linden takes it for granted that not every type of water works, and if one does, its effect can abate as the disease evolves.

One of the issues of venereal disease was the social status of the sick and how the disease affected their public and private relations, which entailed many secret strategies implemented by patients to hide their disease and any identifiable treatment. This was understood by some water doctors, who indicated that venereal diseases could be cured by mineral waters but avoided making them the sole target of that treatment. They typically made use of periphrases and partly veiled notions in their treatises, all of which would have been understood by literate people in search of treatment. Such is the case of the Irish Quaker doctor John Rutty's *Methodical Synopsis of Mineral Waters*. It was published in the same decade as Linden's essay on chalybeate waters, and after several years of intense data-collecting. He quotes his Yorkshire-based fellow physician Thomas Short on Nevill-Holt Spa, keeping the sex-related diseases for the end of the list: 'Dr Short asserts, that among all the varieties of medicinal waters in England he has enquired after, it has no parallel in the bloody urine, bloody flux, vomiting, and spitting of blood, overflowing of the menses, fluor albus (in most of which cases its good effects have been also experienced in Dublin, being a water that bears transportation)'.[77] The 'fluor albus', or the 'whites' – vaginal excretions that were often seen as threatening fertility – could then be conveniently cured at home with bottled water, an welcome expedient in the case of potentially shameful diseases. Rutty then adds: 'it is also effectual in old gleets and seminal weaknesses, and several instances are given of its efficacy in carrying off the relics of venereal disease imperfectly cured by mercurials, and particularly discussing venereal tumors of the testicles by the sole internal use'.[78] The notion of 'relics of venereal disease' is crucial to understand that most diseases did not have an end, and that water treatment, as I will argue shortly, helped patients live with their disease, or with the multiple consequences of previous diseases.[79]

Barrenness remains the most famous sex-related affliction indicated for water treatment. Barrenness, just like venereal diseases, often appeared in a cloud of ailments, some of them venereal or nervous, others entangled in layers of symptoms that had been piling up over the years. As Rose A. McCormack reminds us, female patients visited spas for gynaecological problems, nervous disorders and digestive complaints (cholic, stomach pain or winds).[80] John Rutty's synopsis mentions female barrenness regularly. His comments on the Moffat waters from Scotland does present them as a last-chance therapy, that can restore hope to the childless: 'It is deservedly famous in curing barrenness, even in such as have despaired of having children'.[81] On Dulwich water he writes: 'It cures barrenness, whether from cold and moisture, or heat and dryness';[82] he recommends the 'salino-chalybeate waters' for 'barrenness from too much corpulency or fat'.[83] For the Irish waters of Ballyspellan he indicates 'barrenness depending on obstruction' and in the same vein, the Buxton waters for 'barrenness whether from a constriction or indalatability [sic] of the fallopian tubes'.[84] Unlike venereal disease, Rutty treats barrenness as any other disorder: he simply lists the potential causes, and records the waters and types of treatment.

Medical discourse on barrenness, however, was rarely disconnected from moral injunctions. The relationship between venereal disease and barrenness was regularly emphasised by frustrated doctors who treated the wives for barrenness when they thought they should treat the husbands for contracting venereal diseases in the first place. Linden's development on barrenness in a slightly earlier treatise on the waters of a Welsh spa, *Three Medicinal Mineral Waters at Llandrindod* (1756), illustrates this idea. He attributes barrenness to the spread of venereal diseases, which he ascribes to both sexes: 'Seminal Weakness is too frequent in both Sexes. The causes are various and innumerable. But there is one more fashionable than the rest; which our Ancestors, indeed, were almost Strangers to; I mean the Venereal Disease.'[85] He continues, as many writers did when they dealt with venereal disease or masturbation, blaming both patients and (quack) doctors: 'This, when treated by the Unskilful, weakens some patients, makes other old before their Time; destroys innumerable families, and renders more miserable, both in themselves and in their puny Posterity'.[86] His diatribe ends on a prophetic invitation to be redeemed and reinvigorated by the Llandrindod waters:

> But let such as have seen the Folly of entrusting their Health to the Ignorant, and have any regard for themselves and posterity, dilute, wash away, and purge off, with any regard for posterity, what they have contracted, either by Medicine or Disease, and brace up their flabby weak Muscles again, with the Saline Chalybeate Water: Among which, as the Llandrindod Rock-Water has an equal, if not superior merit to most, on account of the Salts, and those of various sorts, which enter its Composition; I cannot help recommending it, in preference to any other.[87]

The term 'Rock-water' is reminiscent of the expression 'stone juice' I mentioned in the introduction, drawing attention to the solid rather than liquid nature of the water. In this example, it sounds as if the mineral element would transfer some of its density to the patient's body, strengthening his 'flabby' muscles and, by extension, densifying the seminal juices of the patient, opening new possibilities for a healthy posterity. Linden, who was no stranger to the chemical analysis of mineral elements, endows salts with a metaphorical – or magical – agency in the transformation of the body plagued with venereal disease.

Eighteenth-century satirical literature insistently laughed at fertility water treatment. I have argued elsewhere how it triggered the creation of many satirical texts which relied on the 'adulterous woman trope', to use a term coined by Daphne Oren-Magidor. With this expression, she refers to the heavily gendered joke that attributed the success of a cure to the sexual encounter of a supposedly 'barren' woman with a doctor, a rake, a young local peasant or a priest, depending on the situation.[88] In 'A Letter from *Tunbridge* to a friend in *London*', printed in several miscellanies, the narrator pokes fun at watering places, for example, and explains 'The chief Virtue ascrib'd to these Waters are the following two: they very often cure the Greensickness in Maids, and cause Fruitfulness in Marry'd Women, provided they are but properly administred by a young physician'.[89] The sexist rhetoric behind this trope is dual: it shames the impotence of the husband and blames the venereal appetite of the woman. The medical implications were that few treatments for barrenness actually worked, when the great majority of medical discourse argued, on the contrary, that barrenness was rarely incurable, and that patients should never give up hope. Yet, the trope travelled and flourished in the fertile ground of satire, and it worked as a political comment debunking the effect of the numerous spa visits of royal princesses and queens to improve their fertility (Anne, Mary, Mary of Modena, Catherine of Braganza, to name but a few).

The royal visits shaped the identity of Tunbridge, Bath and Buxton: they were recorded in periodicals and remembered in spa guides, which were one of the primary resources used by visitors for medical guidance. Successful case histories of fertility cures extended well beyond the example of monarchs, however. The fertilising virtues of the waters of Scarborough were advertised by the case of a local couple, St Quintin and his wife, who used the waters successfully twice, a foundational case on which the waters' reputation was built. The waters were celebrated for their fertilising effect in a lyrical poem published in the 1733 *Scarborough Miscellany*, 'On the Virtues of Scarborough-Spaw Water':

> If Nature to the wedded Fair
> Denies the Blessing of an Heir,
> These Waters shall her Cares remove,
> And Crown the pleasing Toils of Love.
>
> The Husband dead to Beauty's Charms,
> Whom the faire Wise but faintly warms,

> Shall find his former Fires return,
> and with recruited Vigour burn.[90]

Interestingly, the husband is blamed for his lack of desire and the waters work like an aphrodisiac, restoring his fertility and his sexual appetite. Such reasoning corroborates Jennifer Evans's account of the perception of infertility in early modern medical thought, as she explains how aphrodisiacs were regarded as a treatment for infertility.[91]

One year earlier, the *Scarborough Miscellany* opened with the poem 'Scarborough', which seemed to be praising the virtues of the town:

> Thrice happy Scarborough! of Renown secure,
> The Doctor's Recipe, and Patient's Cure.
> Rival of Bath! whose more prolific Springs
> In hope of Heirs, the sterile Couple brings.
> From Fears of dying Childless, both are eas'd,
> The Man's contented, and the Wife is pleased.

The lyricism at work echoes the numerous encomiums written by water poets in celebration of their cities, placing the poem at the crossroads of a country house poem, a guidebook and an urban poem. It continues, however, with the aforementioned joke that shifts the tone of the poem into a mock-heroic piece:

> For when the Waters fail, there's some will say,
> The Cause has been remov'd ... some other Way.[92]

Relentlessly, poems played with the sexually charged reputation of watering places to counterbalance the medical prescriptions. Barrenness, like most other sex-related disease, was invisible, and thus an easy object of literary imagination. At the opposite end of the spectrum, even if some of them were related to venereal diseases, skin diseases were blatant and unquestionable, but nonetheless a well-known candidate for spa treatment.

Finally, skin diseases naturally called for external water treatment. Some waters paradoxically 'dried' the skin, helping wounds to heal and washing away some of the pus.[93]

John Rutty, whose long comparative survey of mineral waters is scrupulously referenced and annotated, explains the effects of the Westwood vitriolic waters in Derbyshire on a young woman's skin ulcer:

The following is a remarkable instance of its efficacy in healing some of the most stubborn and chronic ulcers, from Dr Short's own observation, viz.:

'I had a servant maid who had, before she came to me, the most frightful and ulcerated leg I ever saw, for five years, prodigiously swelled, livid, and useless: a man might have hid his fist in one ulcer, very foul, of a blackish-green colour. Her parents and she used all means they could possibly procure, but in vain, till I advised her to wash it twice a day with this water, which cured it in three months' time, though she had plied twice as long with Guilswaite spa water and clay to no purpose.'[94]

Skin diseases are most emblematic of chronic diseases, and their visibility, described here in terms of measurability, colour, smell and texture, makes the onlooker cringe. This case highlights how many of the assumptions about mineral waters are incorrect, as pointed out above. First, the patient comes from a poor social background, not from the elite. Secondly, her family gets involved in the search for a cure, taking what is generally assumed to be the role of a doctor as prescriber of water cures. Finally, the medicinal action of the waters over the ulcer is described in all its physicality and chronicity, not in terms of nervous illness or fashionable disease. This case echoes the narrative structure of Linden's case on the twenty-year-old man with venereal disease mentioned above: after several attempts at trying another remedy (Gilthwaite waters in South Yorkshire), a chronic illness deemed incurable gets ultimately cured by specific waters. The borderline between quack rhetoric and medical discourse is often blurred in early modern medicine, and yet in this case, John Rutty, being based in Dublin, has no interest in promoting Westwood waters over Gilthwaite. His comparison between two types of mineral waters implies that his medical reasoning on the effects of the waters differs according to their mineral components.[95]

Many diseases could be added to the list, as we will see in the next chapter, but I have chosen to focus on what seems to me the most prevalent diseases in the case histories of the time. Readers of Montaigne might wonder why the stone and gravel is not mentioned here, for example. Montaigne famously went on a trip throughout Europe to drink the waters in France, Switzerland and Italy, and successfully evacuated some gravel.[96] Although this complaint regularly appeared in the long lists of indications of eighteenth-century mineral treatises, there are not as many case histories as the diseases just mentioned, possibly because the operating techniques were available to a wider range of people, as well as lithontriptics (medicines to dissolve the stone) like Joanna Stephen's powders or Jurin's Lixivium.[97]

The sick rather than the sickness

How did sick people choose to visit one spa over another in particular? Did certain types of water – sulphur, saline, chalybeate, calcareous or sea water – have a specific indication for a certain category of disease? Chalybeate waters, as we have seen, were regularly considered a 'drying' tonic, sulphurous waters were beneficial for skin diseases and rheumatic complaints, and saline or purging waters for digestive ailments and obstructions. The perusal of British medical treatises on mineral waters, however, hardly suggests that a specific type of water should only be prescribed for a specific category of disease, including in the works of medical doctors whose approach to English spas was more systematic, such as Allen, Linden, Lucas, Rutty and Short.[98]

In the introduction to *A Methodical Synopsis of Mineral Waters*, John Rutty reasserts the centrality of chronic diseases in water treatments. He thus relaunched the medical debate around mineral waters towards the middle of the century by attempting to analyse the composition of mineral waters in Britain and on the continent.[99] 'I enlarged my view towards attempting a general history of mineral waters, and being prompted by an earnest desire of seeing something more regular and methodical', Rutty writes, in the spirit of an Enlightened natural historian, 'and more free from intricacy and perplexity than hitherto on this subject as a branch of the *Materia Medica* of great importance in the cure of chronicle diseases.'[100]

As Rutty further explains the effects of waters in the cure of chronic diseases, we get a clearer view on the ways in which waters were expected to work on the body. As he writes about the virtues of the 'nitrous or bitter purging waters' such as Barnet, Holt or Epsom, he declares: 'in habitual costiveness, the foundation of many chronic diseases, as colic, iliac passion, and hernia's; a long course

of these waters, drank before going to bed, excels all remedies'.[101]
Later, he comments on 'the character of iron', the main chemical
component in chalybeate waters such as Tunbridge Wells or Hampstead: 'As an absorbent or sweetener of acids', he writes, 'it is good
in all chronic diseases where an acid prevails, and where an acid is
the cause of obstruction, it removes them'.[102] Following the mechanical
ideas of his age on the circulation of bodily fluids as the basis of
good health, Rutty uses the term 'obstruction' to evoke the diversity
of blockages that can occur in the circulation of bodily fluids like
blood (from arterial blood to menses), digesting juices (such as bile),
or digested food and evacuations all fluidified by the power of iron.
Just as it would be pointless to establish a strict nosology of
eighteenth-century diseases with twenty-first-century correspondences,
the idea that a treatment was strictly prescribed in a specific perimeter
– recommending one particular type of water for one particular
disease – comes much later in the reasonings of hydrotherapy. From
the patient's point of view, other elements were at stake: proximity,
cost, the reputation of the waters, lodgings, and the concurrent
advice of doctors and friends.

As we have seen in Linden's case on the twenty-year-old man
affected by gonorrhoea, the road to treatment was a long-winding
path, scattered with failure and half-satisfactory solutions. Another
way, therefore, to approach the question of specific indications of
the mineral waters is to follow this long-winding road and shift
categories, leaving aside the nosology that roots its reasoning in the
body parts or the organs affected by the disease, and focusing on
its complexity and long-term duration as the main characteristic.
If we shift categories, it appears that rheumatic disorders, nervous
disorders, and venereal and skin diseases have one major characteristic in common with gout: chronicity. They were all long-term
illnesses, disrupting the everyday life of the sick and their friends and
families, evolving in incoherent, sinusoid patterns that distributed
pain, incapacity, tiredness and an array of unexpected symptoms
in uneven and incoherent ways for doctors and sick persons alike.
Although it is hard, and probably pointless, to trace particular types
of water cures for specific diseases, it becomes clear that spa treatment
was primarily concerned with chronic disease, and that chronicity
was at the heart of the theory, representations and practices of the
water treatment.[103]

In the post-surgical medical world of the twenty-first century, chronicity is given increasing attention as many treatments like triple therapy, radiotherapy, chemotherapy and immunotherapy transform what could have been a terminal disease like cancer or AIDS into a long-term, chronic illness with long-term, evolving treatments. This 'change in the paradigm of care', to quote Céline Lefève in the introduction to her book on new approaches to care in the twenty-first century,[104] contrasts with the dominant medical approach of the late nineteenth and twentieth centuries, which was more focused on the resolution of acute diseases through intense hospital care and highly interventionist medicine.[105] The strict opposition between chronic and acute, and the role of mineral waters in the cure of chronic disease, are pointed out at the turn of the twentieth century by Thomas Linn, a medical doctor with international aspirations who published a popular medical survey of the spas of Europe.[106] 'The treatment of acute disease has been much improved in our time', he writes, referring to the development of surgery, 'but neither the *materia medica* nor the newer surgical operations have much value in the relief or cure of those constitutional states called chronic maladies; and for these some of the best forms of treatment are found in mineral waters'.[107] By contrast, chronic diseases, or long-term afflictions, were part of the everyday experience of eighteenth-century bodies: faces scarred by smallpox like Lady Mary Wortley Montagu's, deformed bodies like Alexander Pope's, impaired vision like Samuel Johnson's or incapacitating nervous ailments like James Boswell's, were part of a shared experience across genders and social classes that wealth could accommodate, but did not solve.

For many cases in the eighteenth century, a disease was not just a clear-cut episodic event, with beginning, middle and end, but rather a series of uneven episodes, or a long-winding and disrupting experience, with resurgences and partial recoveries, transformations and degradations. Pope's famous line 'This long disease, my life' captures the relationship between time and disease,[108] and it is crucial to recognise this specific relationship for the water cure, as time is itself part of the remedy. Water cures involved time in many ways: most visits lasted for several days or weeks, and most patients returned for another season, disrupting the usual rhythms of the patient's life. Within the spa town itself, time was often regulated and moni-tored to medical ends, from morning till night, starting with drinking waters early in the morning, then promenade, visits and sociable events at night. A water cure transformed the time of its visitors around the centrality of its waters and activities, dispossessing them of their time as medical institutions do, while paradoxically creating a lot of free time that regularly caused so much boredom.

The journey, the diversions and the 'change of air' were thus an active part of the treatment, as Adam Smith argues in the letter to David Hume cited at the opening of this chapter:

> Change of air and moderate exercise occasion no new disease: they only moderate the hurtful effects of any lingering disease which may be lurking in the constitution; and thereby preserve the body in as good order as it is capable of being during the continuance of that morbid state. They do not weaken, but invigorate, the power of Nature to expel the disease.[109]

This, he supposed, counteracted the potentially dangerous consequences of the medicinal waters, which produce 'violent effects upon the Body'. To Smith, mineral waters worked in similar ways to inoculation: 'It occasions a real disease, tho' a transitory one, over and above that which nature occasions. If the new disease is not so hostile to the old one as to contribute to expell it, it necessarily weakens the Power which nature might otherwise have to expell it.'[110] Although this model was not prevalent in contemporary medical treatises, all medical doctors agreed that a water course was a risky remedy that should not be treated lightly, nor, perish the thought, be self-prescribed.

Notes

1 R. Mankin, 'La maladie comme triomphe de la nature? *My Own Life* de David Hume', in S. Vasset and A. Wenger (eds), "Raconter la maladie au dix-huitième siècle', *Dix-Huitième Siècle* 47 (2015), 181–96.

2 A. Smith, 'Adam Smith to David Hume: Sunday, 16 June 1776', *Electronic Enlightenment Scholarly Edition of Correspondence*, R. McNamee (ed.), Vers. 3.0. University of Oxford. 2018, https://doi-org.janus.bis-sorbonne.fr/10.13051/ee:doc/smitadOU0010201a1c (last consulted 13 June 2020).

3 Smith, 'Adam Smith to David Hume'.

4 Smith, 'Adam Smith to David Hume'.
5 Austen, *Northanger Abbey*, p. 8.
6 Austen, *Northanger Abbey*, p. 42.
7 Austen, *Northanger Abbey*, p. 42.
8 Gout is studied in more detail in the next section of this chapter. For more information see R. Porter and G. Rousseau, *Gout: The Patrician Malady* (New Haven, CT: Yale University Press, 1998).
9 Austen, *Persuasion*, p. 125.
10 Austen, *Persuasion*, p. 125.
11 Austen, *Persuasion*, p. 125.
12 M. E. Fissell, 'Introduction: women, health, and healing in early modern Europe', *Bulletin of the History of Medicine*, 82:1 (2008), p. 8.
13 Austen, *Persuasion*, p. 126.
14 On contemporary reflections on the multiple aspects of care see P. Molinier, S. Laugier and P. Paperman (eds), *Qu'est-ce que le care? Souci des autres, sensibilité, responsabilité* (Paris: Payot, 2009).
15 Hembry, *The English Spa*, p. 97.
16 The spa of Bristol is referred to as both Bristol Hotwells and Bristol Hotwell. Burney, *Evelina*, p. 268.
17 Burney, *Evelina*, p. 269.
18 See for example Rousseau, 'Matt Bramble and the Sulphur Controversy', pp. 577–89; Cossic, 'Fashionable diseases in Georgian Bath', pp. 539–44; McCormack, '"An assembly of disorders"', p. 556.
19 Smollett, *Humphry Clinker*, p. 183.
20 Smollett, *Humphry Clinker*, p. 181.
21 D. W. Linden, *Directions for [the Use] of That Extraordinary Mineral-Water, Commonly Called, Berry's Shadwell-Spaw: In Sun-Tavern-Fields, Shadwell, near London. More Especially, in the Several Distempers Wherein It Has Proved by Experience, of the Greatest Efficacy and Success* (London: printed for the proprietor; and to be had at the Shadwell-Spaw, in Sun-Tavern-Fields, Shadwell; and F. Jones, Mineral Water Purveyor to His Royal Highness the Duke of Cumberland, in Tavistock-Street, Covent-Garden, 1749).
22 Linden, *Directions for [the Use] of That Extraordinary Mineral-Water, Commonly Called, Berry's Shadwell-Spaw*, p. 3.
23 See Hembry's account of Linden in *The English Spa*, p. 168.
24 In the same vein, Peter Borsay argues 'The opportunity to maximise the returns on property holdings provided the obvious stimulus in these cases. For another major group of promoters, medical men, it was the occasion to exploit their professional skills and expand their practices that encouraged them to become heavily committed to

advancing and publicising watering-places; Dr Russel in Brighton, Dr Jephson in Leamington or the apothecary John Livingston at Epsom are examples.' P. Borsay, 'Health and leisure resorts', p. 791.

25 Hembry, *The English Spa*, p. 159.

26 Porter, 'Introduction', p. xi. Porter is referring to one of the articles in Harley's special issue, 'A sword in a madman's hand'.

27 A. Guerrini, '"A club of little villains": rhetoric, professional identity and medical pamphlet wars', in M. Mulvey Roberts and R. Porter (eds), *Literature and Medicine during the Eighteenth Century* (New York: Routledge, 1993), pp. 226–44; M. Pelling with F. White, *Medical Conflicts in Early Modern London: Patronage, Physicians, and Irregular Practitioners, 1550–1640* (Oxford: Clarendon Press, 2003).

28 Cottom, 'In the bowels of the novel', p. 171.

29 Allen, *Natural History of the Mineral-Waters*); Short, *Natural, Experimental, and Medicinal History of the Principle Mineral Waters*; Rutty, *A Methodical Synopsis of Mineral Waters*; Lucas, *An Essay on Waters*; Linden, *A Treatise on the Origin, Nature, and Virtues of Chalybeat Waters*; D. Monro, *A Treatise on Mineral Waters* (London: G. Nicol, 1770).

30 Nicoud, 'Les médecins italiens'.

31 Borsay, *Medicine and Charity in Georgian Bath*. On the history of medical institutions in spas, see for example L. Smith, 'A gentleman's mad-doctor in Georgian England: Edward Long Fox and Brislington House', *History of Psychiatry*, 19:2 (2008), 163–84; M. Brown, 'Medicine, reform and the "end" of charity in early nineteenth-century England', *English Historical Review*, 124:511 (2009), 1353–88.

32 McCormack, '"An assembly of disorders"', p. 557.

33 Herbert, *Female Alliances*, p. 119.

34 Montagu's famous quote on Bath has been analysed by A. E. Hurley and quoted by A. Kerhervé: 'I hear every day of people pumping their arms or legs for rheumatism, but the pumping for wit is one of the hardest and most fruitless labours in the world. I should be glad to send you some news, but all the news of the place would be like the bills of mortality, palsy, four; gout, six; fever, one, &c. &c. We hear nothing but Mr. such-a-one is not abroad today; Oh! no, says another, poor gentleman, he died to-day. Then another cries, my party was made for quadrille to-night, but one of the gentlemen has had a second stroke of the palsy, and cannot come out; there is no depending upon people, no body minds engagement': Hurley, 'A conversation of their own', p. 14; Kerhervé, 'Writing letters from Georgian spas', p. 275.

35 E. Robinson Montagu, *The Letters of Mrs Elizabeth Montagu: With Some of the Letters of Her Correspondents* (London: Wells and Lilly, 1825), p. 141.

36 The notion of animal spirits pervades the popular medical culture of the eighteenth century, and remains anchored in the self-representation of bodies. See S. Kleiman-Lafon and M. Louis-Courvoisier (eds), 'Les esprits animaux: 16e–21e siècles', *Épistémocritique*, 2018, p. 6, https:// epistemocritique.org/category/ouvrages-en-ligne/actes-de-colloques/ les-esprits-animaux/ (last consulted 13 April 2020).

37 Montagu, *Letters*, p. 141.

38 Montagu, *Letters*, p. 141.

39 Montagu, *Letters*, p. 141.

40 Montagu, *Letters*, p. 163.

41 Rose McCormack suggests that the reason might be fertility issues (McCormack, '"An assembly of disorders"', p. 561). The visit mentioned here, however, dates from before her marriage, and fertility problems were rarely referred to as 'illness'.

42 Piozzi, Letter II, 539 (18 December 1798), in Kerhervé, 'Writing letters from Georgian spas', p. 288.

43 These internal conflicts are well described in the context of nineteenth-century French spas by Penez, 'Les stations thermales françaises', pp. 95–115.

44 Walsham, "Reforming the waters,", p. 454.

45 Cossic quotes K. T. Alves in A. Cossic, "The female invalid and spa therapy in some well-known 18th-century medical and literary texts: from John Floyer's "The Ancient Psychrolousia Revived" (1702) to Fanny Burney's "Evelina" (1778)', in Annick Cossic and Patrick Galliou (eds), *Les Villes d'eaux En Grande-Bretagne et En France Aux 18e et 19e Siècles* (Brest: Cambridge Scholars Press, 2005), pp. 115–38.

46 T. Rowlandson, 'The Comforts of Bath', 1798. F. Haslam, *From Hogarth to Rowlandson: Medicine in Art in Eighteenth-Century Britain* (Liverpool: Liverpool University Press, 1996).

47 On the relationship between melancholy and the bowels, see M. Louis-Courvoisier, 'The soul in the entrails: the experience of the sick in the eighteenth century', in R. Barr, S. Kleiman-Lafon and S. Vasset (eds), *Bellies, Bowels and Entrails in the Eighteenth Century* (Manchester: Manchester University Press, 2018), pp. 81–101.

48 Coley, '"Cures without care"'.

49 Porter and Rousseau, *Gout*.

50 W. Cadogan, *A Dissertation on the Gout, and All Chronic Diseases, Jointly Considered as Proceeding from the Same Causes; What Those*

Causes Are; and a Rational and Natural Method of Cure Proposed (London: T. Bradford, 1771).

51 J. Wesley, *Primitive Physick: or, an Easy and Natural Method of Curing Most Diseases* (London: Thomas Trye, 1747). John Wesley, the founder of Methodism, argues that nature abounds in medicines, and his treatise draws on official and folk medicine alike. He recommends fresh air, a quiet mind and cold water. See F. Zanetti, 'Les thérapies alternatives de John Wesley', in M. Cottret (ed.), *Normes et déviances* (Paris: Les Éditions de Paris, 2007), pp. 160–76.

52 Cadogan, *A Dissertation on the Gout*, p. 62.

53 Cadogan, *A Dissertation on the Gout*, p. 62.

54 Porter and Rousseau, *Gout*, p. 54.

55 See Philip Roberts's introduction in P. Roberts (ed.), *The Diary of Sir David Hamilton, 1709–14* (Oxford: Clarendon Press, 1975). On mineral waters and barrenness, see 'Mineral waters as a treatment for women's barrenness in 18th century Britain', in Chiari and Cuisinier-Delorme (eds), *Spa Culture and Literature in England*, 211–31.

56 The curing method of 'packing' was systematically developed in nineteenth-century Malvern; see J. W. Harcup, *The Malvern Water Cure: Or Victims for Weeks in Wet Sheets* (Malvern: Winsor Fox Photos, 1992), pp. 12–15.

57 Smollett, *Humphry Clinker*, p. 172.

58 Smollett, *Humphry Clinker*, p. 172.

59 Smollett, *Humphry Clinker*, p. 172.

60 For an exploration of eighteenth-century medical understanding of the nervous conditions and the nervous system, see H. A. Whitaker, C. U. M. Smith and S. Finger (eds), *Brain, Mind and Medicine: Essays in Eighteenth-Century Neuroscience* (New York: Springer, 2007) and G. S. Rousseau, *Nervous Acts: Essays on Literature, Culture, and Sensibility* (Basingstoke: Palgrave Macmillan, 2004).

61 He is one of the doctors caricatured in *Humphry Clinker* as Dr. L.—n for his obsession with the waters and his praise of their effluvia. Smollett, *Humphry Clinker*, p. 17 and note I, p. 355. See also O. M. Brack's note on Linden in his edition: T. Smollett, *The Expedition of Humphry Clinker* (Athens, GA: University of Georgia Press, 1990), p. 344n).

62 See Phyllis Hembry's account of Linden in *The English Spa*, p. 168.

63 Linden, *A Treatise on the Origin, Nature, and Virtues of Chalybeat Waters*, p. 63.

64 Linden, *A Treatise on the Origin, Nature, and Virtues of Chalybeat Waters*, p. 64.

65 Linden, *A Treatise on the Origin, Nature, and Virtues of Chalybeat Waters*, p. 64.
66 Louis-Courvoisier, 'The soul in the entrails'.
67 Rutty, *A Methodical Synopsis of Mineral Waters*, p. 390.
68 Rutty, *A Methodical Synopsis of Mineral Waters*, p. 390.
69 On nervous complaints, gender and mineral waters see McCormack, '"An assembly of disorders", p. 564.
70 N. Gallagher, *Itch, Clap, Pox: Venereal Disease in the Eighteenth-Century Imagination* (New Haven, CT: Yale University Press, 2018).
71 L. Rowzee, *The Queenes Vvelles That Is, a Treatise of the Nature and Vertues of Tunbridge Water. Together, with an Enumeration of the Chiefest Diseases* (London: Iohn Dawson, 1632), p. 45. 'Parastatae' means the epididymis, a tube that connects the testicle, and the duct deferens which transports sperm.
72 J. Wilmot, *The Complete Poems of John Wilmot, Earl of Rochester* (New Haven, CT: Yale University Press, 1968), pp. 142–9.
73 W. Nisbet, *A Medical Guide for the Invalid to the Principal Watering Places of Great Britain: Containing a View of the Medicinal Effects of Water* (London: Highly, 1804), p. vii.
74 Linden, *A Treatise on the Origin, Nature, and Virtues of Chalybeat Waters*, p. 63.
75 D. W. Linden, *A Medicinal and Experimental History and Analysis of the Hanlys-Spa Saline, Purging, and Chalybeate Waters, near Shrewsbury* (London: John Everingham, 1768), pp. 64–65.
76 'Materia Medica' commonly refers to the array of drugs available from the apothecary through medical prescription.
77 Rutty, *A Methodical Synopsis of Mineral Waters*, p. 301.
78 Rutty, *A Methodical Synopsis of Mineral Waters*, p. 301.
79 I have been made aware of the notion of 'living with one's disease' thanks to the Institute 'The Person in Medicine' at Université de Paris, whose commitment to interdisciplinary approaches to chronic diseases has enlightened my vision of eighteenth-century illness. http://lapersonneenmedecine.uspc.fr/ (last consulted 28 February 2020).
80 McCormack, '"An assembly of disorders"'. My own article confirms McCormack's findings on gynaecology, as I trace how water treatment was prescribed for barrenness – especially female barrenness – and the representations of this treatment in eighteenth-century British culture. S. Vasset, 'Mineral waters as a treatment for women's barrenness in 18th-century Britain', in Chiari and Cuisinier-Delorme (eds), *Spa Culture and Literature in England*, pp. 211–29.
81 Rutty, *A Methodical Synopsis of Mineral Waters*, p. 518.
82 Rutty, *A Methodical Synopsis of Mineral Waters*, p. 171.

83 Rutty, *A Methodical Synopsis of Mineral Waters*, p. 196. On corpulency
    and barrenness see S. Toulalan, '"If Slendernesse Be the Cause of
    Unfruitfulnesse; You Must Nourish and Fatten the Body": thin bodies
    and infertility in early modern England', in T. Loughran and G. Davis
    (eds), *Infertility in History, Science and Culture* (London: Palgrave
    Handbooks, 2017), pp. 171–97.
84 Rutty, *A Methodical Synopsis of Mineral Waters*, p. 610.
85 D. W. Linden, *A Treatise on the Three Medicinal Mineral Waters at
    Llandrindod, in Radnorshire, South Wales* (London: J. Everingham,
    1756), p. 95.
86 Linden, *A Treatise on the Three Medicinal Mineral Waters at Llandrin-
    dod*, p. 95. For a discussion of medical discourse on masturbation, see
    T. W. Laqueur, *Solitary Sex: A Cultural History of Masturbation* (New
    York: Zone Books, 2003); A. Wenger, 'Lire l'onanisme: le discours
    médical sur la masturbation et la lecture féminines au XVIIIe siècle',
    Clio: Femmes, Genre, Histoire, 22 (2005), 227–43.
87 Linden, *A Treatise on the Three Medicinal Mineral Waters at Llan-
    drindod*, p. 95.
88 I tackle this question in two articles: S. Vasset, 'From a specific medical
    case to general definitions: French doctors picturing sterility in the
    1820s', in Loughran and Davis (eds), *Infertility in History*, pp. 311–35
    and in Vasset, 'Mineral waters as a treatment for women's barrenness'.
89 'A Letter from *Tunbridge* to a friend in *London*; being a character of
    the Wells, and company there', in *A Pacquet from Will's* (London: S.
    Briscoe, 1705), p. 1.
90 'On the Virtues of Scarborough-Spaw Water', in *The Scarborough
    Miscellany for the Year 1733* (London: J. Wilford, 1734).
91 J. Evans, *Aphrodisiacs, Fertility and Medicine in Early Modern England*
    (Woodbridge: The Boydell Press, 2014).
92 *The Scarborough Miscellany* (London: J. Roberts, 1732), p. 2.
93 This was the case of the Barèges waters of the French Pyrenees, known
    as 'eaux d'arquebusades'. They were also known and imported – or
    artificially reproduced – in England. See C. Meighan, *A Treatise of the
    Nature and Powers of Bareges's Baths and Waters* (London, 1742);
    J.-C. Sanchez, 'Eaux d'arquebusades et médecine thermale militaire dans
    les Pyrénées centrales (XVIe–XVIIIe siècles)', *Revue de Comminges*,
    (2017) 257–85.
94 Rutty, *A Methodical Synopsis of Mineral Waters*, p. 266.
95 This very question is still at the heart of medical debates in countries
    where spa treatment is reimbursed by the state such as twenty-first-
    century France, as it was the subject of disputes in eighteenth-century
    Britain. See for example G. Weisz, 'Le thermalisme en France au XXe
    siècle', *Médecine/Sciences*, 18:1 (2002), 101–8.

96 Christine de Buzon analyses Montaigne's relationship to health, doctors and to his own pain during the narrative of his therapeutic journey: C. Buzon, 'La Santé selon Montaigne', in C. Buzon and O. Richard-Pauchet (eds), *Littérature et voyages de santé* (Paris: Classiques Garnier, 2017), pp. 181–99.

97 Noel Coley also argues that some waters were accused of provoking the stone and gravel they were supposed to dissolve, as we will see for the Somersham waters, which I will present in chapter 5. Coley, 'Physicians and the chemical analysis of mineral waters', pp. 129–30.

98 See n. 29.

99 This triggered a controversy between John Rutty and Charles Lucas analysed in A. Mason, 'The "Political Knight Errant" at Bath: Charles Lucas's attack on the spa medical establishment in *An Essay on Waters* (1756)', *Journal for Eighteenth-Century Studies*, 36:1 (2013), 67–83. On the question of the treatment of chronic diseases, see for example William Oliver's statement at the beginning of the century: 'Bath is the *Assylum Chronicorum Morborum*, the Refuge for all *Chronical Diseases*; *Scurvies*, *Cachexies*, *Colics*, Old *Aches* and *Pains*, and almost all lingering Diseases that Afflict Mankind, are here very often Cured, *cito*, *tuto*, & *jucunde*, which in all probability would yield to no Course of Medicine out of it'. Oliver, *A Practical Dissertation on Bath Waters*, p. 288. (NB: this Oliver is not the 'bath buns' doctor, who practised later in the century.)

100 Rutty, *A Methodical Synopsis of Mineral Waters*, p. vi.

101 Rutty, *A Methodical Synopsis of Mineral Waters*, p. 69.

102 Rutty, *A Methodical Synopsis of Mineral Waters*, p. 247.

103 I say primarily because fevers and agues were regularly mentioned and some diseases, such as worms or the gleets, are difficult to frame in a binary approach acute/chronic.

104 C. Lefève, J.-C. Mino and N. Zaccaï-Reyners (eds), *Le soin: approches contemporaines* (Paris: Presses universitaires de France, 2016).

105 I thank François Zanetti (Université de Paris) for this analysis which came up during our collaborative study of the medical correspondence of a French spa doctor, Jean-François Delpit.

106 Linn was registered in English, French and American societies of medicine.

107 In a typically late nineteenth-century fashion, he adds 'climatic resorts, sea-baths, and other hygienic therapeutical agents'. T. Linn, *The Health Resorts of Europe* (London: H. Kimpton, 1894).

108 The line is taken from Alexander Pope, *An Epistle from Mr. Pope to Dr. Arbuthnot* (Dublin: George Faulkner, 1735), l.136, p. 7.

109 Smith, 'Adam Smith to David Hume'.

110 Smith, 'Adam Smith to David Hume'.

2

From bog to jug: a risky remedy?

As reflexions on the measurement of risk were developing among eighteenth-century mathematicians, gamblers and insurers, risk management also became an emerging trend of eighteenth-century medical culture. The first attempts at inoculation against smallpox had grown into a widespread enterprise across the country, changing the paradigm of prevention and cure. The new practice of inoculation triggered medical debates on the risk of contracting a fatal version of the disease versus the benefit of lifelong protection.[1] After the passionate disputes following Mary Wortley Montagu's Turkish letters, and the first attempts at inoculating in London, the notion of risk had been introduced in the daily lives of the English people by the mid-eighteenth century, through the initiative of some doctors like the Sutton family who organised nation-wide inoculation campaigns.[2] Taking a chance on your health could now prevent disease in an uncertain future. The evaluation of risk was at the root of the culture of prevention that pervaded medical manuals.[3] One idea behind these manuals was to instruct the sick to evaluate the risks involved in taking specific remedies and identify contra-indications. Many writings on mineral waters include this cautionary principle, and treat them as they would treat any other drug: the waters were potentially dangerous and should be taken cautiously. Were waters dangerous because of their medicinal virtues, or because of lack thereof?

Risk-taking in the context of medicine inevitably raises the question of *pharmakon*. The multiple cautionary directions found in medical treatises to follow medical prescriptions and to prepare the patient's body before taking the waters testify to an overall confidence in the effectiveness of a water treatment, which was a risk in itself because of the strength of the remedy. Conversely, some critics of medicinal spas saw them as a mere cure-all. In medical and satirical literature alike, angry authors recurrently warned their readers against the ill consequences of quack remedies and charlatanism, and mineral waters were not left behind. In that case, another risk lurked underneath the waters – that patients should be ensnared by the dishonest stratagems of nostrum-mongers. The representations of such a risk, however, were often contradictory and should be read within the context of eighteenth-century quack culture. In a final section, I will look at the concerns over the nature of the waters in themselves, and the risk induced by the uncertainty about their path underground and their degree of salubriousness. The inherent murky aspect of some mineral waters made it difficult to distinguish between dirtiness and minerality, especially as the waters came from the bowels of the earth.

Waters as pharmakon

Mineral waters were dangerous. Doctors kept arguing that, as any powerful remedy, they could have damaging effects on the body if they were not properly taken. The idea that waters were understood and experienced as the restoration of balance through the mild and global action of a healthy natural environment, fresh air and whole-some exercise, based on the Hippocratic revival of the eighteenth century, is only partly true.[4] Waters could be found and taken in towns which were not initially spa towns, as the numerous flourishing spas of eighteenth-century London illustrate.[5] They were not neces-sarily set in a rustic environment, and if they were, some of the wells had no pump room, some of the baths no roof. Additionally, the actual process of taking the waters does not resonate as a pleasurable experience to a twenty-first-century reader of eighteenth-century accounts. Mineral waters were indeed first and foremost medicinal and, as such, they were understood to have the double-edged action of any early modern medicine, that is to say a *pharmakon*, inclosing both a healing drug and a foul poison.[6] David Harley's comment on the words of the Restoration physician Patrick Madan, who considered mineral waters to be 'a sword in the *Mad*-Man's hand', corroborates this idea: 'As the image of the knife indicates, there was a recognition that any powerful remedy must be regarded as potentially dangerous'.[7]

William Buchan sums up this ambivalence in his 1786 essay on mineral waters, the appendix to his celebrated *Domestic Medicine*: 'When people hear of a wonderful cure having been performed by some mineral water, they immediately conclude that it will cure everything, and accordingly swallow it down, when they might as well take poison',[8] he writes. Buchan is adamant: 'Without a proper discrimination with regard to the disease and the constitution of the patient, the most powerful medicine is more likely to do harm than good'.[9] Buchan's caution – as said above – is echoed by many contemporary doctors who repeat over and over in their treatises that patients, if not properly monitored in their water intake by a water doctor, expose themselves to great danger. In numerous medical treatises, the medical caution to invalids revolves around three principles: first, their own constitution should agree with bathing (temperament, age and medical history); secondly, they should drink the right dose and bathe for the right amount of time, gradually increasing each; and thirdly, their body should be prepared for the waters by adequate additional prescriptions.

Buchan included sea-bathing in his considerations on mineral waters. 'It is now fashionable for persons to plunge into the sea, and drink mineral waters', he writes, adding that he had not mentioned this treatment in the first version of *Domestic Medicine* and will do so now because 'no part of the practice of medicine is of greater importance, or merits more the attention of the physician, as many lives are lost, and numbers ruin their health, by cold bathing, and an imprudent use of the mineral waters'.[10] Sea-bathing was a form of cold bathing, the only one that Matthew Bramble in *Humphry Clinker* finds useful when he visits Scarborough.[11] In fact, when doctors argue that temperature prevails over minerals as the active principle in bathing treatments, they make little distinction between sea-bathing, mineral waters-bathing and the 'extream cold' springs of common water, as John Floyer calls them at the beginning of the century in *The Ancient Psychrolousia Revived*.[12]

Yet even Floyer, who is set to prove the safety of cold bathing by encouraging parents to immerse their babies in cold water and sick people to plunge into chilly streams, ends his chapter on a series of cautions and directions for the proper use of cold baths. He first warns that the patient's body should be prepared: 'to bleed and purge, and use such proper diet and Medicines, both before and after Bathing, which a Rationale Physician knows to be suitable to the disease, and the constitution of the Patient'.[13] He also sets limits on full-body immersion and advises 'not to stay in the Bath above two or three minutes, as the Patient can easily bear it',[14] reminding the reader that "tis dangerous to go in after drinking and eating'.[15] More than cold water, however, 'the damps', arising from the water themselves, especially in covered baths, threaten the health of those who stay too long. In line with the contemporary attention paid to the emanations of waters into the air, water doctors fretted over volatile gases and subtle particles.

Buchan was not a water doctor, and his reflection, at the other end of the century, echoes the mainstream medical ideas on bathing at the time. Like Floyer, Buchan believed that the body should be fully prepared 'by bleeding, purging, and a spare diet'.[16] Like Floyer, he mentions the ancients, only to rebuke potential readers who would take other people's cure from cold bath as a hope for their own: 'Everyone knows that the same physician who, by cold bathing, cured Augustus, by an imprudent use of the same medicine killed his heir'.[17] The reference to Antiquity, used to channel medical principles to Buchan's educated readers, inscribes the practice of bathing within a long chain of medical knowledge in an attempt to reconcile ancients and moderns around the virtues of waters.

Buchan's writing is built on a series of cases and medical anecdotes which provide a lively illustration of his argument. They also enable readers to identify with the various patients, generating an immediate sense of danger for them when confronted with the consequences of rash behaviour. The anecdotes are also entertaining, as some of them deal with historical or contemporary celebrities. In *Medical Cautions on Cold Bathing*, he inserts a note on the narrow escape from death of the theatre manager George Colman (the elder) after a sea bath. Buchan first presents his own investigation in the matter:

> When I heard of the celebrated Mr Colman's illness, and that it had happened at Margate, I immediately suspected the cause, and mentioned my suspicion to some medical friends; but as none of them could inform me concerning the real circumstances of his case, I should have taken no notice of it, had not the following Letter in the London Chronicle struck my attention.[18]

He links the culture of sociability and medical diagnosis, inviting the reader to enter the intimate sphere of Colman's treatment, as he reproduces the following letter in a footnote, which takes a remarkable space on the page:

> To *the* printer
> 'SIR,
> 'Having seen in your own and other London papers, serious accounts of Mr. Colman's illness, I, who have attended him during the whole time, think it but justice to him and his many friends, to give you a plain and true account of his case and present situation.
> 'Mr. Colman's disorder as a combination of the gout and palsy, the last of which was occasioned by his unadvisedly bathing in the sea at an improper period, which struck in the gout, the consequences, as might be expected, soon became very serious, and his situation extremely dangerous, &c.
> (Signed) JOHN SILVER, Surgeon'
> MARGATE,
> Nov. 5, 1785[19]

According to Rachael Johnson, the rise of the seaside fishermen's village of Margate in the eighteenth century to a major destination for sea-bathing was partly built on its ability to attract theatre celebrities like George Colman.[20] The letter noted by Buchan can indeed be found in the *London Chronicle* in 1785, and presents a recurrent phenomenon in literature on sea-bathing: the patient's stubborn decision of going into the sea in spite of his surgeon's warning. The 'improper period' for sea-bathing mentioned here could either depend on the patient's schedule (going in after eating, for example), or on the actual season (November) that made sea water too dangerous for bathing. The surgeon John Silver implies that the sudden bath affected Colman's gout and transformed it at once into an internal disease, attacking the organs rather than the limbs. Buchan, to justify the insertion of this anecdote, specifies it is meant to protect people 'against some of those errors into which from mere inattention they are apt to fall, and thereby not only endanger their own lives, but bring an excellent medicine into disrepute'.[21] In other words, the better the medicine, the greater the risk in taking it.

Hot baths were no less dangerous, especially for vulnerable constitutions. Diederick Wessel Linden, the Brighton-based Westphalian doctor, insists on comparing mineral waters with other drugs in his 1752 treatise on chalybeate waters:

> There is not one thing in the whole *Materia Medica* that I know of, which can be administered, that is so effectual to penetrate through the small and minute Vessels, and to pass through the whole Machine, without any Disturbance to the Mass of Blood, as the Mineral Spirits of the Chalybeate Baths.[22]

He therefore implies that the volatile spirits – that is to say, micro-elements contained in the water – move away from water into blood through the pores.[23] He then charts the paths of these active mineral elements within the circulatory system during a hot bath:

> Because the mineral Spirits of the Natural Hot Waters are too powerful and heavy for these Patients upon the Nervous system, and promote a too rapid circulation of the Blood, or too violent as, by Means of the extreme velocity occasioned thereby, not only endangers the smaller vessels, so as to Split, but also they force and separate too much *Serum* from the Blood, and oftentimes produce many fatal consequences.[24]

The reason for this velocity remains untold in this description, but the increase of sweating after a hot bath, together with the hot flushes and redness of the skin, were indicative of an altered circulation. Circulation was central to the understanding of health, and nervous maladies were often seen as a weakened condition of the whole system, including of the circulation of the blood.[25] What's more, for many doctors at the time, a subtle and invisible fluid also circulated within the nerves, mimicking the circulatory process of the blood within the nervous system.

Hot bathing was what Bath was famous for, and the renowned Bath doctor William Oliver – who published his *Practical Essay on the Use and Abuse of Warm Bathing in Gouty Cases* only a year before Linden published his treatise on chalybeate waters – wrote that 'Nothing can tend more to enable both Physicians and Patients to judge rightly about Bathing, than a plain and faithful account of the proper and improper methods of using that powerful remedy; and of the usual consequences which attend the one and the other'.[26] Recommendations on Bath would be read by a wider crowd than the Bath visitors, and would serve as a model for other hot springs. According to Oliver, bathing could be beneficial to gouty patients, as long as they followed the modes of 'proper bathing'. Patients had to be well prepared, and gradually exposed to the waters. On the other hand, 'improper bathing', an under-prepared patient suddenly plunged into 'boiling springs', could have fatal consequences: 'a high burning Fever is raised, followed perhaps by a Pleurisy, a Peripneumony, inflammations of the Viscera, or even an Apoplexy; and the patient may justly be said to have died of *improper bathing*'.[27]

In all baths, duration was crucial. William Oliver made it clear: 'It is impossible to say exactly how long the patient should continue in the Bath, because the particular circumstances of each bather can alone determine it. But it must appear from what has been said, that staying in too long must be an error of dangerous consequence.'[28] He fretted over some pragmatic issues in the basins which made the duration of the bath uncertain, a risk which he thought had to be assessed by the bathers:

> This error, I must confess, is sometimes purely the patient's misfortune, and not his fault. The great concourse of bathers is now very disproportional to the conveniences of our baths for their reception. The passages out of them are so few, that a poor weak hysterical creature, who cannot bear the Bath above ten minutes, is often kept in it above half an hour, and sometimes much longer, to the great peril of her life, at least to the irreparable damage of her health. This is so great a grievance, so much, and so justly complained of, that I don't doubt but the Legislature will judge it a matter of higher consideration, and redress, by enabling the corporation to make Baths more safe and useful.[29]

Oliver's appeal to the political and economic structure managing the baths announces the last chapter of Tobias Smollett's treatise entitled 'REGULATIONS proposed to the Mayor and Corporation of BATH', which was to be published the following year.[30] Smollett, like Oliver, connects bodies and politics, demonstrating the ill consequences of political and economic decisions on the bodies of vulnerable patients. The regulation of crowds was becoming a sanitary issue in major spas. In some places, the baths had to open all night, and sick patients sometimes obtained an appointment at two o'clock in the morning if access was too difficult. William Oliver's astute remark on the political implications of the risks taken by patients who could not monitor their time in the water makes bathing a question of public health, to be regulated by law, finance and politics. It transfers the responsibility of failed cures, usually attributed to careless doctors or ignorant patients, to governing bodies. Their decision will have an impact on the quality of care provided to the patients, and their failure to decide might entail deaths caused by an improper management of medical sources.

Another fear among water doctors was the abusive use of the purging waters, which were often 'saline' (containing salts) or 'chalybeate purging', containing both salts and iron. Cheltenham was one of the saline springs that was known for its purgative virtues. It was praised in 1786 by Joseph Smith, an Oxonian medical doctor who took an interest in saline waters and got into a controversy over the composition of the waters with a Cheltenham-based medical doctor, John Barker. Like Linden, Oliver and Buchan, who all belonged to his generation, Smith condemned excess, and complained that patients drank too much too soon:

> [M]any who come from a distance for the sake of these waters, being impatient under their complaints, and desirous of making the best use of their time, drink them to excess; and by so doing, they make the very worst use of it they possibly can. For as the evacuation, by such a proceeding, is generally greater than the constitution can bear, however well-guarded the purgative may be under by the other ingredients, they appetite and strength must necessarily fail; their spirits flag, and not finding in other respect, during the little time they make, all the benefit they expected, they go away disappointed and dissatisfied.[31]

A similar idea can be found in William Oliver's treatise, when he jokes about patients who do not prepare their organs and do not expose their bodies gradually to the hot baths: 'people think that the longer they stay in the water, the sooner they shall be cured, and act as wisely as the poor man did, who was ordered to take three purges in three weeks, but to save time, took them all together'.[32] Oliver's comparison with purging is well chosen in the context of mineral waters, making the reader consider the dangers of hasty self-treatment.

The comic and tragic potentialities of purging were exploited endlessly by critical literature on spas, especially as the triviality of the subject was an efficient counterpoint to the polite aesthetics that surrounded elite spa culture.[33] The satirical letter 'from *Tunbridge* to a friend in *London*' sneers at the eager drinkers mentioned above: 'Some Fools, indeed, thro' their great opinion of the Waters, have made their Bodies such perpetual Aquaducts, that they have wash'd themselves into meer Skeletons', jests the narrator, sketching a *danse macabre* as counterpoint to the pump room.[34] The well-known purging effects of spas gave rise to the much appreciated filthy humour of the time, such as the scene painted in a coarse broadside poem on Islington Spa. It stages a woman about to follow a beau, who is stopped by the immediate effects of inconsequent water-drinking:[35]

> She soon accepts, when of a sudden,
> She shook and Quak'd like any *Pudden*.[36]
> The reason strait I could not tell,
> But soon perceiv'd her Guts Rebell:
> And that which made her Spew before,
> Now through her Tail Work't three times more.[37]

Chamber-pot humour runs through the whole piece, and more waters, of another kind, follow until the narrator's path ends in 'the Womens boghouse'.

Purging is the common denominator of all medical humour, but in the case of the waters, faecal matter becomes a metaphor of the waters themselves, and of their murkiness. Suspicion is thrown upon the origins of the spring, or upon the ways in which it is carried to the bath house or to the pump room. This concern is at the heart of Daniel Cottom's study of the 'new emphasis on the bowels' in eighteenth-century spa culture.[38] Cottom argues that the interest of spa town visitors in visceral matters as well as their 'desire for disgust' were related to a much needed catharsis to purge off the weight of the cannibalistic nature of the social structure they otherwise supported. According to him, the *Beau Monde* enjoyed 'the digestive trope of a social body for which the processes of incorporation and expulsion are necessarily interdependent'.[39] The symbolic and meta-phorical charge of purging is clearly an important aspect of novelistic scenes such as those Cottom studies in the works of Smollett, Austen and Anstey, who were perhaps more targeted towards the middling sort. It is less applicable, I find, to the Restoration broadside poem just mentioned and fails to acknowledge the recurrent representation of the poor who stored up water and gave themselves to excessive drinking, and self-prescribed purging.

In spite of all their efforts, doctors kept encountering many autonomous drinkers in spas of all sizes, some of them using the waters quite independently of any medical supervision or analyses of the waters. Small spas and wells must have been more numerous in eighteenth-century rural areas than the ones recorded in the water treatises. Thomas Short, for example, describes a small spa in Wigglesworth, in North Yorkshire, showing genuine concern for the way in which it is used by the local population:

> Now come to a sulphur water of a very peculiar nature, such as I never met with or heard of in England besides, and deserves to be much more strictly examined and enquired into, viz. Wigglesworth Spaw, near Settle, in the parish of Long-Preston. It has been used time out of mind, and more formerly than at present, because it is little known; rains and drought affect it not. Country people drink four of five pints of it in a morning to vomit them, and six or seven pints to purge them. The water is very black, smells strong of sulphur, has a very small stream, but stagnates not, bubbles not, but springs up, it is always covered with a white scum, dies all in its course white.[40]

Emetics and purges were common remedies, and sometimes even in a preventative action. A gentle purge, to be taken regularly, was a way of maintaining one's health and evacuating the remnants of stagnant food, often called 'vicious matter', which was supposed to clog the digestive system. Short's reliance on local use and his astonishment at the nature of the water are relevant of the relationship that water doctors had with spas. Many spas were discovered through the local folk and their indications guessed through local narratives of cures that had already been performed. The process of medicalisation came later, and much effort was made to try to monitor the medical use of spas that had sometimes been locally used for years.

Short's admonition of reckless use by local people is paralleled by a strong invitation to his fellow physicians to acknowledge the limits of their expertise and let those with an adequate expertise prescribe them to their patients. Short was an advocate of chemistry, and he pushed for a systematic chemical analysis of the waters. He presented the dangers of an improper knowledge of their mineral elements: 'Without we know their vestigable Contents, their Use may do much Harm'.[41] A great responsibility laid in the hands of his fellow physicians: 'Entire strangers to the Nature of Mineral Waters should no more prescribe them, than such as are ignorant of the *Materia Medica* should prescribe Medicines'.[42] Short was thus defending his expertise on waters as an extra-qualification, a training in itself before the advent of specialised medicine in the nineteenth century. Knowledge about spas was in the making, and Short placed himself as a specialist who appealed to doctors outside of spa towns to act responsibly and send their patients to local spa doctors to consult them before taking the waters. Not only should patients find the right type of waters for their constitution, but even then, they should know how to take them, and adjust the treatment to the response of their bodies. This required local monitoring that could not be done by corresponding with one's physician back home.

Such a description of the role of water doctors was at odds with another contemporary representation of them as charlatans at worst, and, at best, as partisan doctors who shared the financial interests of a spa and fashioned their discourse to promote it.

A cure-all?

Scholars of the history of mineral waters are often confronted by a set of questions on therapeutics which are difficult to answer, yet valuable, as they also represent contemporary concerns. Were mineral waters just another cure-all, a miracle treatment, and were they perceived as such or, even worse, as potentially harmful quack medicines? Were they understood as an early form of placebo, a harmless common water, whose effects relied solely on the power of the imagination? Confronted by the volume and variety of medical publications on waters in the eighteenth century, one is tempted to rush to the conclusion that the recurrent bickering of their authors, the long-winded descriptions of miraculous cures and the endless lists of applicable diseases were all signs of their belonging to the protean realm of quack medicines. In all cases, such questions required that attention be paid to the risk of taking such medicines, whether their lack of efficiency let the course of the disease worsen, or whether their unknown components entailed unwanted secondary effects and pointless loss of money. Quackery is a complex question that needs cautious historical reading and awareness of the common use of the term. Contemporary accusations of quackery were part of wider politics of eighteenth-century medicine. In the writings of eighteenth-century doctors, a quack is an impostor who offers medical services or fake drugs even though unskilled and untrained in medicine. Quack rhetoric, as it is now understood, is built on the emphasis of the wonderful effects of the treatment advertised, and the accumulation of false cases appealing to the emotions of the reader. And yet, such rhetoric pervaded many types of medical discourse, from popular treatises to medical dictionaries. To discuss this notion, I will focus on one particular spa town, Malvern, which developed in the middle of the century. The reputation of the pure and light waters of the holy well at Malvern, originally known as St Ann's Well, grew after the investment of local landowners, as Phyllis Hembry explains.[43] The waters were analysed, and contemporary medical discourse on the Malvern waters is a good example of the ways in which medical indications intertwine with a type of rhetoric that stems from the rich and disturbing prose of charlatans. Quackery was also connected with the idea of fashion, from fashionable resorts to fashionable disease and remedies, and the section will end with an analysis of the interaction of the two notions which pervaded the representations of water medicine.

One of the common ideas attributed to mineral waters stems from a belief that they do not, in fact, differ from common water and are no more effective in treating diseases than simple water. An epigram about the Malvern waters sums up the idea:

> The Malvern Waters, says Dr Wall
> Is famed for containing just nothing at all.[44]

This epigram, quoted in 1953 in an article on the history of the Malvern waters from the *Proceedings of the Royal Society*, has since had a long legacy in spa literature, and has even been mentioned in Malvern touristic publications.[45] It was a familiar theme to eighteenth-century readers. Endangering a patient by attempting cures with common water rather than proper medicine was a long-lived literary trope which was revived in Alain-René Lesage's popular satire *Gil Blas*, published in France between 1715 and 1735.[46] In this French picaresque novel, the hero is trained as an apprentice to Dr Sangrado, whose quack dealings and dogmatic statements recall the stock character from the Commedia dell'Arte, *Il Dottore*. Sangrado cures by bleeding and regular intakes of common water: 'Drink, my children', Sangrado tells Gil Blas when he gets sick, 'health consists in the suppleness and great humectation of the parts, drink water in great abundance, it is a universal menstruum that dissolves all kinds of salts. When the course of the blood is too languid, this accelerates its motion, when too rapid, checks its impetuosity.'[47] This lively translation was undertaken by Tobias Smollett, whose medical knowledge must have helped him in the task.[48] Sangrado's words are only a slight variation from some of the medical treatises on mineral waters which Smollett must have read, having written one himself.

Here I must pause, and examine Smollett's opinion on the medical use of mineral waters before returning to the Malvern waters, as his ideas reflect a whole trend of thought that cast doubt on the effect of mineral waters. Smollett would play around with some of Sangrado's ideas without naming them when he ironically endorsed the role of a water doctor himself in the only medical treatise that he ever published, *An Essay on the External Use of Water*. Many scholars have quoted Smollett as an example of contemporary suspicions on the action of the minerals of Bath waters on the bodies of bathers ('external use'). He starts his essay by claiming that the minerals have little or no effect on the patients' bodies compared with that of common water. The only power they have, he explains, lays in the belief of doctors and patients alike in this very power. He then illustrates what we would today call the placebo or psychological effect with the Catholic tradition of 'touching' children suffering from scrofula, which he attributes to 'the power of the imagination'.[49] In the same vein, he attributes the benefit of bathing to the temperature of the water alone, quite independently of its mineral component: 'I am inclined to believe, that the Mineral Principles in Hot Springs have often, in the cure of Patients by bathing, usurped that praise and reputation which was due to the simple element', he writes, 'and that the external use of common Water; properly warmed, would have the same, or nearly the same, effect in the gout, which an ingenious Physician attributes to the *Saponeous* and *Sulphureous* Particles with which the Waters of Bath are impregnated'.[50] Smollett's attack on the numerous treatises dedicated to the chemical analysis of waters is laden with irony. The chemical terms in italics, together with the sarcastic reference to the physician's 'ingenious' qualities, sheds a sardonic light on the new branch of chemistry as a science. And yet, Smollett's view on mineral waters cannot be reduced to this passage only. He was convinced of their impact on the bodies of drinkers – in internal, rather than external use – as well as of the existence of volatile particles carried by the vapours into the lungs of bathers.[51]

In spite of Smollett's reflection on their external use, mineral waters were commonly accepted to differ from common water, even the crystal-clear Malvern waters. Notwithstanding, they were regularly perceived as quack remedies. They certainly shared a number of characteristics with quack medicines, including long lists of indications and edifying narratives of miraculous cures. Unlike quack remedies, however, which were usually advertised by a single 'doctor' who reaped the benefits of selling them, mineral waters were often reviewed, analysed and advertised by several physicians, and their analyses were digested, published and discussed by others. To continue the case of the Malvern waters, a 1762 treatise which, like Linden's treatise on the Shadwell waters, was 'printed for W. Owen, and sold at his mineral water warehouse', compares the waters of Pyrmont, Spa and Seltzer with those of Malvern. It is based on John Wall's second edition of his *Experiments and Observations on the Malvern Waters*. At the beginning of the treatise, the author gives a list of the medicinal virtues of the Malvern waters:

> *Their* Virtues
> In all Diseases of the Skin or cutaneous Distempers these Waters are the most powerful and effectual Remedy ever yet found out; since they not only remove all Eruptions and Foulnesses of the Skin, but have perfectly cured even the most confirmed Leprosies; as appears by the most undoubted Testimony. They are also of the utmost Benefit in all scrophulous Cases, Tumours and glandular Obstructions, also in scald Heads; in all old Sores, and even in Cancers; and there is undeniable Proof, that they have perfectly restored to Health many Persons, who have been afflicted with Kings-Evil in the most miserable Manner; They are of prodigious Service in all Inflammations and other Diseases of the Eyes.[52]

Such a list recalls the inflating rhetoric of quack remedies. It does not lack coherence, since all distempers belong to a cluster of skin diseases, as they were understood in the eighteenth century (many cancers and tumours were thought to be a disorder of the skin or membranes). The list goes on, however, with further therapeutic indications related in no manner to skin conditions:

> they have also been found very beneficial in the Gout, Stone, Scurvy, and all cachectic bilious and paralytic Cases; in inveterate Disorders of the Head, and also where the natural Discharges of the Sex are deficient, which they assist by procuring a due fluidity of the Humours.[53]

The medical logic changes as this new family of diseases seems to find its cause in the improper circulation of the humours, broadly understood as encompassing all bodily fluids. These fluids, when obstructed, were thought to provoke a variety of disorders by accumulation. Stones in the kidneys or gouty toes were thus assimilated to the 'deficient discharges of the Sex', to be fluidified by the solvent powers of the Malvern waters. The author ends on a warning inferred from several cases presented in John Wall's treatise: '– There is one Disorder, however, in which these Waters are found not to agree, which is the Cardialgia or Heartburn'.[54] As we have just seen, such cautions were usually perceived as further confirmation of a remedy's potency, and therefore contributed to render other indications more authentic. Readers will easily identify elements of quack rhetoric-based emphasis and accumulation, yet the text retains some ambivalence, as it is strongly linked to Wall's treatise, which had been discussed and reviewed in respectable medical journals.

The original treatise by John Wall, on which this list is based, is void of any similarly emphatic list: is the effect of quack rhetoric only due to Wall's ideas being condensed and clarified for the layperson, or can the quack rhetoric be traced back to the original treatise? John Wall had already published extensively – and sometimes controversially – on several medical subjects and was likely to have been known as one of the most successful physicians around town: his practice was based in Worcester, only a three-hour walk from Malvern.[55] After the success of the first edition in 1756, Wall added a long appendix to his small twenty-one-page treatise, topped up with an additional one in the following edition. As the title *Experiments and Observations on the Malvern Waters* clearly suggests, Wall relied on received medical rhetoric strategies. On the one hand, he gave a detailed account of complementary experiments on the mineral waters of Malvern, which required applying the methods of chemistry in the vein of the German doctor Friedrich Hoffmann, whose work was praised by British doctors like John Rutty and Thomas Short.[56] (As I argued in the introduction, the status of chemistry changed throughout the eighteenth century and gradually gained credit among medical doctors, mathematicians and natural historians.[57]) On the other hand, Wall commented on multiple case histories. The accumulation of case histories, or *Observationes*, dates back to Renaissance medicine and was first used as a way to strengthen one's town practice by emphasising therapeutic success, as Giana Pomata explains in her study of the evolution of this medical genre.[58] Having said that, the high level of Wall's entrepreneurial spirit is beyond doubt: he later became the head of a porcelain company in Worcester. Wall's self-promotion and the successful attempt at becoming a scientific authority on the medical use of Malvern waters must have played a part in his treatise.

The accumulation of successful case histories in Wall's book reminds the reader of similar quack rhetoric found in tracts and pamphlets for miracle cures of the time. The 1756 edition opens with the case of a tradesman:

> A considerable Tradesman of this Town had, when a Boy, several sinuous Ulcers above and below the Elbow, which communicated through the Joint; the Bones were much enlarged and foul, and the Arm much emaciated. He had been long attended by two eminent Surgeons who thought the Case desperate and had proposed Amputation. He was reduced to the last Degree of Weakness; but by the Use of this Water a few Months, all the Ulcers except one below the Elbow were heal'd. This continued to discharge a small Quantity till He returned again to the Well the next Summer, when He obtain'd a compleat Cure, and has continued well ever since. After he first began upon the Waters, He never used any other Application to the Sores, but Linnen Rags dipt in the Water. This Cure was perform'd several Years ago.[59]

No proper explanation is given for the healing action of the waters, yet both the method and the description of symptoms are very similar to the type of cases found in the *Observationes* of the times. And yet, the perfect cure and the desperate case presented here evoke the miraculous cases narrated in the broadsides and pamphlets selling quack remedies. Delineating quack rhetoric in eighteenth-century medicine as a specific discourse or style that would stand independently of the rest of medical discourse is virtually impossible, especially when a remedy was at stake. In this case, the waters do represent a last-chance therapy and the successful cure is a clear invitation to readers suffering from a similar illness to go to Malvern and try the waters. Reducing the treatise to a scam, and the Tradesman's case to a fictional account, would however be a mistake, as they would be disconnected from the cultural representation of health and sickness in the eighteenth century. Although rare and often partial, cures did occur, and recovery ensued. The measure of that recovery is hard to trace, since the extent of the physical damages performed by diseases on bodies, with few means of barring their evolution, was as dramatic as the ulcerated arm described in the case of this young boy with foul bones, who was threatened with amputation.

One of the last cases in the appendix to the third edition narrates the medical history of Mrs Cotton, from Newberry. Mrs Cotton's case is related by the author – John Wall's medical persona – with epistolary excerpts that give the reader access to two other narrative voices on top of his: those of the patient's son and her doctor. The letters describe her miserable condition at the beginning of the story, and her miraculous recovery at the end. Mrs Cotton was first brought to Malvern lying in a cart at full length, with a 'most frightful' leprosy: 'The Scabs were very thick and foul, with deep Fissures, from which issued a putrid Matter extremely fetid. She was also paralytic, scarce able to speak properly or intelligibly, or to walk across the Room.'[60] Her son writes that 'she has to very little purpose taken several medicines'.[61] Dr Collet's letter gives a detailed account of her medical history, reminding his colleague that considering Mrs Cotton's age – she is sixty-six years old – she would be content with 'a partial cure, if She *can* but get a partial Cure; so as to make the Remainder of her Life a little more comfortable to herself and her Friends'.[62] This request is in line with the above-mentioned notion of recovery, and doctors' and patients' expectations alike: a complete cure was not necessarily expected from the treatment. Temporary relief was desirable enough to be transported lying down in a cart from Newbury to Malvern, seventy-eight miles away.

Wall's account shows the marvellous success of her treatment, since 'the sole Use of Water had her Skin clear'd of all these Foul Eruptions'.[63] He describes the dramatic effects of the water on the patient: 'And what was very remarkable, She was not *only cured of her Leprosy, but her paralytic Disorders also*. She recover'd her Speech and Memory tolerably well, and was able to walk without Assistance twice or thrice the Length of the Terrace, which is several hundred Yards.'[64] He then comments on the case by relying on the notion of acrimonious fluids circulating in the entire body 'From whence it appears that the same Acrimony which had fouled her Skin, had also affected the Brain and Nerves; and that when this was washed away by the Water, they again recover'd their Natural Functions'.[65] Water naturally 'washes away' the noxious fluids, though no mention is made of the volatile spirits described earlier in the book. He adds two other letters from Dr Collet that testify to Mrs Cotton's recovery, and concludes with a personal visit to that doctor and a permission to publish the story, a common mark of authenticity in such treatises: 'Mrs *Cotton* thought her cure so very extraordinary, that She desired it might be made publick, and permitted me to mention her Name'.[66] Such methods are in no way dissimilar to the commercial strategies of quacks and the lists of 'authentic' patients who benefited from miraculous cures thanks to the likes of an anodyne necklace, venereal bolus or universal pill.[67]

Wall's treatise is thus built on rhetorical strategies that quacks may well have copied from competent doctors as much as the reverse: he starts with incurable conditions and desperate cases, remarks on the inefficacy of other cures, suggests a sense of authenticity, narrates radical changes in the constitution of patients, adopts a miraculous yet non-religious tone and concludes on a successful cure with an array of medical explanations.[68] The notion of charlatanism and quackery needs therefore to be taken with critical distance, as such traits of commercial rhetoric were commonly shared between what we would now call official medicine and non-official health practitioners. Historians of medical treatment have reassessed the concept of charlatanism, which divides the world of eighteenth-century doctors too simply, with retrospective notions of science according to a binary system of what is scientific and what is not.[69] Although promotion clearly played an important part in treatises like those of John Wall, the long-term economic development of spas like Malvern also relied on their capacity to bring relief to those who came to take the waters. In this context, what can be made of cases like Mrs Cotton's, or of the young boy's ulcerous elbows? True or not – an unresolved yet valid question – the presence of such cases in a medical treatise is a sign of the great expectations patients and doctors placed on mineral waters. In that sense, a risk of disappointment was taken by all those who tried a new course of the waters. These cases also reveal that eighteenth-century medical culture strongly integrated promotional discourse.[70] The descriptions of the sick before the cure remain edifying narratives of diminished bodies and desperate cases, standing among the darker prospects of eighteenth-century lives, when diseases would push a body to the limits of what it could bear.

Another reason for considering water treatment as a cure-all was that spas and seaside resorts were the epicentre of 'fashionable diseases', a term which suggested potential quackery. What did the phenomenon of fashionable diseases bring to spa culture, and how did it play out in the perception of waters as a cure-all? Fashionable diseases such as bilious disorders, vapours, nervous disorders, the hyp, consumption, gout and rheumatism permeated the discourses on spas in fiction, popular writings and medical publications. Anita O'Connell examines such discourse in her analysis of the character types representing the sick and their friends in late eighteenth-century literature. She mentions Lady Gertrude, a self-styled 'Lady Doctor' in Ann Gomersall's 1790 novel *The Citizen*, who spends much time 'discussing illnesses with the fashionable company', giving medical advice and prescribing treatment to her friends.[71] 'Such characters had become so ingrained in the satirical fabric of spa literature', she writes, 'that, more than simply a woman fainting from vapours or nerves, or a gouty man attempting to lead a young lady out to dance at a ball, numerous as these are, characters such as Lady Gertrude depict the hypochondria of fashionable society'.[72] Satire, she argues, acted as the counterpoint to the culture of 'overmedicalisation' spreading in watering places:

> While the letters and medical records of patients who visited the waters reveal genuine concern for the health of their friends and faith in the water treatment as a genuine cure, literary satires take issue with the larger cultural shift of medicalisation at the watering-places at a time when they were becoming intensely popular centres of fashion.[73]

O'Connell's article stems from a research project dedicated to a thorough interdisciplinary study of the phenomenon of fashionable diseases in the long eighteenth century that relies on the distinction between the discourse of fashion and the experience of diseases – as Clark Lawlor remarks: 'Diseases which, however painful to the sufferer, rise into fashion through popularity in medical texts, advertising, literature and social circles'.[74]

O'Connell and Lawlor explain how the role of the medical market is not 'merely a way of gulling people' but also 'a manifestation of demand'.[75] The medical marketplace shapes the discourses of fashionable disease, and is shaped in return by the coping strategies of individuals who experience sickness in various degrees: 'The more a fashionable disease appeared in various literary "templates", which narrated how it might be experienced, and where and in what social circles, the more people were likely to identify it as, to deploy the philosopher Ian Hacking's useful phrase, "a way to be a person"'.[76] O'Connell and Lawlor's argument weaves together medical consumerism and the individual experience of illness. This approach can be transferred to the question of quackery and spa treatment: mineral waters were invested as an object of consumption by patients and health practitioners, and several elements of contingency made some waters more successful than others. Fashion and promotion were certainly among them, but the investment of the town, neighbouring philanthropists, the quality of the waters and their local reputation, the genuine relief they could procure to the sick and the building of a community around the waters were also crucial to their success or failure. What's more, while the role of fashion was crucial to establish the reputation of towns like Harrogate, Buxton, Tunbridge, Scarborough, Moffat, Bristol and Bath in their efforts to reach out to the wealthy, tradition and the interaction between local communities were more powerful agents for places like Llandrindod in Wales, Ilkley in Yorkshire, or even Liverpool.[77] Taking the waters was a phenomenon strongly connected to processes of fashion, but can in no way be reduced to them.

Interestingly, the term 'fashionable disease' was popularised in medicine by the controversial physician James Makittrick Adair in his 1786 essay *Medical Cautions, for the Consideration of Invalids; Those Especially Who Resort to Bath: Containing Essays on Fashionable Diseases*.[78] Adair's essay focuses primarily on bilious and nervous disorders, and targets excessive purging remedies, which he contrasts with a more beneficial 'course of the Bath Waters'.[79] He mentions his practice at Bath and acknowledges therefore that Bath is a favourite destination for the fashionably diseased. Adair's main criticism does not lie in the Bath waters themselves. Rather, he condemns the diagnosis of the (fashionable) disease and the course of treatment that patients with such diagnoses will follow, which he understands to be either self-prescribed or directed by a 'fashionable' doctor. If a proper course of waters is followed and prescribed by a reasonable doctor – unsurprisingly, himself – the effects can help restore health when it had been put in danger by improper diagnosis and treatment. Adair thus condemns fashionable diseases while keeping the reputation of the waters safe. His treatise is not devoid of the very commercial interest he imputes to fashionable doctors. Such is the way with quackery: the quack is the other, as well as the one who initially called him such.

The term 'cure-all' and other denominations of mineral waters that imply a certain degree of quackery cannot be rejected altogether. I certainly care to avoid being swallowed in the vortex of opposing genuine and non-genuine remedies in the eighteenth-century medical marketplace. And yet, the notion of quackery, with which many authors played and used against each other, brings an element of ambiguity to this book's focus on the murkiness of mineral waters. Acknowledging that quackery, which was part of the medical culture at large, was present in spas in many forms, ranging from the exploitation of 'fashionable diseases' to the over-statement of previous cures in medical treatises, helps us understand the general feeling of uncertainty that revolved around medical cures. As they navigated through the supply of potential treatments, sick people had recourse to several measures and references. The advice of family, friends and doctors was mitigated by other means of information; the perusal of medical treatises was restricted to the knowledgeable elite, but their ideas were distilled and discussed in periodicals, popular medical manuals and literature. In all these texts, the recurrent presence of quackery was a potential threat that lurked in any treatment option, including mineral waters. Travelling to the waters was thus a risk taken by the sick: they could spend a lot of money for almost no effect, take the further risks of submitting to a potentially dangerous treatment, as we have seen, or, as I will now explain, find themselves in a much filthier place than expected.

Brine, mud and dung

In *The Register of Folly*, the anonymous author calling himself 'An Invalid' depicts his first impressions on arriving at the pump room of Bristol Hotwells:

> But first of water I will give you a sketch
> That seems to arise from a deep filthy ditch

Yet the spring is so bright, so exceedingly fine,
That many who drink it prefer it to wine.[80]

The waters were known indeed for their purity and Celia Fiennes noted in her journal that they were 'exceedingly clear and warm as new milk and much of that sweetness'.[81] The contrast between the clear waters and the 'deep, filthy ditch', evoking infernal underground waters or simply sewers, shows how ambivalent the image of mineral waters could be.[82] Even when clear and sweet, which was rare enough to be worth noticing, they are relegated to their murky origins beneath the ground.

Most mineral waters were far from being clear and fine. The glasses served at the pump room were not always made of glass, but when they were, the water inside was often revealed as cloudy. The materiality of the thick, tepid, salty and sometimes bubbly water expressed its minerality, not to mention the 'balmy' or 'oily' wells such as the one near Edinburgh.[83] Some waters like Malvern could be clear and agreeable to the taste, but they were rare. There was a fine line between brackish and dirty. Brine, mud and dung were at one end of a continuum in the imaginary of mineral waters, with clear waters at the other. Readers were always reminded of the waters' minerality, of their association with stone, gas and peat, as authors narrated the genesis of a spa. They also read about the potential dirtiness of watering places and mismanagement of the baths. Eighteenth-century ideas about salubriousness did not necessarily associate dirt and contamination, but recurrent representation of spas as insalubrious and potentially noisome to the bathers and drinkers showed that a real concern revolved around their proper management. Basins and conduits had to be maintained, and behaviours of the bathers and drinkers monitored.

Where did the water come from? Writing about Cheltenham, the Oxonian Doctor of Medicine Joseph Smith captured its path in one sentence: 'As water percolates through the bowels of the earth, it cannot fail being impregnated with those fossil matters it happens to meet with in its course, that are all soluble or suspendible in it'.[84] The idea of an element coming from or moving through the underground viscera was usually associated with mining and, in urban spaces, with sewers. In fact, both mines and sewers had a certain degree of connection with mineral waters. The image of galleries and paths underneath the ground permeated eighteenth-century culture.[85] In nature, it challenged natural historians who developed observational methods to track them. One of the most striking passages on the traceability of the old sulphur well of Harrogate, Tuewhet Well, is to be found in Thomas Short's 1766 *General Treatise on Various Cold Mineral Waters in England*, which I will quote at length.[86] The narrative follows the ways in which water is deployed along the path from a bog to the well. This excerpt comes early in Short's treatise and works like an initiation into the nature of mineral waters, their physical properties, their composition, their movement and their origin.

Short shows the dynamic process of the water and its evolution. This passage invites the reader to follow the meanders of the waters and the twisting lines of its movement through the ground. It takes note of the quality of the ground, and the variations of the landscape are correlated with the mineral elements of the water (in italics in the quote).[87] At the same time, the quality of the ground is related to its history through cultural references to Antiquity, which illustrate a sense of *longue durée* raised by geological observations (underlined in the quote). Finally, the water is described in multiple sensory terms with a strong prevalence of smell (in bold characters). It contrasts the stinking bog with the crystal-clear spring that is found in the 'basons', a basin-shaped stone in which the water settles. The meandering rhythm of the text is 'sliding along' the path of the water.

About five hundred yards south of the Sulphur Wells lies the **stinking,** *sulphureous,* or *vitriolic* Bog before mentioned, two or three yards long, but not so broad, with its mixture of fresh, common, and *vitriolic,* **black, thick, foetid** waters, which meeting and mixing together on the surface or the middle of the Bog, on a sloping descent of *gravelly* earth, may give some idea of the **horrible** <u>Stygian lake of the poets,</u> for **smell, colour,** and **consistence.** Its **stench** is so strong that travellers going that way, and the wind in their face, may perceive it at a good distance. This place, <u>antient times,</u> was a vast forest of wood, and here stood <u>*great iron forges.*</u> This Bog is compared on all sides by dry, small *rising grounds,* so as no other springs can get into it, and it has only one outlet from it. These mixed waters in it glide gently *on hard ground,* which has an *ascent* on each side, that prevent all ingress of other springs or drains getting into the Bog water. It runs softly along an easy, hard, *gravelly descent* where it is lost, or swallowed up under a hedge, at the head of some inclosed fields, which on each side rise up into two *dry, steep hills* of seven or eight yards perpendicular. There the water falls into the *crannies* of two sorts of *stone* (one a bastard *lime-stone and free-stone*, the other *greyish and lighter*, somewhat soft) through the *chinks and fissures* between the layers of those stones, shut up in these two hills. It is probably this very water (for it seems *filtered* for five or six hundred yards,) [that] springs in a very little vale below, between three or four small eminences, into four *basons* covered over-head, and in its *chinks* leaves fine *yellow sublimed flowers of sulphur*, especially under the *basons*, which have been taken up twice in my time. The water (probably that from the Bog) rises up into the *empty basons*, crystal clear, sparkles, bubbles in a glass, tho' it contains much *muriatic salt, sulphur*, and a very *little calcareous earth*. But this crystal clear water, set to stand some hours in the open air, turns a **pearl whitish, muddy**, and **loses its smell**, and, as it springs up, loses all its appearance of *iron* or *vitriol*. Before the spring comes to the Day, it sends off some small branches, which meetings with oozings of common water, weaken them before they reach their respective basons, yet all the basons are within four or five yards of one another. Tho' the water springs up thus clear, yet when any is spilt or thrown out on the pavers about the well, it turns **black** and **thick** as in the Bog, or in the *gutters* in the *pavers*; or by standing there, it leaves a **bluish, black, slimy sludge**, soon covered with *white rags*, like thick *hoard frost*, or as *sulphur* and *vitriolic, chalybeate* Bilge waters mixed. These *white rags in the gutters*, dried slowly, and laid on red-hot iron, *burn like sulphur*. From Bilton, Knaresburgh, and Harrigate, to Storra, five or six miles, have outbreaks of *sulphur* and *chalybeate* waters, all from the same principles, viz. a range of the *pyrites*, which breaks into dies of the colour of **brown sugar-candy**, and **smells strong** of *sulphur*; and near the head of the Bog it lies within a foot or two of the surface.[88]

Short's comments on dried up 'white rags' make minerals in the water visible and palpable: even when the water is crystal clear, active principles hide inside it. The traceability of the water is drawn from bog to rags, and its repulsive smell and slimy aspect are proof of its healing properties.

This water narrative contrasts with the pastoral representation of nature associated with spas and with the poetisation of the countryside.[89] The water finds its force in a repulsive bog, hidden within the woods, and mineral waters are associated with early forms of industrial work: forging and mining. Tracing the path of the waters within the earth was impossible, except through the work of miners, who regularly discovered waters in their digging, as often happened in Yorkshire. Thomas Short's account of the Tuewhet Wells is further documented by the neighbouring coal pit:

> The late Mr. Ker of Carhead had a lease of this forest, from the late Earl of Burlington to get coal or iron. He said, that, in digging near the Sulphur Wells, the first stratum was corn or grass mould; the next a marley lime-stone, so abraded by acid and salts, that when dry, some of it was a mere sponge. [90]

In another area of Yorkshire, Short comments on the Wigglesworth waters mentioned in the previous section for their excessive purging effects on the local population. He explains their effects by the presence of 'turbaries, or peat mosses, whose standing waters abounding with sulphur, are most foetid, so is the peat or turf dug out of them'.[91] Short's insistence on associating earth and water can be explained by his constant investigation into natural processes of chemistry that enriched the waters under the ground. He argued that the components of the waters could be found 'by ransacking the bowels of the earth, and finding out the materials used in the operations of nature, which will be found plain and simple, without force or violence'.[92] By force or violence, Short means the various techniques of chemistry with which components can be revealed: 'What great surprising works are carried on to perfection', he writes, 'by a natural laboratory, in the dark recesses of the earth, often without fires or furnaces, by so simple menstrua as air, water, and acid spirit, assisted by motion, friction, and abrasion'.[93] Short takes the stance of an anatomist, 'ransacking the bowels' to understand the invisible coction, decoction and fermentation processes at work in the transformation of the fluids. His description includes slimy mud and stinking sludge, but Short does not consider this filthy, nor repulsive. Smell and sludge are the tangible signs of the 'natural laboratory' at work within the bowels of the earth. The same sensations are familiar to the surgeon anatomist, whose interest in human bowels predominates over any reaction of repulsion.

Daniel Cottom argues that 'an immemorial trope had hot springs such as those at Bath originating in "the very bowels of the earth"' since the twelfth century.[94] For Cottom, the meaning of this trope had evolved, however, 'for the world whose bowels were in question

was no longer what it had formerly been'.[95] Thus, in the context
of eighteenth-century elite visits to Bath and Tunbridge, the bowels
trope should be seen as a wider digestive trope which acts like a
catharsis of the consumption culture. Cottom's reading can be
convincingly applied to the context of wealthier spa towns and
privileged spa-visiting. He puts to the fore the sick bodies of the
wealthy, and integrates the visceral processes and representations
abounding in novels and caricatures into a wider cultural context,
finding coherence between the culture of mud and the culture of
politeness and elegance, rather than focusing on their opposition.
And yet this reading is restricted to Bath, Bristol and Tunbridge
while second-rank places like Harrogate, and minor watering places
like Wigglesworth, are not mentioned. In these places, the bowels
trope might be interpreted in various ways, some of them, as we
have just seen, relating to the anatomy of the water and grounds
while other interpretations simply focused on filth and repulsion
with few signs of the cultural process described by Cottom.

Filth and insalubriousness, like quackery, were recurrent objects
of accusation for spa critics. The quality of air played a crucial role,
as air was seen as an active agent of cure in spa towns. In a letter
about Thorp-Arch, in Yorkshire, Thomas Short is surprised by the
exceptional clarity of the air: 'This vale and rapid river causes a
constant current of air; and as all the adjacent country is champain
ground, free from any morasses, fens, or putrid waters', he writes
– champain ground meaning mildly hilly –; 'we are not troubled
with any unwholesome damps or vapours, but enjoy a more clear
and salubrious air than in most other situations'.[96] Short, as we
have just seen, knew the waters of Yorkshire. His mention of 'other
situations' implies that the air is rarely salubrious in many other
spas, mostly because of the damps. The presence of marshes and
bogs around some of the spas played a part in concerns on the
quality of the air. The phenomenon was not restricted to Yorkshire
spas, and the proximity of marshy grounds and healing waters was
one of the stakes of starting spa towns such as Bristol in Pennsylvania.
Writing about the development of the colonial spa in the eighteenth
century, Vaughn Scribner explains that

In 1768 the Swiss-born physician Dr. John De Normandie presented
Philadelphia's American Philosophical Society with a tract analyzing

how the citizens of Bristol, Pennsylvania, had transformed their small village from 'its natural state' – an 'unhealthy' environment (allegedly) plagued by 'diseased ... low marshy grounds' – into 'one of the healthiest spots in America'.[97]

The making of the spa into a respectable health resort implied purifying the air, which involved transforming the very ground in which the waters were rising. Spa towns failing to do this had little chance of improving their reputation.

Wholesome air was one of the advantages of seaside spas, which combined sea-bathing and water-drinking. The seaside town of Scarborough in Yorkshire had chalybeate waters, so did Weymouth in Dorset, Aberystwyth in Wales and Liverpool, then in Lancashire, and in the Regency era Brighton integrated a drinking station of artificial mineral water called 'The German Spa'. Seaside resorts are the target of Jane Austen's satirical comments on water treatment in her unfinished novel *Sanditon*. Mr Parker, who has heavily invested in the bathing and housing facilities of the village of Sanditon, keeps praising the place to his new friends, the Heywood family. Parker's conversation is lively and enthusiastic, if not single-minded, as he always returns to his favourite subject, Sanditon, which he contrasts with a neighbouring seaside village, Brinshore:

> But Brinshore, Sir, which I dare say you have in your eye – the attempts of two or three speculating people about Brinshore this last year to raise that paltry Hamlet, lying, as it does between a stagnant marsh, a bleak Moor and the constant effluvia of a ridge of putrefying sea weed, can end in nothing but their own Disappointment. What in the name of common Sense is to *recommend* Brinshore? A most insalubrious Air – Roads proverbially detestable – Water Brackish beyond example – impossible to get a good dish of Tea within three miles of the place.[98]

Parker contrasts this ghastly portrait with the salubrious Sanditon, in possession of the 'finest, purest Sea Breeze on the Coast' and 'no Mud – no Weeds – no slimey rocks'.[99] The term 'effluvia' denotes a conception of potentially toxic airborne particles that are reminiscent of the miasma theory, associating marshes and epidemics.[100] Parker's attack on Brinshore relies on medical principles, transforming the competing health resort into a potentially toxic environment. Brinshore is a risky remedy, not because of its powerful effects, but because of the noisome environment and the poor quality of the waters, endangering the health of its visitors.

The natural environment was not the sole agent of filth in watering places. Many factors, beyond the inevitable moisture present in the facilities, could create a dirty environment: the plumbing system, insufficient bathing structures, a lack of ushers or staff in the facilities, dense crowds and irregular cleaning made many sick patients recoil from the bath and restrict their visits to the pump room. A famous passage in Smollett's *Essay on the External Use of Water* pictures the materiality of the Bath waters after they had been in use for a few hours: 'a gross, *unctuous* matter was found floating upon the water, and might have been taken off with a spoon'.[101] As Amanda Herbert explains, the bath was regulated by early hygienic principles, and it was emptied three times a day. She also analyses a picture by Thomas Johnson representing bathers at the end of the seventeenth century in the King's and Queen's baths.[102] The picture shows children, assistants, women and men swimming or walking in the water, some resting by its side, in a rather dense crowd. The pump room was just as promiscuous, and there could be long queues to drink from a glass distributed by 'a pumper' who drew the water out of a tap, or simply 'dipped' the glass into a bucket of freshly drawn water.

One of the most scurrilous satires of Bath blames the town for bringing disease rather than curing it, primarily due to overcrowding both in the pools and in the pump room. The following sketch depicts the experience of taking the waters, or attempting to take them, in the midst of a pressing crowd:

> By patient squeezing to the Pump I get;
> There roughly thrust next to some Clown I wait;
> Who, when he 'as rudely swilled his Potion up,
> Leaves me the slobber'd favour of his Cup
> Glad at all rates t'obtain the healing Draught,
> I take the Glass with all his Drivel fraught:
> The Pumper dips it, fills; and I (convinc'd
> By the foul Finger-prints, the Glass is rinc'd)
> Attempt to drink: when by my next Fool prest,
> The slipping Bicker pours along my Breast.[103]

The narrator's use of terms like 'Clown' and 'Fool', usually associated with lower social status, is a way of linking social mix and dirt. The joke in parentheses, annotated on the same page '*Imit. see.

Boileau', comes from the first book of the French poet's *Satires*
published in 1666:

> On a porté partout des verres à la ronde,
> – Où les doigts des laquais dans la crasse tracés –
> Témoignaient par écrit qu'on les avait rincés.[104]

In Boileau's satires, written in the vein of Juvenal, bodily filth is a
way of making social relationships visible, which is the case in this
sketch. One of the striking effects of such rhetoric in the context
of the waters is that the fingerprints of the pumper are a metonymy
for the general effect of the waters: they foul what they should have
cleansed.

The culture of filth, at the heart of satire, expanded in every
direction with little limit to its expression. The ambivalence of the
term 'waters' was the subject of many puns, as the joke in the 1714
Tunbridge and Bath Miscellany: 'The chiefest compliment among
Women is, *I hope the Waters pass well with your Ladyship*; which
is, in plain *English*, I hope, Madam, you piss well'.[105] Some broadside
poems, like *May Day: Or, The Original of Garlands*, went so far
as supposing that the spa water was partly made of piss, in this
case, the London Spa, which became famous at the beginning of
the seventeenth century.[106] Although urinotherapy came much later
in Britain, and urine was not so much in use in eighteenth-century
remedies, the trope of urine and faeces being used as components
of drugs was a sign of a general suspicion cast on the apothecary's
workshop.[107] Similarly, the salts contained in mineral waters were
an object of phantasmatic projections on their provenance, and the
transfer from the bowels of the earth to human bowels was an easy
image at the service of satire.

Scatological humour stepped into the theme of the 'bowels of
the earth', and scurrilous pamphlets like *The Grand Mystery, or
Art of Meditating over an House of Office* used the context of the
waters to revel in mucky metaphors. The pamphlet, wrongly attributed
to Swift,[108] is a proposition for the establishment of public houses
of office modelled on the corporations of mineral waters. To make
the matter clearer, the front page mentions that it is 'recommended
to all Persons that drink the Mineral Waters of Pyrmont, Bristol,
Bath, Tunbridge, Epsom, Scarborough, Aton, Dullidge, Richmond,
Islington'.[109] It targets the much satirised physician and natural

historian John Woodward and his ideas on purging and vomiting. The pamphlet may have been a late response in a wider controversy between Woodward and the royal physician Richard Mead, on the relevance of emetics in smallpox treatment.[110] It develops an elaborate art of 'sh-ting' and several proposals for the erection of public offices of ease.

An earlier Restoration pamphlet with a different target, *An Exclamation from Tunbridge and Epsom against the Newfound Wells at Islington*, runs a similar scatological tone. It criticises the new craze for Islington in a long complaint from its rival spa towns from the London area. The suspicion of the provenance of the waters mentioned above is made clear, as subtlety is not the main characteristic of the poem, which rejoices in excremental visions: 'That the juice of a few *cowturds* mixed with a sham of *steeldust* and steeped into a *Newvamp Well*, that in all likelyhood was an old *House of Office*; can be effectual as our *Wonder-working Fountains* that taste of *Cold Iron* and breathe pure *Nitre* and *Sulphur*'.[111] Disgust and coarseness run through the poem, which suggests a continuity between the wells and the house of office, mocking the pride of the older spa and mocking the pretentions of the new one. For example, the poem depicts the nightmen who emptied the cesspits to sell their contents as manure to neighbouring farmers: 'Strangers from remote regions came in *Guilt Coaches* to DUNG our barren *Heaths* for us, at their own charge, and having given 3. or 4. pounds for a Supper over-night, returned us the substance of it, with an overplus, next morning *Gratis*'.[112] Excrements become a commodity, and the water business is investing in excremental processes, which, thanks to the purging effects of the waters, seem entirely profitable with no production cost.

Were patients conscious that they were taking a risk when they decided to travel to the waters, or to walk to a nearby spa town? In any remedy, the certainty of sickness was counterbalanced with the hopes for a cure, and every cure had a physical and financial cost. For mineral water treatments, the risk was threefold: they could have damaging secondary effects on the patient's body; they could be another quack medicine, expensive and inefficient at best, toxic at worst; and the quality of water itself could either be lied about or endangered by poor maintenance. The waters were not just physically dirty: bad company, promiscuity and lewd manners were often associated with the spa towns that had built social premises. The dirty waters paradigm did not end at the scatological imagination, but could sink deep into the murky waters of scandal.

Notes

1 On inoculation and its consequences in culture, see S. S. Gronim, 'Imagining inoculation: smallpox, the body, and social relations of healing in the eighteenth century', *Bulletin of the History of Medicine*, 80:2 (2006), 247–268; and more specifically on the question of risk, see C.-O. Doron, 'The experience of "risk": genealogy and transformations', in A. Burgess, A. Alemanno and J. Zinn (eds), *Routledge Handbook of Risk Studies* (New York: Routledge, 2016), pp. 35–44.

2 See S. Vasset, 'Prévention et paratexte', in S. Vasset, *Décrire, prescrire, guérir: médecine et fiction dans la Grande-Bretagne du xviiie siècle* (Paris: Hermann, 2013), pp. 133–63; M. W. Montagu, *The Letters and Works of Lady Mary Wortley Montagu* (Cambridge: Cambridge University Press, 2011).

3 The most famous medical manual was William Buchan's *Domestic Medicine* (1769). Buchan's work was modelled on the popular medical manual of the Swiss doctor Samuel Auguste Tissot – S. A. D. Tissot, *Avis au peuple sur sa santé* (Lausanne: J. Zimmerli, 1761) – but domestic manuals had started earlier in the previous century, especially for women and children's diseases, and a lot of eighteenth-century editions included some guidance on inoculation.

4 See for example O'Connell's statement on the medicinal effects of waters in the eighteenth century: 'Spas and seaside resorts were originally intended to provide fresh air, relaxation and water treatment, which were believed to restore balance to a diseased body'. O'Connell, 'Fashionable discourse of disease', p. 572. Similarly, Cossic suggests that 'Bathing was therapeutic and pleasurable, because also voluptuous'. While all the sexual connotations associated with bathing she underlines are justified, very few primary sources, if any, mention the experience of bathing as genuinely pleasurable. Cossic, 'The female invalid and spa therapy', p. 131.

5 See chapter 1, n. 43. Borsay's geographic investigation into the *rurs* and *urbs* is helpful in approaching the question on a larger scale: P. Borsay, 'Town or Country? British spas and the urban–rural interface', *Journal of Tourism History*, 4:2 (2012), 155–69.

6 For a more complete analysis of the ambivalent notion of pharmakon, see L. Totelin, 'The Pharmakon: concept figure, image of transgression,

poetic practice', *Bulletin of the History of Medicine*, 93:3 (2019), 453–4; J. Derrida, 'La pharmacie de Platon', *La Dissémination* (Paris: Seuil, 1972), pp. 162–3; R. Girard, *La violence et le sacré* (Paris: Grasset, 1972).

7 Harley, 'A sword in a madman's hand', p. 52.

8 Buchan, *Cautions Concerning Cold Bathing*, p. 18.

9 Buchan, *Cautions Concerning Cold Bathing*, p. 18.

10 Buchan, *Cautions Concerning Cold Bathing*, p. 5.

11 Smollett, *Humphry Clinker*, p. 183.

12 J. Floyer, *The Ancient Psychrolousia Revived: or, an Essay to Prove Cold Bathing Both Safe and Useful* (London: Walford, 1702), pp. 24, 90.

13 Floyer, *The Ancient Psychrolousia Revived*, p. 29.

14 Here Floyer means 'as much as the patient can bear', a notable attention paid to each patient's reaction to the medicine.

15 Floyer, *The Ancient Psychrolousia Revived*, p. 29.

16 Buchan, *Cautions Concerning Cold Bathing*, p. 13.

17 Buchan, *Cautions Concerning Cold Bathing*, p. 6. This cure is mentioned in Floyer's treatise: '*Augustus* was cured of his defluxions, as Suetonius relates, by Cold-Bath', but no mention is made of his heir. Floyer, *The Ancient Psychrolousia Revived*, p. 162. Cassius Dio reports that Antonius Musa, the emperor's physician who cured Augustus by cold bathing, applied the same method to no avail to the emperor's nephew and son–law, Marcellus, who died of a fever (Cassius Dio, Book 53:30).

18 Buchan, *Cautions Concerning Cold Bathing*, p. 13.

19 Buchan, *Cautions Concerning Cold Bathing*, p. 13.

20 Johnson, 'The Venus of Margate'.

21 Buchan, *Cautions Concerning Cold Bathing*, p. 12.

22 Linden, *A Treatise on the Origin, Nature, and Virtues of Chalybeat Waters*, p. 58.

23 On the absorption of micro-elements through the pores of the skin, see Vigarello, *Concepts of Cleanliness*.

24 Linden, *A Treatise on the Origin, Nature, and Virtues of Chalybeat Waters*, p. 59.

25 See for example my chapter on circulation, 'La circulation des fluides', in Vasset, *Décrire, prescrire, guérir*, pp. 31–61, or C. H. Flynn, *The Body in Swift and Defoe* (Cambridge: Cambridge University Press, 1990).

26 W. Oliver, *A Practical Essay on the Use and Abuse of Warm Bathing in Gouty Cases* (Bath: Hawes and Co., 1751).

27 Oliver, *The Use and Abuse of Warm Bathing*, p. 74.

28 Oliver, *The Use and Abuse of Warm Bathing*, p. 74.

29 Oliver, *The Use and Abuse of Warm Bathing*, pp. 74–5.

30 T. Smollett, *An Essay on the External Use of Water* (London: M. Cooper, 1752) was appendixed with '*Particular Remarks upon the Method of Using the Mineral Waters at Bath, and a Plan for Rendering Them More Safe*'. The regulations in question are not an original proposition of Smollett's. They created a major controversy around the position of the surgeon Archibald Douglas, who had presented them a few years earlier, to the Bath corporation. Smollett supported Douglas in the pressure he put upon the corporation to improve the baths, which led to a medical and political controversy. A. Borsay, '"Persons of honour and reputation": the voluntary hospital in an age of corruption', *Medical History*, 35:3 (1991), 281–94.

31 J. Smith, *Observations on the Use and Abuse of the Cheltenham Waters* (Cheltenham: Harward, 1786), p. 12.

32 Oliver, *The Use and Abuse of Warm Bathing*, pp. 74–5.

33 Further developments on the medical, aesthetic and political function of the discourse on bowels can be found in Barr, Kleiman-Lafon and Vasset (eds), *Bellies, Bowels and Entrails*.

34 'A Letter from *Tunbridge* to a friend in *London*', p. 4.

35 On the persistence of filthy humour in the eighteenth century, see S. Dickie, *Cruelty and Laughter: Forgotten Comic Literature and the Unsentimental Eighteenth Century* (Chicago: University of Chicago Press, 2011).

36 'Pudden': pudding (hence the shaking), meaning either dessert, or guts.

37 *A Morning Ramble or Islington Wells Burlesqued* (London: George Croom, 1684).

38 Cottom, 'In the bowels of the novel'.

39 Cottom, 'In the bowels of the novel', p. 162.

40 Short, *A General Treatise on Various Cold Mineral Waters in England*, p. 73.

41 Short, *A General Treatise on Various Cold Mineral Waters in England*, p. 4.

42 Short, *A General Treatise on Various Cold Mineral Waters in England*, p. 6.

43 Hembry, *The English Spa*, pp. 250–51.

44 John Wall was the physician that analysed the Malvern waters and published his findings in *Experiments and Observations on the Malvern Waters* in 1756. W. H. McMenemey, 'The water doctors of Malvern, with special mention to the years 1842 to 1872', *Proceedings of the Royal Society of Medicine*, 46:1 (1953), p. 5.

45 See for example, Osborne and Weaver, *Aquae Britannia*, p. 207; Denbigh, *A Hundred British Spas*, p. 176. The epigram is quoted to illustrate the narrative of John Wall's reflection on the purity of the waters in his 1756 publication that contributed to making the Malvern waters famous. It is said to have circulated at the time, yet there is little evidence of a primary eighteenth-century source for this joke: the earliest occurrence I have found comes from the 1865 *Book of Epigrams*: 'Those waters, so famed by the great Dr Wall / Consist in containing just nothing at all'. J. Booth *Epigrams, Ancient and Modern* (London: Booth, 1865), p. 120. Such a time lag between the publication of John Wall's treatise and of the epigram can be explained by the posthumous writing of the epigram: although water treatment was the target of much satire in the 1750s, mineral waters were not so easily assimilated to common water as they would later be.

46 A.-R. Lesage, *Histoire de Gil Blas de Santillane* (1715–35; Paris: A. Colin, 2002).

47 'Il nous disait quelquefois: Buvez mes enfants, la santé consiste dans la souplesse et l'humectation des parties. Buvez de l'eau abondamment, c'est un dissolvant universel. L'eau dissout tous les sels. Le cours du sang est-il ralenti? Elle le précipite: Est-il trop rapide? Elle en arrête l'impétuosité.' Lesage, *Gil Blas de Santillane*, p. 12. The translation comes from the 1747 edition of Smollett's translation, *The Adventures of Gil Blas of Santillane. A New Translation, by the Author of Roderick Random*, book I, ch. 3 (London: Rivington, 1747), vol. 1, p. 131.

48 Tobias Smollett was a physician who had also been an apprentice to a surgeon in Scotland. See the section 'Scottish surgeons' in S. Vasset, *The Physics of Language in* Roderick Random (Paris: Presses universitaires de France, 2009), pp. 160–3.

49 Smollett, *An Essay on the External Use of Water*, p. 10. The power of the imagination was more commonly invoked for pregnancies – a theme that also appeared in Smollett's novels *Roderick Random* and *Peregrine Pickle*. See B. C. Southgate, '"The power of imagination": psychological explanations in mid-seventeenth-century England', *History of Science*, 30:3 (1992), 281–94; P. K. Wilson, '"Out of sight, out of mind?" The Daniel Turner–James Blondel dispute over the power of the maternal imagination', *Annals of Science*, 49 (1992), 63–85.

50 Smollett, *An Essay on the External Use of Water*, p. 23.

51 Smollett's idea on the uselessness of chemical particles is later contradicted within the same treatise. His suspicion of the effect of the mineral particles in mineral waters is in fact limited to their external use for bathing, while fomentation, as he calls it, or vapour, and,

implicitly, internal use, differs so greatly from the one of common water that it can lead to undesirable effects.

52 *A Treatise on the Nature, Properties, and Medicinal Uses of the Waters of Pyrmont, Spa, and Seltzers. Also of the Malvern Waters, from Dr. Wall's Observation* (London: W. Owen, 1762), p. 27.
53 *A Treatise on the Nature, Properties, and Medicinal Uses of the Waters,* p. 27.
54 *A Treatise on the Nature, Properties, and Medicinal Uses of the Waters,* p. 27.
55 J. Lane, 'Wall, John (bap. 1708, d. 1776), physician and a founder of the Worcester Porcelain Company', *Oxford Dictionary of National Biography*.
56 Hoffmann's work on mineral waters was translated and commented upon in the 1730s by the Scarborough doctor, Peter Shaw: F. Hoffmann, *New experiments and observations upon mineral waters: directing their farther use for the preservation of health, and the cure of diseases* (London: J. Osborn and T. Longman, 1731).
57 I am aware that this is a quick and reductive sketch of the evolution of chemistry. See for example R. G. W. Anderson (ed.), *The Cradle of Chemistry: The Early Years of Chemistry at the University of Edinburgh* (Edinburgh: John Donald, 2015) as well as C. Hamlin and N. Coley's articles mentioned in this book.
58 Pomata explains how gathering observations was a common practice among medical doctors and folk healers in early modern Europe: 'Far from being an isolated case, Cardano's *curationes* are strongly reminiscent of the "cure testimonials" when they applied for a permit to practice. Often undersigned by the patients, the testimonials listed successful cures and the composition of the remedies used.' Pomata, 'Sharing cases', p. 213.
59 Wall, *Experiments and Observations*, p. 18.
60 Wall, *Experiments and Observations*, p. 141.
61 Wall, *Experiments and Observations*, p. 142.
62 Wall, *Experiments and Observations*, p. 144.
63 Wall, *Experiments and Observations*, p. 144.
64 Wall, *Experiments and Observations*, p. 145.
65 Wall, *Experiments and Observations*, p. 144.
66 Wall, *Experiments and Observations*, p. 147.
67 See R. Porter, *Quacks: Fakers and Charlatans in English Medicine* (Stroud: Tempus, 2000). Further work has been done on the subject of quacks and rhetoric since Porter's survey of British charlatanism (see n. 70).
68 On quack rhetoric, see L. Forman Cody, '"No cure, no money", or the invisible hand of quackery: the language of commerce, credit, and

cash in eighteenth-century British medical advertisements', *Studies in Eighteenth-Century Culture*, 28 (1999), 103–30.

69 D. Gentilcore, *Medical Charlatanism in Early Modern Italy* (Oxford: Oxford University Press, 2006); Porter, *Quacks*; M. A. Katritzky, *Women, Medicine and Theatre, 1500–1750: Literary Mountebanks and Performing Quacks* (Aldershot: Ashgate, 2007); B. Dhraief, E. Négrel and J. Ruimi (eds) *Théâtre et charlatans dans l'Europe moderne* (Paris: Presses Sorbonne Nouvelle, 2018).

70 In chapter 4, I will also examine the persistence of a culture of miracles that was associated with water treatment, as this plays an undeniable role in the narrative of miracle cures, be they medically acknowledged as they are in Wall's treatise.

71 O'Connell, 'Fashionable discourse of disease', p. 577.

72 O'Connell, 'Fashionable discourse of disease', p. 578.

73 O'Connell, 'Fashionable discourse of disease', p. 578.

74 O'Connell and Lawlor, 'Fashioning illness', p. 492. The notion of 'fashionable diseases' is a recurrent cultural trend in eighteenth-century medicine and fiction, as shown by the studies of the Leverhulme programme on that subject directed by Clark Lawlor. Half of the articles in this issue of the *Journal for Eighteenth-Century Studies* are devoted to watering places and seaside resorts: Cossic, 'Fashionable diseases in Georgian Bath'; O'Connell, 'Fashionable discourse of disease'; Johnson, 'The Venus of Margate'; McCormack, '"An assembly of disorders"'.

75 O'Connell, and Lawlor, 'Fashioning illness', p. 492.

76 O'Connell, and Lawlor, 'Fashioning illness', p. 496.

77 Reaching out to the wealthy did not necessarily bar the lower classes from accessing the waters, as we will see in chapter 5.

78 J. Makittrick Adair, *Medical Cautions, for the Consideration of Invalids; Those Especially Who Resort to Bath: Containing Essays on Fashionable Diseases; Dangerous Effects of Hot and Crowded Rooms; Regimen of Diet, &c. An Enquiry into the Use of Medicine During a Course of Mineral Waters; an Essay on Quacks, Quack Medicines, and Lady Doctors* (Bath: R. Cruttwell, 1786).

79 Adair, *Medical Cautions*, p. 22.

80 The Invalid, *The Register of Folly: Or, Characters and Incidents at Bath and the Hot-Wells, in a Series of Poetical Epistles, by an Invalid* (London: F. Newbery, 1773), p. 56.

81 Fiennes, *The Illustrated Journeys of Celia Fiennes*, p. 193.

82 In *Humphry Clinker*, Bramble confronts Lewis at Bristol Hotwells on the 'exhalations arising from such a nuisance', and their potential toxicity. As a response, Lewis launches himself into a long dissertation on the origin of the term 'stink' and the cultural perception of stench. The passage is worth noting for the history of sensations, as well as

medical anxieties around water and air. Smollett, *Humphry Clinker*, pp. 17–18.

83 See John Andrews's 1797 map of mineral waters, Figure 0.1.

84 Smith, *Observations on the Use and Abuse of the Cheltenham Waters*, p. 47.

85 See G. Thomas, 'The belly and the viscera of the capital city' and A. Guillerme, 'The intestinal labour of Paris', in Barr, Kleiman-Lafon and Vasset (eds), *Bellies, Bowels and Entrails*, pp. 23–43, 44–62.

86 The well is more commonly known as 'Tewitt' or 'Tuewhit' Well, allegedly because it reproduced the call of lapwings coming to drink the waters there.

87 No word is underlined in italics in the original excerpt, a rare fact for an eighteenth-century text.

88 Short, *A General Treatise on Various Cold Mineral Waters in England*, pp. 5–8.

89 See for example Borsay, 'Town or country?', or Katherine Glover's article, 'Polite society and the rural resort', in which she writes about Moffat spa, explaining that its visitors 'should expect to gain a sense of well-being from the time spent in a sublime yet refined setting' (p. 68). In other words, rural spas offered the topoï of the countryside and sublime settings at the crossroads with a specific, health-oriented small-town environment.

90 Short, *A General Treatise on Various Cold Mineral Waters in England*, p. 8.

91 Short, *A General Treatise on Various Cold Mineral Waters in England*, p. 76.

92 Short, *A General Treatise on Various Cold Mineral Waters in England*, p. 10.

93 Short, *A General Treatise on Various Cold Mineral Waters in England*, p. 9.

94 Cottom, 'In the bowels of the novel', p. 158.

95 Cottom, 'In the bowels of the novel', p. 158.

96 Short, *A General Treatise on Various Cold Mineral Waters in England*, p. 54.

97 Scribner, '"The happy effects of these waters"', p. 409. Scribner quotes from John De Normandie, 'An analysis of the chalybeate waters of Bristol, in Pennsylvania', *Transactions of the American Philosophical Society*, 1 (Philadelphia: R. Aitken & Son, 1771).

98 Austen, *Sanditon*, p. 327.

99 Austen, *Sanditon*, p. 327.

100 Miasma theory existed before the nineteenth-century cholera epidemics. See for example Lucinda Cole's account of the role played by moisture

in early modern theories of contagion: L. Cole, 'Of mice and moisture: rats, witches, miasma, and early modern theories of contagion', *Journal for Early Modern Cultural Studies*, 10:2 (2010), 65–84.

101 Smollett, *An Essay on the External Use of Water*, p. 62.

102 'Figure 1: Thomas Johnson, "The King's and Queen's baths at Bath, looking West," c. 1675', Herbert, 'Gender and the spa', p. 363.

103 *The Diseases of Bath: A Satire* (London: J. Roberts, 1737), pp. 13–14.

104 *Œuvres complètes de Boileau Despréaux* (Paris: Firmin Didot Frères, 1851), p. 188.

105 *The Tunbridge and Bath Miscellany for the Year 1714* (London: E. Curll, 1714), p. ii.

106 *May-Day: Or, The Original of Garlands. A Poem* (London: J. Roberts, 1720).

107 J. Armstrong advocated it in early twentieth-century Britain, but the practice is also found in ayurvedic medicine. See A. Sahai et al., 'Urine therapy: from the ancient remedy of Shivambu Kalpa to modern times', *British Journal of Urology International*, 103 (2009), 52–52.

108 On the wrong attribution to Swift, see A. B. Bricker, 'Who was "A. Moore"? The attribution of eighteenth-century publications with false and misleading imprints', *Papers of the Bibliographical Society of America*, 110:2 (June 2016), pp. 181–214.

109 *The Grand Mystery, or Art of Meditating over an House of Office, Restor'd and Unveil'd; after the Dublin Edition: Published by the Ingenious Dr. S-Ft* (London: booksellers of London and [Westminster], 1726).

110 For more information on Woodward and Mead see my article, S. Vasset, 'Medical laughter and medical polemics: the Woodward–Mead quarrel and medical satire', *Revue de la Société d'études Anglo-Américaines Des XVIIe et XVIIIe Siècles*, 70 (2013), 109–33. On Woodward, see J. Levine, *Dr. Woodward's Shield: History, Science, and Satire in Augustan England* (Ithaca, NY: Cornell University Press, 1977).

111 *An Exclamation from Tunbridge and Epsom*, p. 2.

112 *An Exclamation from Tunbridge and Epsom*, p. 1.

3

Waters of desire: promiscuity, gender and sexuality

Watering places offered a variety of entertainment outlets. Not only were they justified by the prolonged presence of patrons in need of distraction, but they were also repeatedly validated by the medical literature of the times. In his comments on the use of mineral waters, for example, William Buchan prescribed exercise for drinkers and bathers: 'The best kind of exercise are those connected with amusement. Everything that tends to exhilarate the spirits, not only promotes the operation of the waters, but acts as a medicine.'[1] This injunction was quite common in the preventative medicine of the times. Inspired by Hippocrates and Galen, the idea of *Medicina Gymnastica* flourished throughout the eighteenth century.[2] Buchan further encouraged patients to socialise and be merry:

> All who resort to the mineral waters ought therefore to leave every care behind, to mix with the company, and to make themselves as cheerful and happy as possible. From this conduct, assisted by the free and wholesome air of those fashionable places of resort, and also the regular and early hours which are usually kept, the patient often receives more benefit than from using the waters.[3]

Good company was thus rationalised into treatment, and diversions encouraged. Many watering places seemed to offer a balanced alternative to the isolation of countryside retreat for some and to the social pressure and suffocation of business and industry in foul-aired cities for others.

As early as 1704, social life at Bath was regulated by the efforts of its local celebrity, Beau Nash, the famous master of ceremonies. In imitation of Bath, the supervision of entertainment and social spaces was better planned in other watering places in the country.[4] Local forces tried to introduce new rules and enforce some regulations in the larger spa towns – especially those closer to London – to counter the excessively cheerful patrons, spurred by the possibilities of entertainment and promiscuous gatherings available on site. This chapter offers an exploration of the dangers of the unmonitored and ephemeral sociability Beau Nash was claiming to fight against. Spa towns lived on seasonal time, and their visitors socialised around entertainments – walks, horse-riding, breakfast, tea, dinner parties, games, concerts, theatre and dancing. This bubbly leisure life combined with two other elements to make spa towns specific places in the eighteenth-century imagination. First, the omnipresence of the medical context rendered bodies more accessible. The imagined nudity of women in the bath, for example, is a recurrent trope of spa poetry. Secondly, most visitors stayed for a few weeks only – at best for a whole season – and were not attached to the society of spa towns by long-lasting social bonds. Many novels played with this idea, and had some characters suddenly leave town, reinvent themselves or hide their identity. As a consequence, the imagination of spa culture tended to foster seduction, sexuality and transgression.

The centrality of health remained crucial in questions of sexuality and debauchery, as Thomas Shadwell's early Restoration comedy, *Epsom Wells*, exemplifies. The second scene opens on a conversation on the way Bevil and Raines, both confirmed rakes, have been spending their young lives and endangering their health:

BEVIL: Yet your dull, splenetick sober Sots will tell you, we shorten our lives, and bring Gouts, Dropsies Palsies, and the Devil and all upon us.

RAINES: Let 'em lye and preach on while we live more in a week, then those insipid temperate fools do in a year–

BEVIL: We like subtle Chymists extract and refine our pleasure; While the like Fulsom Galenists take it in gross.

RAINES: I confess, a disorder got by Wine in scurvy company, would trouble a Man as much as Clap got a Baw'd; but there are some Woman [sic] so beautiful, that the pleasure would more than balance the disaster.

BEVIL: And your honest Whore-master makes haste to his cure only to be at it again, so do we take Pills and Waters to prepare us for another heat.

RAINES: For my part I hate to hoard up a great stock of health, as Miser do Gold, and make no use on 't: I am resolv'd to lay it out upon my Friends as far as 'twill go; and if I run myself out, I'll be a good Husband for a while to lay it out again when I have it.[5]

Like London – or worse, Paris – spa towns were thought to be inhabited by uncontrollable sexual mercenaries, putting visitors at a higher risk of contamination of venereal disease, as well as general debauchery and drinking. The insolent and rash behaviour of the rakes reveals deeper cultural anxieties over the potential danger of visiting watering places. Raines intends to enjoy life to its fullest with little regard for the consequences it might have on his body – not to mention other people's health. Meanwhile, Bevil's absurd use of preventatives for the clap, taking 'Pills and Waters to prepare us for another heat', echoes contemporary criticism of spa visitors, whose copious dinners and excessive drinking cancelled the purgative glasses taken at the wells in the morning. Bevil and Raines embody the intricate and entangled relationship of disease and desire.

Spa towns, as places of health and diversion, stood at the crossroads of disease and desire, healing and contagion. Their ambivalence is also omnipresent in novels, from encounters of heroes and heroines with dangerous rakes or fortune-hunters, to their initiation to dancing, gaming and licentiousness. What's more, bathing required a lighter form of garment, and its wet delineation of female body shapes gave way to the imagination of nudity and dishabille. Visual satire and literature showcase the body in contradiction with the various strategies implemented to hide it. Easier access to female bodies was a constant theme for the literature of spa towns, which were referred to as places of the marriage market and adultery, prostitution and promiscuity. Such was the central theme of several comedies staged in Bath, Tunbridge or Epsom, from the Restoration to the end of the eighteenth century. The inherent theatricality of watering places was put forward by their use as a setting for a play. As self-contained, seasonal microcosms between town and country, spa towns were sometimes depicted as real-life theatres in which everyone played their part in what young Jerry Melford called 'the farce of life' when he described the pump room in Smollett's *Humphry Clinker*.[6]

In these comedies, the waters served as pharmaceutical solvent not only to maladies but potentially also to social and gender norms.

The stage presence of beaux and belles, macaronies and manly wives highlighted gender roles and gender play, made more visible to the audience. Watering places were depicted as hazardously attractive and playful. In a trip to improve one's health, young men and women could altogether better their condition, or altogether ruin it. The murky waters of local power dynamics, performed through seduction, gossip and performance, presented both a danger and an opportunity, and were perceived as such. This chapter will explore the ways in which watering places were a privileged setting for the transgressive imagination of the body. The spectacle of nudity regularly surfaces in poems and caricatures as a mode of representation of female bodies under the male gaze. The imagination of accessible bodies and the celebration of desire cultivated a culture of seduction that spanned from the libertine culture staged in Restoration comedies to the well-known marriage market represented in Austen and Burney's novels. At the same time, the sexual opportunities depicted in poems and plays largely questioned gender norms, with the overwhelming presence of female beaux and manly widows.

Nudity

When imagining life at watering places in eighteenth-century Britain, two major visual references come to mind. On the one hand, most of the Jane Austen adaptations on screen have depicted Bath as a polite Georgian resort catering to well-behaved and clean company,[7] which rarely include drinking and even less bathing.[8] On the other hand, the satirical prints of Rowlandson, *The Comforts of Bath*, reveal sick bodies and social promiscuity, from the baths to the pump room.[9] The plate *The King's Bath* depicts large men and women in full clothing and feathered hats seemingly in pain, struggling in the waters and hot vapours, in close proximity to each other's sick bodies. One ageing man on the left-hand side is bending over his oversized body, with gouty hands at his sides. Another plate entitled *The Company at Play*, also depicting in the front left corner a body deformed by illness and placed on a wheelchair, shows that much of the gambling happening in the room is based on seduction. Perhaps less crowded but more voyeuristic is Rowlandson's later series on Margate composed of three prints, each of them, when considered

as a tryptic, gradually focusing in on the naked female body in
the water. It plays with the apparatus of sea-bathing – the bathing
machines – and the absence of privacy on the beach which made
visible what was fantasised about in the literature of spa towns.

In seaside towns, the growing practice of sea-bathing also fuelled
visual representations of nudity. In *Summer Amusement at Margate,
or a Peep at the Mermaids*, a group of older, rather unattractive
men in the foreground point monoculars at a group of naked women
in the background. The men are standing behind a wooden fence
on the beach, with one woman with a small parasol trying unsuccessfully to beat her husband into looking away. The spectacle consists
in a steady flow of fully clothed women entering bathing machines
to jump into the sea at the other end, their bodies distinctively naked
yet too small for us to enjoy the level of detail offered by the men's
ocular devices. The second plate, *Venus Bathing, A fashionable Dip*
(Figure 3.1) shows the naked body of a woman plunging into the
sea with her head already in the water; groups of people are standing
on the beach and on the cliff above in the background – the spectator's
gaze is no more mediated by other onlookers in the picture, and
the disembodied viewpoint is much closer, hitting the side of her
faceless body.

In *Side Way or Any Way, Venus's Bathing (Margate)* (Figure 3.2),
a woman is swimming naked in the foreground with her back to a
group of men just as far in the background, atop the very same
cliffs; she is looking lasciviously at the viewer, fully exposed.[10] The
ironic reference to Titian's *Venus of Urbino*, as she is lying in the
same position – her swimming is unconvincing – creates a playful
erotic aesthetic which Rowlandson mastered. Interestingly, the second
picture addresses the external viewer instead of the peepers on top
of the hill, as if the image of nude women in health resorts was a
particular attraction of watering places, a presence observed and
fantasised from afar. Rachael Johnson's article on fashion and disease
at the seaside starts on these two caricatures in close-up, explaining
that, as one would expect, they were excessive in their representation
of nudity. Female bathers generally wore a bathing suit, and 'these
works sexualized the sea water cure, using the sea as a setting for
romantic encounters'.[11] Johnson insists on the sea water cure as a
place for the sick, and underlines that women bathing in the sea
were not a likely feature of the English coast: 'Indeed, even when

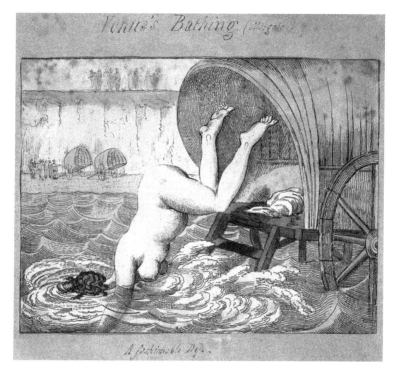

Figure 3.1 T. Rowlandson, *Venus Bathing, A fashionable Dip*, c. 1800

swimming in England emerged as a popular pastime, from the 1830s it remained a predominantly male preserve. Furthermore, although men often bathed naked, women typically wore flannel gowns while illustrations showed them without clothes.'[12]

The actual occurrence of nude bathing at spa towns and seaside resorts remains to be determined. Surely, bodies in spa towns tended to circulate closer to each other than in other towns or even than within the domestic spaces of the privileged. There were several reasons for this proximity: sickness and care, bathing and fashion. Sick bodies at the spa were a constant object of care: wheelchairs were pushed, the sick were carried from one place to another, ushered, helped in various ways by their friends, families and servants. In bath houses, bath guides, who were organised in corporations in some of the main spas, helped you find your way in the water, and bath women sold goods in the water.[13] Even smaller wells offered

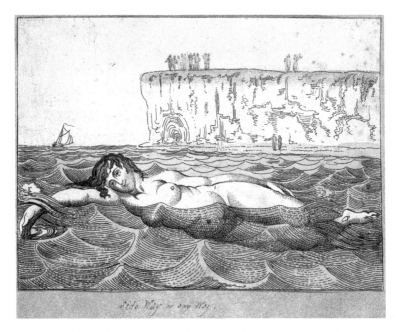

Figure 3.2 T. Rowlandson, *Side Way or Any Way, Venus's Bathing (Margate)*, c. 1800

assistance: in Floyer's *Psychrolousia*, an early eighteenth-century treatise praising the virtues of cold water, a letter from a 'former Cambridge fellow' describes the bathers at Honwick Wells and mentions 'the officious women at the Well' who dip the children in cold water and 'are active in rubbing their back'.[14] While promiscuity was constitutive of water cures, it was not necessarily sexual, as Rowlandson's caricature *The King's Bath* also suggests.

Did men and women bathe together, as the caricature portrays? Daniel Cottom and Penelope Byrde both mention the 1737 imposition by the Bath corporation on men over ten years old to wear 'a pair of Drawers and a Waistcoat' and on women a 'decent shift on their bodies'.[15] They infer from this ban that inappropriate clothing or nudity were a recurrent and undesirable practice, common enough to be punished with a fine of 'three shillings and four dimes', that would be 'committed to and for the use of the Poor of the said City [Bath].'[16] For Amanda Herbert, this question remains to be solved. She notes contradictory testimonies, some of which express surprise at seeing men and women in the same bath, sometimes naked, while the seventeenth-century English traveller Celia Fiennes's account of the pools in Bath shows that they were 'rigidly segregated'.[17] In other large spa towns like Tunbridge and Harrogate, further investigation is needed: there were several baths, some private, some owned by the town corporation, and their admission and bathing rules differed. Regulations must have been looser in a small spa like Honwick Wells, where 'the Well is so little, that they are forced to take it up in pitchers, to fill a Vessel large enough to bathe in', as Floyer's correspondent N. Ellison explains. Free access to the wells implied some degree of free bathing, especially as, before leaving the well, 'the Healthful that go in for pleasure, put on their Cloaths, and go to their Business for diversion',[18] which suggests that they must have taken them off before.

As Penelope Byrde explains in her article on bathing costumes, there were specific garments to be worn at the bath: the head was covered with 'linen caps', 'night caps' or 'chip hats',[19] and the body was covered with 'loose-fitting shifts, high to the neck with long sleeves'.[20] She also quotes Celia Fiennes's detailed description of bathing habits at Bath in 1687:

> The Ladyes goes into the bath with Garments made of fine yellow canvas, which is stiff and made large with great sleeves like a parsons gown; the water fills it up so that its borne off that your shape is not seen, it does not cling close as other lining, which Lookes sadly on the poorer sort that goes in their own lining.[21]

Fiennes's account reveals the paradoxical qualities of bathing clothes, which both covered and revealed – by clinging – shameful body parts, an exposure that women of the higher classes were spared through a complex ritual of going in and out of the bath.[22] Byrde's analysis is based on Bath, however, and little can be concluded on other watering places of second and third rank, that did not have the same facilities and staff to usher bathers or hide them from the view of others. Even at Bath, the very structure of the baths enabled voyeurism, as the King's Bath, for instance, was exposed to the view of drinkers in the pump room.

Fact or fantasy, the male gaze on female bathers is unquestionably a recurrent motif in visual and literary representations of bathing. In the 1735 *Bath and Bristol Miscellany*, the poem 'On a Lady

Bathing' celebrates this very spectacle. It starts with classical tones and ethereal bodies which Barbara Benedict aptly describes as a 'neo-classical nostalgia for the Golden Age':[23]

> When *Caelia* bath'd, how did I trembling gaze!
> Her eyes sent forth innumerable Rays;
> Those Rays restor'd me to my self again,
> Converting into Pleasure all my Pain.[24]

Staging the object of his desire against a lyrical background styled in the Renaissance trope of pleasure and pain, the (male) poet continues to compare Celia's body to the '*Cyprian* Queen, When naked from her wat'ry Bed she rose'.[25] 'Celia', however, is more modest than Venus, and the poet despairs:

> But *Celia* carefully conceal'd the Part,
> Which might have thaw'd a frozen Hermit's heart.[26]

Here the tone of the poem breaks, and although mythological figures remain, they mediate a rape fantasy clearly asserted by the speaker:

> Had I a *Triton* been with *Argos'* Eyes,
> I wou'd have seized *Love's Fortress* by Surprize.[27]

The poem therefore turns into a much bawdier piece than it set out to be, as in 'her kind embrace', the poet would 'take the Jewel, and she keep the Case',[28] robbing chaste 'Celia' of her virginity had she not been modest in her bathing dress and 'conceal'd the Part'. Eighteenth-century rape culture thus triumphs in mock-lyrical extravagance. As the rules of courtship command, this fantasy seems to be spurred by Celia's very modesty and by her refusal to bathe naked, unlike her mythological counterpart. The tension between modesty and the imagination of nude bodies triggering sexual encounters was the very fabric of which popular spa poetry was made.

In the *Scarborough Miscellany* of that same year (1734), the editor apologises for including a poem on Bath: 'we think an excuse for inserting the following verses, though they were produced in a different scene'.[29] Indeed, the Scarborough waters were cold, and the poem, 'writ with a Pencil, and sent to *Lady* * * * * while she was Bathing at Bath', talks of hot waters. Watering places were in regular contact with each other, and miscellanies were a channel to mediate this dialogue. As above, the poet couches his lewd undertones in a neoclassical overture: 'Flumine dum meditor Flammas extinguere; Flumen Fervet, & in medio Flumine Flamma fui. [While I am thinking on how to extinguish the flame with water, the waters boil, for she is the flame with the water.]'[30] The use of Latin contrasts with the inspiration on the spur of the moment which the use of a pencil suggests. The poem thus presents itself as a *pièce d'occasion* – occasional poetry written in the mundane circumstance of everyday life – as well as a learned piece abounding in Latin references, inserted in multiple notes at the bottom of the page. It is built on the opposition between hot and cold, and starts with scientific undertones:

> The Cause, which makes these Waters hot;
> The Cause – my *Celia*, in vain is sought
> In Sulphur, or Chalybeate,
> Or other principle Innate.[31]

Although this piece cannot be attributed to the rising genre of scientific poetry, the playful use of mineral elements to evoke desire introduces a discrepancy between the poetic appeal to the object of desire and a mock analysis of their mineral component.[32] The tone evolves as the poet is aroused by the spectacle of Celia bathing:

> 'Tis only now the *uxorious* wave
> Does your divine Perfection view
> That he does *swell* – does *pant* – does *heave*
> Does *own* his flame and *Wonder* too.
>
> 'Tis only now, the *officious* wave
> Does his *own Flame* and *Wonder* too
> Does *swell* – does *pant* – does *groan*, does *heave*
> Whilst *happy* in *caressing* you. [33]

As the poem insists on the immediacy of the experience, the waters become a metaphor for his growing desire, giving leave to express the physical experience of sexual arousal in his masculine body – panting, groaning and swelling as he gazes on the female bather. The waters of desire surrounding Celia do not, however, manage to provoke similar passion in her body, and the poem ends on the trope of the frigid beauty: 'The nymph who does these feats – is cold'.[34] Again, the imagination of nude women bathing is bridled by the impossibility of enjoying any pleasurable encounter other than hidden observation. This prime example of water poetry expresses

the longing for a culture of courtship deeply connected with a wider
sense of nostalgia linked with spa towns: the unrequited love of the
poet only reinforces his desperate desire.

Beyond the pure nudity of neoclassical statues pictured in mythological settings, lighter dress was regularly evoked as a common
trait of watering places, linking more relaxed fashion codes with
alleviated social protocols. In the ballad 'The Humours of New
Tunbridge Wells at Islington', also published in 1734, the poet scans
the promenades, waters and assembly rooms of Islington, which
became fashionable enough at the turn of the century to be considered
a rival to Tunbridge and Epsom.[35] The poem was written by John
Lockman, whose work as a translator of French might explain why
each stanza ends on the French term 'dishabille', the revolving point
of the poetic depiction.[36] The use of the French word sexualises
what was mostly understood as a lighter form of dress, or 'undress'
– a dishabille is simply a nightgown, a negligee, but also means
'undressed'. The ballad starts by celebrating the 'brighter charms'
of the Ladies:

> No Homage at the Toilette paid,
> (Their lovely Feature unsurvey'd,)
> Sweet Negligence her Influence lends,
> And all the artless Graces blends,
> That form the tempting Dishabille.[37]

The 'features unsurvey'd' evoke the body shapes of women revealed
by the absence of stays, or lighter stays or 'jumps' worn by women
when they were unwell, levelling the distinction between the sickness-
induced intimacy and more seductive one, in which 'Negligence'
would indicate desire rather than tiredness or unease. The 'artless
Graces' of women, who are less made up than they would be in
town, triggers the poet's imagination as he peers at shapes otherwise
hidden in dress codes. The ending inflection of each stanza makes
the dishabille a *raison d'être* of spa towns, from the 'Manners in
high Dishabille' to the disappointing bareness of bread and butter
with 'no Napkins, Tongs' or, I will explain below, the 'Equestrian
deshabille' of riding women. Later in the poem, as one would expect,
the poet launches into a targeted chase of 'Chloe':

> I'd fly to clasp the Magic Shade
> And kiss away the Dishabille.[38]

The glory of Islington had just been revived by the regular visits of George II's daughters, Princess Amelia and Princess Caroline, who took the waters at Islington in 1733.[39] The day trippers following the court enjoyed the entertainments provided by the London suburbs, a competitor to the Vauxhall pleasure gardens, and Lockman's poem was adapted into song, reprinted and illustrated in *The Musical Entertainer*, a series of musical sheets illustrated by the engraver George Bickham the Younger.[40] Bickham's engraving has a woman facing the viewer looking at a short gentleman or boy, while leaning invitingly on the balustrade of the wells (Figure 3.3). In parallel, the illustration of another publication of Lockman's poem pictures a crowd of men and women happily mingling around the well, holding hands, in close conversation, while a caricature of goddess Hygeia standing in a chariot pulled by a grasshopper and a butterfly blows bubbles onto the dense crowd from above (Figure 3.4). In both scenes, one can sense the light, relaxed atmosphere of social mixing and joyful drinking. Other engravings and literature of seaside-bathing go far beyond the enticing notion of 'dishabille' to present bolder pictures of crude and literal undress, which became the object of many a comic scene in the literature of the second part of the century.

At watering places on the seaside, the literary trope of men standing on the beach watching women bathing in the sea started much before Rowlandson's caricatures on Margate at the turn of the nineteenth century. In fact, several poems published as early as those mentioned above in the *Scarborough Miscellanies* of 1732 and 1733 mention women bathing in the sea, caught by the poet's gaze. The piece of occasional poetry, for example, entitled '*On a Sight of the* LADIES *bathing in the Sea*', starts on the self-reflective wonderings of the poet, unsure as he is of his capacity to distinguish fact from fiction:

> But when amid the gentle Main
> A Troop of lovely Nymphs I view,
> I grow enamour'd with the Strain,
> And think the pleasing fiction true.[41]

He rejoices that he alone can be a witness to the scene and enjoy it with pure thoughts:

> Here no indecent Sight allures
> The bold Access of lewder Eyes,

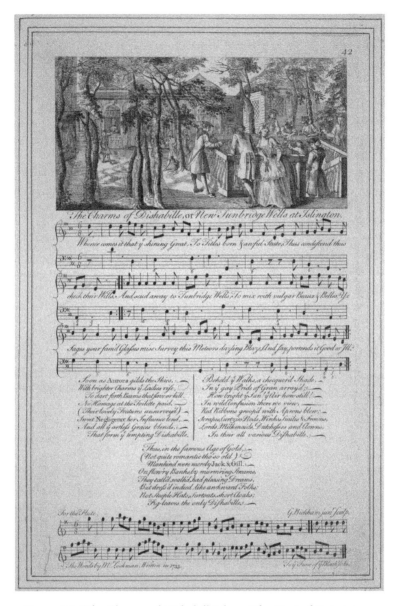

Figure 3.3 'The Charms of Dishabille' from *The Musical Entertainer*, 1733

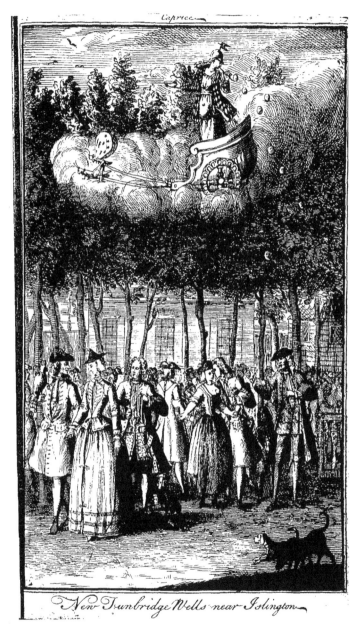

Figure 3.4 Frontispiece to 'The Humours of the New Tunbridge Wells at Islington', 1734

> A spreading Vest the Nymph secures,
> And every prying Glance defies.[42]

Of course, the mere evocation of a 'prying glance' places both poet
and reader in a position of indecent watching in spite of all claims
to decency, which may be why the speaker ends his description by
bidding the 'Rash Gazer' to 'Fly from the Nymphs'.[43] In the same
miscellany, a short piece entitled 'Scarborough-Spaw, a Song' repeats
the same wave metaphor as in the poem previously mentioned on
the hot waters of Bath:

> When she bath'd I have seen the Salt Wave
> Seem eager the Fair-One to meet;
> Each wantonly strove, which should have
> The Pleasure of kissing her Feet.
> But now the Sea, sullen and rough,
> In murmurs retires from the Shore,
> Ye Waves you've had Pleasure enough,
> In clasping the Nymph I adore.[44]

The poem's hackneyed theme is yet another embrace by proxy of
a woman bathing whom the sea in its bold and brave moves reduces
to feet and fair traits.[45]

Comic scenes of nudity contrast with the adoring poets' suffering
over the unattainable – and objectified – naked bodies of their
nymphs. Comedy forces nudity out of the classical ideal of the
unattainable nude as it turns to the more terrestrial and awkward
naked body. Rachael Johnson gives an account of *Adam and Eve,
A Margate Story*, a tale in which a newly married couple bathe,
only to find that their clothes have been robbed on the shore, and
they must reveal themselves naked to the world. This tale is the
Margate version of earlier scenes set in Brighton or Scarborough.[46]
In John O'Keeffe's comedy *The Irish Mimic; Or Blunders at Brighton*,
for example, the Irish character Parrots complains of an unexpected
sea bath:

PARROTS: Bathing! Oh a blessed affair happen'd to me, the very day
I arrived, I was so afraid of nobody coming to hear me, that I was
about to go back to London; so I took my place in the machine, but
instead of a stage coach, they put me into a wooden closet, and
dragg'd me into the sea: Hallo! Says I, let me out! Off with your
cloaths, says the fellow, and tumble out here headlong.[47]

Parrots's unexpected plunge, the misunderstanding and forced undress feminise his position in this situation. So does his cry 'let me out!' which, instead of fighting, gives him the status of a ridiculous wuss. At the opposite end of the comic spectrum, Humphry Clinker's brave plunge into the sea to save his master is imbued with powerful masculinity verging on the grotesque:

> One morning, while he was bathing in the sea, his man Clinker took it in his head that his master was in danger of drowning; and, in this conceit, plunging into the water, he lugged him out naked on the beach, and almost pulled off his ear in the operation. You may guess how this achievement was relished by Mr Bramble, who is impatient, irascible, and has the most extravagant ideas of decency and decorum in the oeconomy of his own person.[48]

Unlike Parrots, Clinker plunges. Unlike Parrots, Bramble fights. Yet they are both overwhelmed by fear: fear of drowning for Clinker, and fear of ridicule for Bramble. Their nudity is exposed in both cases, and renders them vulnerable, in contrast to their initial plunge in the sea.

Therapeutic baths tapped into a visual imaginary of female bathing. Nude nymphs inhabited the classical scenes of local poetry, turning into erotic scenes of female privacy invaded by a male gaze, or in pastoral scenes of naturalist sea-bathing. Such tropes were a fertile ground for visual satire around bathing. By contrast, male bathing was an object of grotesque comedy or farce, in which men alternatively found themselves exposed and confounded, or revealed in their potency. It is hard to tell whether the imaginary of nudity in spa towns made them more attractive to those in search of a partner. Nonetheless, the recurrence of images of nudity in literature and visual culture, as well as the prevalence of the marriage market, created of a prosperous culture of courtship in spa towns.

A stage for the marriage market and adultery

In literature, spa towns hit a remarkable narrative balance between town and country. Town folks would go to a watering place for their health as one goes to the countryside, seeking the benefits of fresh air and isolation, while country people would expect their medical query to provide the social life and entertainment opportunities of the town. It made spas a convenient setting for the marriage market, as they were an opportunity to introduce new characters. There was also an opportunity for comic encounters between the rural conduct of country visitors and the urban manners of those who came from town. Marriage was the essence of the plots of novels and of comedies. 'Spa comedies' became a prolific subgenre[49] abounding with *mise en abyme*, given that the very theatricality of spa towns fed the genre. Every middle-sized spa town had its theatre, from Buxton to Brighton. Some spas, like Sadler's Wells near Islington, were joined to a theatre, and their existence is mentioned in more eighteenth-century songs and short plays than in medical treatises. Theatre-going was part of spa schedules and plays were announced on week nights or late afternoons, together with balls and games, while mornings were reserved for drinking the waters.

On stage, spas were an alternative setting to London, which probably raised specific expectations if the action of the play was located in Bath, Scarborough or Islington. Sheridan's *A Trip to Scarborough* (1781) insisted on the distance between London and Scarborough and on the smallness of society there, while George Colman's 1776 comedy *The spleen, or, Islington Spa* played on its proximity to London. Spa towns themselves were seen as a fertile ground for social performance. The recent architectural developments of many spa towns gave them a particular, sometimes almost interchangeable, look reminiscent of theatrical settings. The promenades, pump rooms and ballrooms were spaces of social display, ephemeral encounters and comic social confrontations with the theatricality of the everyday life of health resorts. Young John Melford in *Humphry Clinker*, for example, writes to his friend in a stoic manner on the ridicule and clumsy interactions in the pump room at Bath, directly pointing at the theatricality of the place: 'I cannot account for my being pleased with these incidents, any other way, than by saying they are truly ridiculous in their own nature, and serve to heighten the humour in the farce of life, which I am determined to enjoy as long as I can'.[50] 'The farce of life' fashioned the farce on stage, and was spun into love intrigues that ranged from the classic stingy guardian aspiring to marry his ward, to scenes of adultery and even prostitution in the true spirit of Restoration comedies.

The spectacle of negotiating supply and demand on the marriage market of spa towns is best embodied by the bold Hillaria, a provocative character in Thomas Baker's *Tunbridge-Walks: Or, the Yeoman of Kent*, the most famous of Baker's plays at the turn of the eighteenth century, which was performed and published regularly until the 1760s.[51] It narrates the story of Reynard, 'a gentleman who lives by his wits' and dresses up as a yeoman to seduce Belinda's conservative rural father Woodcock, get his approval and keep his daughter's dowry, even though he has already married her in secret. Reynard's sister Hillaria is presented as a 'railing, mimicking lady' who engages in battles of wit with the men who court her. Having provided wholesome advice to her sister-in-law – she's the one who comes up with the idea of a peasant costume for her brother – Hillaria remains on stage alone to reveal her own plan for her Tunbridge stay:

> HILLARIA: Now for my own Matters – – This Musick, Rambling, Tea, and Scandal, are very pleasant, but all don't secure the Main Chance, and that must be done before I leave *Tunbridge*: for faith, I'm so damnably in Debt, I daren't show my Head in Town, till I have got some body to clear Scores – – ere comes *Woodcock*, if I coul'd trap the old Fellow now for a Husband, what Variety of young Lovers wou'd his Estate purchase – – Sure no Body in this World had ever greater Occasion for a Fool than I have at present.[52]

Hillaria cleverly connects the dots between money and marriage by clearing her credit history and becoming solvent again. Marriage is reduced to an economic transaction whose added benefits involve maintaining lovers, just like rich men keep mistresses. As Florence March explains in her study of marriage in Restoration comedies, the legal status of marriage was unstable until the Marriage Act of 1753. The multiple ways in which a marriage contract could be ratified made it easier to sign than to terminate, and therefore a potential source of profit for fortune-hunters, who seemed to be proliferating.[53] Little difference is there, from this perspective, between marriage and prostitution, with the advantage however of less hazard to one's health, better long-term economic security and the absence of social stigma. Hillaria adds to the list of benefits the titillating perspective of her potential enjoyment of male prostitutes – lovers she would 'purchase'.

The setting of the spa comedy is a fitting background for Hillaria's playful reverse of gender roles – in this case, turning the trope of the penniless rake seducing an older dowager to her advantage. Her lively inversion of gender roles is further illustrated as, chatting with Belinda, she interrupts herself in her speech upon meeting her brother with a group of friends: 'But here come the He-things',[54] she says, comically objectifying them. The scene happens at 'the Tunbridge Walks', also the title of the play, which refers to the shopping area of the town better known as the pantiles. This paved alley of shops had just been refurbished as the reputation of Tunbridge grew with numerous royal visits of Anne when she was still a Princess of Denmark. The pantiles were emblematic of the modernity of the town. Hillaria's assessment of the upcoming men as 'he-things' suggests the Walks are an extension of the pantiles' shopping shelves, and the men its consumable goods. As display shelves for the marriage market, the Walks exclude those economically unfit for consumption, and threaten with ridicule the established couples who would not be the target of adultery: 'Good Mr. *Loveworth*', Hillaria tells her suitor, 'don't mention marriage at *Tunbridge*, 'tis as much laugh'd at as Honesty in the City; This is a Place of general address, all Pleasure and Liberty; and when we happen to see a marry'd couple dangle together at the Knife and Fork, they are a Jest to the whole Walks'.[55]

Literary representations of sexual freedom in spa towns seem to vary according to the time and place, and were certainly not all as provocative as Baker's Tunbridge scenes. In 1781, William Fordyce Mavor wrote a sequel to Christopher Anstey's 1766 *New Bath Guide*, which had become a satirical reference for spa culture. Mavor set his sequel in Cheltenham and evinced adultery from Anstey's narrative, even though the whole plot of his *Cheltenham Guide* revolves around the marriage market. The characters of the B—R—D (Blunderhead) family are kept in this new adaptation; they all accompany Prudence on a trip to Cheltenham, where she is to be cured of her religious melancholy induced by 'Roger', her Bath lover and preacher. All three principal characters, Prue, Jenny and Simkin, are determined to settle their condition and find a proper lifelong companion. The tone of the work does not match Anstey's vigorous earlier satire, as Mavor, a botanist, biographer and school director, was more turned towards educational satire than scathing laughter. Everything works according to plan in the pure air of Cheltenham:

What events unforeseen often rise to our view,
When objects quite diff'rent we meant to pursue!
I came here for my health, and my blood to refine;
And PRUE to forget her convential whine:
She has pick'd up a parson last night at the ball;
I am fall'n in love, *over head, ears, and all.*
Jenny soon will be married – a fine expedition!
All likely to *change*, if not *mend* our condition.[56]

Mending one's condition and mending one's body are presented as one, provided by the soothing atmosphere of polite Cheltenham. The rural spa repairs the devastating effects of Bath social life described in the *New Bath Guide*. Tristram, the narrator, even talks of Prudence's melancholy as a 'Bath-caught disease',[57] which soon abates with the drinking of the Cheltenham waters:

O bles'd be this fount! it in mercy was giv'n
And the pigeon that shew'd it came wing'd from heav'n!
It surely to cure ev'ry ill was design'd,
To heal the weak frame, and pour balm on the mind!
For PRUDENCE more chearful and rational grows,
Nor prates about ROGER and screws up her nose.[58]

The poet refers to the legendary discovery of the waters by local people who saw in their meadows a flock of pigeons pecking in the grass for crystal salts after a flood. It emphasises the pastoral setting, which is an ideal context to cleanse one's past and find new purity. The healing virtues of the waters combined with quiet rural life seem to be able to cure unrequited love and religious melancholy. They heal the young girl of past passions and transform her into a fresh item on the marriage market.

Both sides of the coin are evoked in a dialogue between Mrs Rubrick and her sister Mrs Tabitha in George Colman's *The spleen, or, Islington Spa* (1776), an adaptation of Molière's *The Imaginary Invalid*, set in a spa town near London. Mrs Tabitha refuses to accompany her sister to Islington on the grounds that it is a debauchee's den: 'as to watering places, I'm told nobody goes there, that's fit to go anywhere else. – Cripples, and sharpers! Phthisicky old gentlewomen, and frolicksome young ones! Married ladies that want children, unmarried ladies that want sweethearts, and gentlemen that want money! Newgate out of town, the London

Hospital in the country, sister!'[59] All spa stock characters are captured in Mrs Tabitha's derogatory view of Islington, which was
then being revived by John Holland's 'genteel tea garden', growing
ever more notorious among London's middling sort.[60] Her sister,
on the contrary, sees the spa as a wonderful pool of would-be
husbands for younger girls: 'the watering places are the only places
to get young women lovers and husbands',[61] to which her sister
replies: 'Ay, they got lovers, oftener than husbands, I fear, sister'.[62]
Mrs Tabitha's remark on the role married women played in the
dangerous speculation of the marriage market, highly beneficial
to the market of adultery, targets her sister. Indeed, Mrs Rubrick
is getting ready to go to the spa independently of her husband's
commute between London and Islington, a rather common trait of
novels and spa comedies. As Ronald Cooley points out: 'a recurrent
motif in spa literature is a wife's independent visit to the spa, either
in advance of, or in the absence of her husband, who remains in
town to attend to business'.[63] Such independent visits, largely driven
by friendship rather than marriage or adultery, have been confirmed
by historians Amanda Herbert and Alison Hurley in their research
on eighteenth-century spaces of female sociability.[64] In chapter four,
I will examine how alternative modes of sociability participated in
creating political atmospheres that were spa-specific. In this chapter on
scandal, I would like to turn to the place of adultery in the collective
imagination of spas and the relaxed atmosphere associated with
watering places.

The presence of independent women in spas naturally introduced
one of the most ancient figures of comedy: the ignorant cuckold.
In Colman's play on Islington, young Jack Rubrick depicts Old
D'Oyley's ignorance of the amorous dealings of his wife-to-be (Jack's
sister) as he goes on his horse-ride, an exercise often prescribed to
patients after their morning drinking at the well:

> JACK: Ha! yonder's old D'Oyley on horseback. – Let us make
> haste to the Spa! He is just returning from his constant exercise.
> His is as regular as the clock, as exact as a Time-Piece, and the
> good housewives roast their meat by him. He enjoys the air of the
> New Road every day, takes a whet at Mother Redcap's, trots up to
> Hampstead, crosses the Heath, comes down Highgate Hill, and so
> through Holloway, back to Islington. This is Cuckold's Round, as they
> call it![65]

The connection between D'Oyley's regularity and his cuckolding is telling, as the whole town was regulated by a schedule which told visitors when and where they could meet, and conversely, when their companions would be busy. Jack Rubrick elaborates on the witty geography of cuckoldry, revealing how adultery is dependent on time and place. Spa towns, with their regulated time schedules and organised spaces, were a perfect setting to imagine and stage adulterous relationships.

The short poem 'The Unfortunate Blow' is another variation on the theme of cuckolding, enlivened by a slapstick ending. It appears in *Summer Amusement*, a compilation of poems published in 1772 by the local Canterbury writer John Burnby and addressed to 'the frequenters of Margate, Ramsgate, Tunbridge Wells, Brighthelmstone [Brighton], Southampton, Cheltenham, Weymouth, Scarborough'. The omission of Bath and Bristol is worth noting here, along with the priority given to spa towns in Kent. The poem is reminiscent of Hillaria's sarcasm on married couples dangling on the Walks. It starts with a domestic quarrel performed in a public space, as 'Cleora the Gay' is 'parading the rooms' at Margate with her 'dear on her side':

> Madam broke out loud in a fit of ambition,
> 'no woman of spirit, whate'er the condition,
> will ever be confined to one place for the season,
> So begged that her Deary would hearken to reason,
> And fly to partake of diversions she saw,
> At Tunbridge, at Weymouth, and Scarborough Spa.[66]

The irony in Cleora's use of the verb 'confined', a striking term to any post-2020 reader, is heightened by the fact that pregnant women were systematically confined to their house before and after delivery. By contrast, Cleora's 'confinement' is an abusive term, not related to any pregnancy but only to the urge to travel from one spa to another, an early form of the fear of missing out that might have affected eighteenth-century people of fashion with the multiplication of cultural centres. Unsurprisingly, the trope of the dominant wife which pervades the poem is complemented by the husband's submissive response:

> The dotard consent to humour his wife,
> As fools always do in conjugal life,

> Then with arms wide extended he ran to enfold her,
> When the bailiff clapped spousy a blow on the shoulder.[67]

The mistaken bailiff's blow is both literal and figurative, as the reader realises that he is not the man that is usually seen with Cleora in these assembly rooms. The presence of the bailiff in the assembly rooms of Margate, though, signals the local governing body's attempt at regulating manners in their town, an attempt which the anecdotical poem proves vain and hopeless.

Rakes are far from being the only sexual predators in spa towns. Medical men are recurrently pictured in dangerous proximity to their patients' bodies. A scene mixing medicine and seduction taken from Colman's comedy *Spleen, or, Islington Spa*, published four years later, exemplifies the sexualisation of doctor–patient relationships. Old D'Oyley's wife-to-be is said to have been seduced by D'Oyley's new doctor:

> ASPIN: The Doctor's the matter. He has been feeling the pulse of your wife that was to be, examining too closely her constitution, Mr. D'Oyley.
> D'OYLEY: I don't understand you.
> ASPIN: You are the only person in Islington that don't. It is the common topick of the Wells, that there is too strict an understanding between Eliza and this young Practitioner.[68]

Dr Aspin is spurred by jealousy. His new rival, 'Dr Anodyne', is in fact Eliza's female friend, Laetitia, dressed up as a doctor, but he doesn't know that. Aspin, as D'Oyley's regular doctor, is prone to believe in Anodyne's lecherous intentions because he knows the temptations of his own profession. Aspin thus depicts Anodyne's seduction of Eliza and insists on his patient's ridiculous exposition as the ignorant cuckold in the whole spa town, hoping to find an ally in his determination to destroy the growing reputation of a dangerous rival.

The sexual undertones of medical examination were already cause for concern in an earlier and racier play by Thomas Rawlins, the *Tunbridge-Wells: or A days Courtship* (1678), almost a century before Colman's comedy on Islington. As in many early Restoration comedies, the play features common prostitutes, humorously named Brag and Crack, who try to improve their status by marrying gullible older men. In an early scene, Brag is pretending to be a 'Person of

Quality drinking the Waters at their lodgings' while Crack is posted at the entrance, monitoring the comings and goings of men passing by. Dr Outside, the quack in the play, comes to visit her:

> OUTSIDE: Madam, I cou'd not take my round, without certifying myself of the intrisical operation of your Ladyships waters.
> BRAG: They pass but dully.
> OUTSIDE: Do you ponderate them, according to prescription?
> CRACK: Alas! She has not discharged (saving your Worships reverence) the demi-quantity she drank.
> OUTSIDE: Some viscous obstruction latent, but I'll prescribe an apperative: I profess they should be drank at the Well, least they evaporate their volatile Salt.[69]

The visit is both a pretext to proceed to further examination, as is made clear by the succession of men coming to the lodgings, as well as the opportunity to talk of Brag's guts –and throw in some scatological humour within the bawdy setting. Dr Outside's services, however, are requested somewhere else as Lady Parret, 'parcel Midwife, parcel Bawd', interrupts the scene 'in a heat' to complain that her friend Mrs Paywel is being ill-used by the doctor: 'You are a worshipful dispatcher indeed, t'have had a Lady under your hands these five weeks for the common cause, when I have known more good done in five minutes'.[70] Outside's protest that 'The Husbands old and defective' quickly informs the spectator that Mrs Paywel is barren, and has come to Tunbridge in hopes of a cure, which Lady Parret expects will be provided by Dr Outside:

> PARRET: Were you not imployed to supply those defects? Do we not call the Phisician to help th'infirmities of Nature? And were not you called (as they say) by my advice, I thought you an able Man, but you approve yourself a Man of weak practice, and feeble parts.
> OUTSIDE: Be pacified, what's within the power of Man I'le effect.
> PARRET: What's within the pores of Man may do much by a right application, I know't by experience, I beg your Ladyships pardon that I borrow your Doctor for an hour.[71]

The adulterous woman trope could not be made clearer: not only does Outside have leave to approach Paywel as her physician but her husband, like Cleora's 'dear', is indulgent and submissive.[72]

In the archetypal plot of adultery, a necessary complement to the ignorant cuckold is the unsatisfied, lecherous wife. Such is the case with Mrs Paywel, described as a 'pampered Alderman's wife who employs more of her husband's Estate in Lewdness than in Charity'.[73] One of the scenes is directly staged at the wells, an uncommon feature in spa comedies. It was illustrated on the frontispiece to the play: a pastoral scene of courtship around the wells shows men drinking to each other's health, three of them flanked by women at various stages of courtship (Figure 3.5). In the corresponding scene in the play, the characters drink the waters and engage in an exchange of playful puns and jokes, which is spurred by one of the protagonists, the beautiful and spirited Lady Courtwit:

> WILDING: I would not have you put a constraint upon yourself; you have beauty and youth sufficient to heighten love without such artifice.
>
> COURTWIT: I cannot digest this compliment without a glass of Water, Lets to the Well.
>
> *They walk towards the Well, and the Alderman and Mrs* Paywel, Outside *and* Parret *advance, follow'd by an Old Woman with Water.*
>
> ALDERMAN: Give me the other glass; these Waters are so cold, I profess th'l hardly down.
>
> DR OUTSIDE: Stir Mr. Alderman, motion warms, and gives the Waters just operation.
>
> MRS PAYWEL: By my truly, if they don't satisfy my longing for a Boy, I can scarce applaud them.[74]

In the context of the previous dialogue between Outside and Parret, the doctor's advice to 'stir' the waters takes on a double entendre on his impotence, which is confirmed by his wife, Mrs Paywel, as she publicly acknowledges her frustration and desire. The waters become a metaphor for each character's sexual interaction: they help the clever ingestion of compliments by Courtwit, make up for the cold lack of motion in the Alderman's genitals, and hardly satisfy Paywel's sexual hunger.

On the continuum of seduction that pervaded the collective imaginary of Restoration and early eighteenth-century Britain, prostitution is only an extreme form of the levity of manners. The spas mostly associated with various forms of sex work or unlawful sexual relationships were located in London, including 'The London Spa', and in nearby villages such as Islington, Sadler's Wells and Hampstead, as well as within a day's distance of London such as Tunbridge Wells, Epsom and Richmond. In the broadside poem 'An

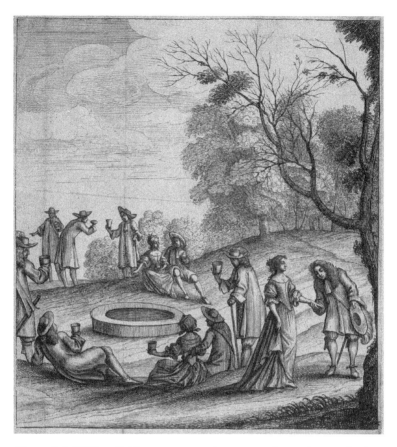

Figure 3.5 William Faithorne, Frontispiece to Rawlins's play *Tunbridge-Wells*, 1678

Exclamation from Tunbridge and Epsom against the Newfound Wells at Islington', for instance, the nostalgic voice ironically regrets the glorious times of Tunbridge and Epsom when they were not threatened by their new competitor from London: 'Here [in Tunbridge and Epsom] the over-fraighted *strumpet* (undone by doing, or ruin'd, like some improvident *Shopkeepers*, by grasping at too great a Trade) puts in to *New-Wash*, Carreen, and Tallow; and so returns a fresh and blooming *Virgin*'.[75] The sex worker is thus compared to a ship going to the shipyard, to get repaired and tallowed, and ready for the next cruise. In the same vein, the broadside ballad entitled 'Hampstead Wells' assigns sexual intentions to spa visitors:

> And Ladies never scruple, but Undress.
> What else makes wanton R——ge with softn'd Grace,
> Sweep all the WALKS, and set her dimpled Face,
> To Catch the first promiscuous Embrace.[76]

R——ge's dimples are marks of the pox, and a promise of contagion for her next embrace. Brag and Crack, the two common prostitutes in Rawlins's play *Tunbridge Wells*, were not the only examples of prostitutes trying to improve their station in spa towns, helped as they were by the general atmosphere in which one could reinvent oneself. The epilogue to Shadwell's play, Epsom Wells, closes the play as it began, with a discussion between the 'cheating, sharking, cowardly bullies' Kick and Cuff, who comment on the drinking women in the opening scene. Kick asserts: 'Many a London Strumpet comes to Jump and wash down her unlawfull Issue, to prevent shame? But more especially charges.'[77] The 'unlawful issue' – the result of adultery, possibly a child, more probably venereal disease – is also to be washed away in the waters. A similar idea is exposed in the provocative poem *Hampstead Wells*, as the waters mingle with the sickly fluids from venereal disease:

> Here, in vile Hack, the viler Punk comes down,
> Seeking thy Streams her inbred Fires to drown,
> Through whom the WATERS with loud Hissings pass,
> And one Green-Gown burns up the friendly Grass.[78]

The 'inbred fires' of the prostitute infect every other bather, and the image of contagion, symbolised by the 'green gown', a gown stained by amorous play in the grass, makes the Hampstead waters murkier than ever. In her study of venereal disease in literature, *Itch, Clap and Pox*, Noelle Gallagher analyses how eighteenth-century literature and art expanded on the metaphor of venereal disease to address wider social issues – race, gender, class and immigration. In the context of spas, venereal disease is certainly connected to social promiscuity, and the multiple traps on one's way to signing a suitable marriage contract. As I will now show, a certain degree of uncertainty as to people's identities lurked in the ephemeral social relationships that were entertained for one season. Spas were often represented with elements of a carnivalesque culture where one could reinvent oneself, come clear of one's past, usurp someone else's identity, and lie about one's wealth, status and gender.

Gender roles and gender fluidity

The marriage market and the game of adultery were strict conceptual frames within which the dance of gender roles could be executed with many entertaining diversions. Adultery and prostitution were constitutive of a society ostensibly built on polite courtship and religious marriage. Each gender was ascribed its part to play. Spa culture, however, disrupted the application of such codes and its murky waters became an imaginary locus for the representation of gender fluidity. Nudity on the beach most strikingly, but also bathing, exercising and modes of socialising that diverged from the gendered norms of everyday life, created visions of gender widely expressed through satire and criticism.

'One of the most striking characteristics of resorts was the female profile of their population', writes Peter Borsay.[79] Recent scholarship has confirmed Borsay's remark. Alison Hurley has emphasised the role of spas in epistolary conversations of the bluestockings.[80] Amanda Herbert has shown how they fostered female friendships and shared activities such as confectionary-making.[81] Rose McCormack has noted a trend of prescription for spa waters specifically addressed to female patients.[82] To Ronald W. Cooley, the feminisation of spas expands to the urban space itself. He explains that 'gendered representations of Tunbridge Wells extend back to the town's seventeenth-century foundations and to its very different early reputation as a spa and summer resort for the fashionable denizens of Restoration and eighteenth-century London'.[83] The association of space and sexual identity makes an interesting entry into the issue of spas and gender, for if a spa town like Tunbridge was feminised as a town, or at least associated with feminine occupations and taste, it could then be perceived as a place that might contaminate its visitors.

Perhaps because spa towns were mostly frequented by women, female beaux and 'macaronies' pervade the satirical writings of spas. Conversely, spa town settings often staged women experimenting with new modes of dress and new gender roles for the length of the season. Cooley establishes a connection between women's gendered roles in eighteenth-century narratives and the identity of the urban spaces of the watering place:

> What these divergent treatments share is the feminisation of space and place – a feminisation that is sometimes merely conventional, but is often distinctive and historically specific. It is as if the history of the town's representation in English discourse were constructed around a stereotypical narrative of a genteel woman's life, from blushing debutante, to a competitor in a cutthroat sexual marketplace, to frustrated spinster or complacent matron.[84]

The narrative of the town thus delineates gendered types and the performance of gender on the walks, in the pump room, the concert rooms, or in the baths. The urban space of the spa as represented in literature framed the constructions of gender while at the same time creating spaces for gender crossings.

The first threat to the heterosocial order is the bath itself. In the satirical letter published in the *The Guardian*, already mentioned in previous chapters, the narrator, Nestor Ironside, expresses his surprise at seeing both sexes in one pool:

> My fancy was diverted to the Water, where the Distinctions of Sex and Condition are concealed; and where the Mixture of Men and Women hath given Occasion to some Persons of light Imaginations, to compare *The Bath* to the Fountain of *Salmacis*, which had the Virtue of joining the two Sexes in one Person; or to the Stream wherein *Diana* washed herself, when she bestowed Horns on *Acteon*.[85]

Rather than pointing to the promiscuity denounced elsewhere, the narrator focuses on the grotesque disappearance of gender markers. The reference to Salmacis, the nymph of the fountain who transforms Hermaphrodite as she attempts to ravish him, is an interesting variation on the previously mentioned waters caressing the bodies of nude women. It introduces a powerful female figure, the sexually aggressive nymph (she will later inspire the term *nymphomania*), making a bath in the waters potentially threatening to the bathers' gender specificity. The waters, often presented as a solvent in medical discourse, become a solvent of gender identity in the tableau of mixed bathing portrayed in the learned and jocose tone of Nestor Ironside, who acknowledges, *de facto*, being among those who contemplate such scenes with 'light imagination'.

Whether on the walks or in the pump room, traditional masculinity is represented in spa literature as threatened by the fops, men whose taste for fashionable clothes, good manners and knick-knacks was the target of anxious and aggressive satirical poems, prints and plays. This phenomenon soared at the end of the seventeenth century; the culture of the Restoration was often accused of being influenced by continental fashion, as the Italian word 'macaroni' conveys. As cultural successors to the fops and beaux, who embodied similar characteristics in the first part of the eighteenth century, macaronies were a cultural construction of effeminate, witty masculinities, highly concerned with high fashion, gossip and self-care, regularly presented in literature as a threat, since their attractive visual performance and seductive wit provided them with influential social power.[86] They remained present in spa cultures throughout the eighteenth century, which is another sign of the nostalgic culture of spas and their connection to the Restoration, even towards the end of the eighteenth century.[87] The late *Register of Folly: Or, Characters and Incidents at Bath and the Hot-Wells* (1773), for example, has a whole epistle dedicated to the excesses of 'Bath Macaronies', in which the narrator laments a general loss of masculinity in the whole city of Bath:

> So that of female I write you I mean
> All the male to include; – scarce a man to be seen![88]

The narrator continues with a long description revelling in the details of their fashionable attire:

> Such fantastical fops, that (between you and me)
> They all foreigners seem, with air *je-ne-sçais-quoi*
> Take their figure and dress, *a-la-mode-de-Paris*;
> French coats without skirts, pudding sleeves and long waists,
> Dutch breeches, short waistcoat, cut back with such taste!
> With silver-clok'd stockings and buckles of paste.[89]

The foreign paraphernalia of fashion turns the fop into a one-man parade. He becomes the object of the poet's male gaze. By mocking each part of the fop's costume with the exact and appropriate sartorial name ('Dutch breeches', 'silver-clok'd stockings'…), the poet reveals himself a connoisseur of fashion whose ambivalent disdain betrays a certain degree of attraction for the 'fantastical' fop. Such visions belonged to a larger fascination for a culture of performance in which gender crossings were one extravagance among many in playful sartorial creativity. This is the case in the whimsical struggle for fashion depicted in Burnby's *Summer Amusement* in 1772, for example. The poem 'On Seeing a Lady with a large head-dress at a concert',[90] in which the speaker bemoans the disasters of fashion, is followed by the 'Lady's Answer', which blames the macaronies for the disproportionate wigs they must wear to outwig them:

> But you modern monkeys
> Some call Macaronies
> Who hours sit under the Tonsors
> Sure were born in a den,
> You're so far unlike men,
> You feminine-masculine monsters.
>
> When you sit in your chair
> For your delicate Hair
> To be dress'd in the tip of the fashion
> If not scented and greas'd,
> Then your spirits are teaz'd,
> And like Fribble you fly in a passion.[91]

Wigs and frizzles are a metonymy for the competition between women and macaronies. The juxtaposition, within Burnby's miscellany, of the initial poem mocking large head-dresses with the 'Lady's Answer' transfers the stakes of the wigs in a competition of wit. The monstrosity of the macaroni and the trouble cast by his gender-bending is thus countered by the woman's anxious reclaim of her own attributes, and her call for the accepted gender codes to be reinstated.

If we leave the assembly rooms and head towards the wells, we find gender-bending to travel along with spa-goers. A popular song on Harrogate in the first half of the century claims, not unlike Nestor Ironside in *The Guardian*, that the relationship between spa towns and gender-bending fashionable dress codes can be found in the waters:

> The grave they turn gay, the stupid make witty,
> The fools they make wise, and the plain all quite pretty;
> Give youth to old age, of a clown make a beau,
> In the ton of high taste of gay Harrogate Ho!

> *Alamode* and polite here each parson so grown is,
> Th' apostles you'd think were all turn'd macaronies:
> For wonders more fam'd than old Jordan shall flow,
> Thy sulphureous fountains sweet Harrogate Ho![92]

The transformational powers of the waters create a carnivalesque society for a season, exploring the potentials of the other side, whether age, class or gender. Such portrait of the transformational powers of the waters, already presented as changing the sick into the sound, is 'a charismatic meditation on human possibilities', as Terry Castle puts it.[93] Barbara Benedict calls spa miscellanies 'printed carnivals' which 'popularize freedom, leisure, and play, but do so within the context of reproduced fashionable verse'.[94]

The theatres were perhaps the best place in town to encounter the most accomplished form of transvestism. The ultimate example of cross-dressing in this case is the character rightfully named 'Maidenhead' in Thomas Baker's play *Tunbridge-Walks*, who acknowledges that he enjoys dressing as a woman in public places:

> LOVEWORTH: But if you neither read, study, nor converse with Men, how do you employ your superfluous Hours?
> MAIDENHEAD: Why, Sir, I can Pickle and Preserve, raise Paste, and make all my own linen: Then I love mightily to go abroad in Woman's Clothes: I was dress'd up last Winter in my Lady Fussock's Cherry-colour Damask, sat a whole Play in the Front-Seat of the Box, and was taken for a Dutch Woman of Quality.[95]

Maidenhead is careful to sit in the front seat, displaying his elaborate feminine looks to the whole audience. This metatheatrical moment in the play establishes a parallel between the feminine domestic crafts and the ability to be admired in a theatre, as if pickle and preserve-making, which were restricted to female circles, were preparation for sitting in the front row of the box in the comfort of a 'fussock' (a large cotton coat).

Gender-bending representation was not the privilege of male characters, and women held their equal share of playful cross-dressing. The narrative poem 'The Female-Beau: Or, The Beau-Female', published in *The Bath and Bristol Miscellany* for the year 1735, is a rare example of cross-dressing in both sexes. The poem, or song, probably inspired by the sea shanty culture of Bristol Harbour, starts on the mating season in the 'Merry month of May'. 'The genial salts arising', an expression suited to the spa town yet applying to 'jolly, young, and gay' Mira's rising desire, move her to start looking for a companion. The whole poem is built on the metaphor of piracy, an alternative to hunting for narratives of seduction:

> She, like Man, dressed *Cap-a-Pie*
> Now prepares for Privateering
> *Strephon*, cloath'd contrary way
> Steer'd his course a Buckaneering.[96]

The expression 'Cap-a-Pie', in use for soldiers or duels, comes from the French and refers to being dressed up from head ('cap') to foot ('pied'). In parallel, Strephon's buccaneering requires that he be dressed up as a woman ('the contrary way') to hide among other women and get closer to them. Such accoutrement provokes Cupid's appetite for pranks and he gives 'Strephon Mira's eyes / To Mira Strephon's heart'.[97] The poem concludes on a mischievous question after the two cross-dressed protagonists go to bed:

> Say you learn'd in the Law
> Ye *Casuist* deride,
> Without Error of Flaw,
> Who Bridegroom was, who Bride?[98]

The song does not comment on the mutual homosexual attraction of the lovers, which might have been made more acceptable by their original gender. The inability to tell bride from groom echoes *The Guardian*'s depiction of bathers where 'Distinctions of Sex and Condition are concealed', leaving the reader to imagine a third gender, or a possible situation in which the inability to ascribe strict gender identification does not hinder life from following its course.[99]

The country walks and thereabouts of the spa town were another space of gender-bending practices. Mira's figure of the armoured woman, ready to fight and dressed up as a privateer, could be a reference to the execution of Mary Read and Anne Bonny a decade earlier, but in the context of spa towns, it rather brings to mind a familiar image of poems and lampoons, of the woman in a riding habit.[100] Riding was regularly prescribed by doctors after taking the waters in the morning, as it was a form of exercise that was understood to set the fluids in motion. In the 1714 poem 'A Lady in a riding Habit', the speaker complains of the loss of femininity and the frustration of the male gaze such riding habits entailed:

> Now in Revenge, behold the Brightest Fair,
> Who conquer most, the Manly Habit wear,
> And try to hide beneath the Male Attire,
> Those Charms, for which a thousand Youths expire.[101]

As Cally Blackman explains, a riding habit was but a dress that tended to follow the style of men's clothing, the over-gown was often patterned on a military vest – with pockets – and it was perceived as extremely masculine: 'While the habit jacket aped men's coats in almost every detail, both it and the skirt always followed the currently fashionable female silhouette, being worn over habit-stays, or jumps, and hooped petticoats or pads in order to achieve this'.[102] As the century moved on, it was more frequently worn for other types of exercise such as walking or travelling, and the dress was a form of informal wear.[103] The 'denaturing' effect of the riding habit was a trope present in many poems, most of which I found in *The Scarborough Miscellany*, such as 'To *Florelia*, upon seeing her in a riding habit at Scarborough', which is followed by another poem, 'Upon seeing Miss B— in the same habit', a repetition further warning the reader of the dangers of this new fashion:

> Forsake, *Dear Nymph*, this awkward Dress;
> For who in Prudence can
> Divest the loveliest Goddess,
> T'assume the *mimic* Man.
> The Rival Ladies out of Spite
> Or envy, soon will say
> The person is Hermaphrodite
> That's seen in such an array.[104]

Florelia stands out as a troubling gendered presence, provoking an ambivalent feeling of 'envy' – jealousy or desire – in persons of her own sex.

The riding habit was not the only way in which women could display masculine attributes; several other instances of manly women are found in spa literature. The 1734 *Scarborough Miscellany* opens on 'A view of the Long-Room, by Mr. C.'. The speaker scans the Assembly in the Long Room in a critical glance, which makes the poem sound like a long inventory of stereotypes. After praising

'B— C—' for her wit and beauty ('You set a pattern – and in all you please'), Mr C. turns to her direct opposite:

> Not so, when *Tom-Boy-Flavia* I survey
> Drest like some vain Sir *Fopling* of the Play.
> The Peruke, Beaver, – the pert manly Mien,
> Raise my Disgust, provoke my very Spleen,
> Were she as *Venus* Fair, as Pallas Wise,
> I'd loath her in that masculine Disguise;
> 'Twere an *Italian* Taste t'indulge Desire,
> No, – Let the Fools she imitates admire.[105]

Although the expression 'Tom-Boy' is an entry in dictionaries of the English language as early as 1650, it is recorded in few printed literary works. Here, the presence of the term in popular literature is a sign of its use. Thomas Sheridan's *Dictionary of the English Language* (1789) defines the term as referring to a 'Wild Coarse Girl'.[106] As Cally Blackman explains, 'part of the problem had to do with where the habit was worn' – in this case, in an assembly room rather than outdoors.[107] The presence of a tomboy as one of the stereotypes of the Long Room is evidence that gender-crossing was not restricted to the male sex. The speaker's disgust draws a strict parallel between Flavia's tomboyish dress and a fop's feminine manners, establishing in spite of himself a continuum of gender, and a meeting point on this continuum, implying that gender fluidity is one of the dangerous possibilities of spa societies.

Other forms of tomboyishness could be more invisible to the eye, to be found out in conversation and manners, rather than dress. The locales of conversation in spas were numerous, ranging from the pump room and assembly rooms to the common rooms of pensions and inns or the private salons of wealthier individuals. I have explained how, in Frances Burney's *Evelina*, the heroine was convinced by her tutor to accompany a spirited and generous widow, Mrs Selwyn, to Bristol Hotwells in spite of her tutor's unease with the society Evelina would meet there.[108] The reason for such defiance lies in Selwyn's masculinity, as is plainly exposed by Evelina:

> Mrs. Selwyn is very kind and attentive to me. She is extremely clever; her understanding, indeed, may be called masculine; but, unfortunately, her manners deserve the same epithet; for, in studying to acquire the knowledge of the other sex, she has lost all the softness of her own.

In regard to myself, however, as I have neither courage nor inclination to argue with her, I have never been personally hurt at her want of gentleness; a virtue which, nevertheless, seems so essential a part of the female character, that I find myself more awkward, and less at ease, with a woman who wants it, than I do with a man. She is not a favourite with Mr. Villars, who has often been disgusted at her unmerciful propensity to satire.[109]

Although Mrs Selwyn differs greatly from the depersonalised 'Flavia' in the previous poem, she provokes the same disgust in Evelina's tutor, evoking an early form of gender trouble. The definition of a tomboy – a 'wild coarse' girl – applies to Selwyn's manners in Evelina's perception, and her masculinity is a touchstone for the narrator's femininity. While she is 'personally hurt' at this eighteenth-century version of an angry butch woman whose defence is based on satirical attack, Evelina betrays her fascination for Selwyn's intelligence, reminiscent of Courtwit's or Hillaria's sharpness in Restoration comedies and unmatched by other characters. Selwyn will be Evelina's watchdog at the spa, protecting her when she is harassed by the unruly Lord Merton and his rake friend on her way to the pump room, till one of them asks: 'is that queer woman your mother?',[110] a question that resonates to twenty-first-century readers as stemming from the trouble raised by Selwyn's freedom with gender codes. Selwyn is the one who offers to take Evelina with her to Bristol Hotwells when she falls ill, as she is a regular visitor of watering places. She shows a great familiarity with the spa and enjoys all the opportunities it has to offer in terms of sociability and conversation, moving with ease among the various assemblies. To persuade Evelina to stay longer, she argues that they should accept Mrs Beaumont's invitation to stay at Clifton Heights because 'she has always a house full of people, and though they are chiefly fools and coxcombs, yet there is some pleasure in cutting them up'.[111] Her castrating conversation and her quick-spirited comments attract much hatred from Sir Clement, one of Evelina's suitors who, in a conversation with her, expresses the same irritation as her tutor for Selwyn's masculine behaviour:

'Mrs. Selwyn, indeed, afforded some relief from this formality, but the unbounded licence of her tongue–'
'O Sir Clement, do *you* object to that?'

'Yes, my sweet reproacher, in a *woman*, I do; in a *woman* I think it intolerable'.[112]

In Evelina's teasing question and Clement's insistence on gendering wit, Burney unveils Sir Clement's defence mechanism. He oversexualises Selwyn's wit, decrying its 'unbounded licence', a term usually reserved for libertine behaviour, and then resorts to strict categorisation when faced with trouble and uncertainty – and, as Evelina hints, unwanted competition.

The stage remains the central site for crossing the boundaries of gender, and the epilogue to George Colman's *The spleen, or, Islington Spa* is one of the most elaborate rewritings of gender roles. D'Oyley, the old man whose role is modelled on Molière's imaginary invalid, is astonished by Laetitia's revelation of her gender as she is confronted with the accusation of having seduced D'Oyley's ward under the usurped identity of Dr Anodyne. D'Oyley is disturbed by the retrospective sexual proximity suddenly revealed by the medical gestures he let her perform on him when he thought she was a man: 'Wha! Have I been bled and blistered, and purged and pickled by a female physician?'[113] The exclamation suggests farcical indignation for having thus been woman-handled, rather than astonishment at a female doctor's skills. In the epilogue to the play, which differs greatly from the enthronement of the invalid as a doctor in the Molière play, Mrs King, the actress who performed the part of Laetitia, came back to the stage and addressed the audience thus:

> A female doctor, sirs! And pray why not?
> Have men from Nature a sole Patent got?
> Can they chain down Experience, Sense, and Knowledge
> (Like madmen in straight waistcoats) to a college?
> Let us prescribe! Our wholesome Revolutions
> Would quickly mend your crazy Constitutions.[114]

The monologue is provocative and satirical, yet the satire targets the absurdity of restricting access to medicine to males – what we now call sexism – much more than the pretensions of women, a usual trait of eighteenth-century satires on learned women. In fact, by contrast with the 'straight waistcoats' of academia, the patent of nature might appear as a sensible choice to the audience. The 'revolution' implied, ten years before the writings of Mary

Wollstonecraft in England or Olympe de Gouges in France, is not restricted to the realm of medical knowledge. It extends to all the governing bodies, law, politics and religion:

> Invest a female with a Reverend Cassock–
> What spruce Divine, woul'd more become the Hassock;
> Or robe her in a Lawyer's gown and band,
> What judge so sweet a pleader could withstand?
> Into St Stephen's Chapel let us go!
> What power our Aye would have, what force our No!
> Try us in all things – there are very few,
> We Women could not do, as well as you.[115]

The qualifications 'sweet pleaders' and 'spruce Divine' feminising the professions at stake, are the expected mark of the times. They are to be contrasted with the expression 'what force our No!' which gives agency and power to the vision of women in governing bodies. Spoken by an actress, one of the rising professions for women, the monologue was a case in point, and could give some credit to the feminist visions it triggered. In the context of spas, where gendered identities and gender roles could be questioned by the visible presence of alternative models, Mrs King's epilogue to the *Imaginary Invalid* opens up new possibilities of defining genders, however distant, playful and unrealistic at the time, that were initially triggered by the care of the sick.

From the imagination of nudity to the possibilities of transgression, it is tempting to conclude that spas were early examples of what Michel Foucault called 'heterotopias', spaces in which otherness could be experienced, other forms of the self, and other modes of relationship.[116] As mentioned in the introduction to this book, Foucault talks specifically of holiday resorts, beaches and cafés that could be reminiscent of the seasonal activities of spa towns, and the alternative modes of sociability found in these sites of short-term visits. I have tried to explore in the last section of this chapter the singular connections between the urban spaces of spa towns and the possibilities of playing with one's identity. The murky waters of desire, debauchery and gender play were part of the literary imaginary of spa towns, making them a dystopic place of libertinism as a counterpart to the architectural ideals of health utopias.

Notes

1 Buchan, *Cautions Concerning Cold Bathing*, p. 18.
2 See for example F. Fuller, *Medicina Gymnastica: Or, a Treatise Concerning the Power of Exercise* (London: Knaplock, 1705).
3 Buchan, *Cautions Concerning Cold Bathing*, p. 18.
4 See Eglin, *The Imaginary Autocrat*.
5 T. Shadwell, *Epsom-Wells: A comedy* (London: H. Herringman, 1673), p. 3.
6 Smollett, *Humphry Clinker*, p. 49.
7 See A. Hudelet, D. Monaghan, and J. Wiltshire, *The Cinematic Jane Austen* (London: McFarland, 2009).
8 To my knowledge, only two screen adaptations of Austen's novels have interesting bathing and drinking scenes: the 2019 mini-series *Sanditon* (Red Planet Pictures, ITV, Masterpiece Theatre, 2019), and the 1987 adaptation of *Northanger Abbey* (British Broadcasting Corporation (BBC), A+E Networks, 1987).
9 T. Rowlandson, *The Comforts of Bath*, 1798. Watercolour painting, 18.6 × 12.4 cm, Yale Center for British Art.
10 T. Rowlandson, *Venus Bathing, A fashionable Dip*, c. 1800. Etching with hand colouring on woven paper, 13.6 × 18.6 cm, Wellcome Library, London, ICV no. 20451; T. Rowlandson, *Side Way or Any Way, Venus's Bathing (Margate)*, c. 1800. Etching with hand colouring on woven paper, Wellcome Library, London, ICV no. 20452; *Summer Amusement at Margate, or a Peep at the Mermaids*, 1813. Etching with hand colouring on woven paper, 24.5 × 34.8 cm, Wesleyan Collection.
11 Johnson, 'The Venus of Margate', p. 587.
12 Johnson, 'The Venus of Margate', p. 587.
13 See A. Herbert, 'Creatures of the bath: transformations at the early modern British spa' in Chiari and Cuisinier-Delorme (eds), *Spa Culture and Literature in England*, pp. 117–34.
14 Floyer, *The Ancient Psychrolousia Revived*, p. 133. According to Floyer and the author of the letter, N. Ellison, Honwick is near St Mungo's Well, in Scotland (south Ayrshire).
15 Cottom, 'In the bowels of the novel', p. 167; P. Byrde, '"That frightful unbecoming dress": clothes for spa bathing at Bath', *Costume*, 21:1 (1987), p. 50.
16 Byrde, '"That frightful unbecoming dress"', p. 50.
17 Herbert, 'Gender and the spa', p. 50.
18 Floyer, *The Ancient Psychrolousia Revived*, p. 134.
19 Byrde, '"That frightful unbecoming dress"', pp. 51–2.
20 Byrde, '"That frightful unbecoming dress"', p. 55.

21 Fiennes, *The Illustrated Journeys of Celia Fiennes*, p. 46.

22 Celia Fiennes's account of Bath spa shows a process that enabled wealthy bathers to hide from voyeurs by waiting in warm rooms to be guided into the bath. Fiennes, *The Illustrated Journeys of Celia Fiennes*, p. 46.

23 Benedict, 'Consumptive communities', p. 207.

24 'On a lady bathing', in *The Bath, Bristol, Tunbridge and Epsom Miscellany* (London: T. Dormer, 1735), p. 8.

25 'On a lady bathing', p. 8.

26 'On a lady bathing', p. 8.

27 'On a lady bathing', p. 8.

28 'On a lady bathing', p. 9.

29 *The Scarborough Miscellany for the Year 1734* (London: J. Wilford, 1734), p. 67.

30 *The Scarborough Miscellany*, 1734, p. 67.

31 *The Scarborough Miscellany*, 1734, p. 66.

32 On the rise of scientific poetry, see H. Marchal (ed.), *Muses et Ptéro-dactyles. La poésie de la science de Chénier à Rimbaud* (Paris: Seuil, 2013).

33 *The Scarborough Miscellany*, 1734, p. 67.

34 *The Scarborough Miscellany*, 1734, p. 68.

35 I have already quoted in the previous chapter from the poem *An Exclamation from Tunbridge and Epsom against the Newfound Wells at Islington*, witnessing the growing fame of Islington and the competition between the spas within a day's travel of London.

36 The original French word is *déshabillé* and all possible inflections of the term (dishabille, déshabille, deshabille ...) exist in English.

37 J. Lockman, *The Humours of New Tunbridge Wells at Islington: A Lyric Poem* (London: J. Roberts, 1734), p. 2.

38 Lockman, *The Humours of New Tunbridge Wells*, p. 9.

39 See McKellar, 'Peripheral visions', p. 501; Denbigh *A Hundred British Spas*, p. 57.

40 G. Bickham the Younger, 'The Charms of Dishabille, or the New Tunbridge Wells at Islington', 1733.

41 *The Scarborough Miscellany*, 1733, p. 26.

42 *The Scarborough Miscellany*, 1733, p. 27.

43 *The Scarborough Miscellany*, 1733, p. 27.

44 'Scarborough-Spaw, a Song', *The Scarborough Miscellany*, 1733, p. 44.

45 More poems can be found on the subject with very similar titles in the Scarborough Miscellanies: 'On seeing the Ladies bathe at Scarborough', *The Scarborough Miscellany*, 1732, p. 15; 'On the Ladies bathing in the Sea, at Scarborough', *The Scarborough Miscellany*, 1734, p. 28.

46 Johnson, 'The Venus of Margate', p. 597.
47 J. O'Keeffe, *The Irish Mimic; Or Blunders at Brighton* (London: T. N. Longman, 1795), p. 12.
48 Smollett, *Humphry Clinker*, p. 185.
49 More research should be conducted to properly define spa comedies as a subgenre, but some elements for generic reflection can be found in Sandor L. Weingrod's doctoral dissertation, *Spa Drama from Shadwell to Sheridan* (Brandeis University, 1990).
50 Smollett, *Humphry Clinker*, p. 49.
51 O. Baldwin and T. Wilson, 'Baker, Thomas (b. 1680/81), playwright and journalist', *Oxford Dictionary of National Biography*. Baker's interest in the theatrical possibilities of spa towns is reflected in his second play, *Hampstead Heath*, which was the rewriting, in the setting of a London spa, of his most provocative play, *An Act at Oxford*. The play set in Oxford was judged too racy to get the approval of censorship. Baker softened its tone and transferred the action to Hampstead Heath, as if the setting of a spa town allowed for more liberty than its initial Oxford setting. See A. Marshall, *The Practice of Satire in England, 1658–1770* (Baltimore, MD: Johns Hopkins University Press, 2013), p. 168.
52 T. Baker, *Tunbridge-Walks: Or, the Yeoman of Kent* (London: B. Lintott, 1703), p. 39.
53 F. March, 'La Mise en scène du mariage dans la comédie de la Restauration: vide rituel et anti-rites', *Revue de la Société d'études Anglo-Américaines des XVIIe et XVIIIe siècles*, 62 (2006), p. 55.
54 Baker, *Tunbridge-Walks*, p. 20.
55 Baker, *Tunbridge-Walks*, p. 22.
56 Mavor, *The Cheltenham guide*, p. 98.
57 Mavor, *The Cheltenham guide*, p. 19.
58 Mavor, *The Cheltenham guide*, p. 24.
59 Colman, *The spleen, or, Islington Spa*, p. 3.
60 Denbigh, *A Hundred British Spas*, p. 58.
61 Colman, *The spleen, or, Islington Spa*, p. 3.
62 Colman, *The spleen, or, Islington Spa*, p. 3.
63 Cooley, '"Sexy in a 'Tunbridge Wells' sort of way"', p. 94.
64 Herbert, *Female Alliances*; Hurley, 'A conversation of their own', pp. 1–21.
65 Colman, *The spleen, or, Islington Spa*, p. 16.
66 J. Burnby, *Summer Amusement: Or, Miscellaneous Poems: Inscribed to the Frequenters of Margate, Ramsgate, Tunbridge Wells, Brighthelmstone, Southampton, Cheltenham, Weymouth, Scarborough* (London: J. Dodsley, Pall-Mall, 1772), p. 22.

67 Burnby, *Summer Amusement*, p. 23.
68 Colman, *The spleen, or, Islington Spa*, p. 27.
69 T. Rawlins, *Tunbridge-Wells: or A days Courtship* (London: H. Rogers, 1678), p. 15.
70 Rawlins, *Tunbridge-Wells*, p. 15.
71 Rawlins, *Tunbridge-Wells*, p. 16.
72 There are other examples like this in Spa comedies, such as Dorothy Fribble's justification in *Epsom-Wells* for her husband leaving her alone: 'Ay, that's because the Air's good to make one be with Child, and he longs mightily for a Child; and truly Neighbour, I use all the means I can, since he is so desirous of one'. Shadwell, *Epsom-Wells*, p. 23. On barren women and spas, see chapter 1 'A catalogue of diseases', p. 00.
73 Rawlins, *Tunbridge-Wells*, p. 1.
74 T. Rawlins, *Tunbridge-Wells: or A days courtship* (London: H. Rogers, 1678), p. 23.
75 *An Exclamation from Tunbridge and Epsom*, p. 2.
76 *Hampstead-Wells* (London, 1706).
77 Shadwell, *Epsom-Wells*, p. 1.
78 *Hampstead-Wells*.
79 Borsay, 'Health and leisure resorts', p. 795.
80 Hurley, 'A conversation of their own'.
81 Herbert, *Female Alliances*, p. 117–40.
82 McCormack, '"An assembly of disorders."'
83 Cooley, '"Sexy in a 'Tunbridge Wells' sort of way"', p. 93.
84 Cooley, '"Sexy in a 'Tunbridge Wells' sort of way"', p. 93.
85 *The Guardian*, 174, p. 501.
86 On macaronies and fops, see P. McNeil, 'Macaroni masculinities', *Fashion Theory*, 4:4 (2000), 373–403; and A. Rauser, 'Hair, authenticity, and the self-made macaroni', *Eighteenth-Century Studies*, 38:1 (2004), 101–17.
87 On the connection with Restoration culture, see B. Benedict: 'This Restoration heritage shapes the rhetoric of later spa literature. Both drolleries and resort compendia are titled after places of pleasure to signal the escapism their verses supply, but this printed utopia is as ordered as the social utopia of spa or playhouse. Similarly, spa literature celebrates a spontaneous, physical nature opposed to the disciplined middle-class body, even while they also represent an ideal society appropriated by Restoration political discourse.' Benedict, 'Consumptive communities', p. 216.
88 The Invalid, 'Epistle IV', *The Register of Folly*, p. 44.
89 The Invalid 'Epistle IV', *The Register of Folly*, pp. 47.

90 Burnby, *Summer Amusement*, p. 11.
91 Burnby, *Summer Amusement*, pp. 12–13.
92 *Trifles from Harrogate* (Harrogate: Hargrove, 1797).
93 T. Castle, *Masquerade and Civilisation: The Carnivalesque in Eighteenth-Century English Culture and Fiction* (London: Methuen, 1986), p. 51.
94 Benedict, 'Consumptive communities', p. 209.
95 Baker, *Tunbridge-Walks*, 26.
96 'The Female-Beau: Or, The Beau-Female', in the *Bath, Bristol, Tunbridge and Epsom*, p. 14.
97 'The Female-Beau', p. 14.
98 'The Female-Beau', p. 15.
99 *The Guardian*, 174, p. 501.
100 Mary Read and Anne Bonny were women privateers and companions of John Rackam, also known as Calico Jack; see M. Rediker, 'Liberty beneath the Jolly Roger', in M. Creighton and L. Norling (eds), *Iron Men, Wooden Women: Gender and Seafaring in the Atlantic World, 1700–1920* (Baltimore, MD: Johns Hopkins University Press, 1996), pp. 1–33.
101 *The Tunbridge and Bath Miscellany for the Year 1714*, p. 6.
102 C. Blackman, 'Walking Amazons: the development of the riding habit in England during the eighteenth century', *Costume*, 35:1 (January 2001), p. 48.
103 Blackman, 'Walking Amazons'.
104 'To *Florelia*, upon seeing her in a riding habit at Scarborough', in *The Scarborough Miscellany*, 1734, p. 65.
105 'A view of the Long-Room, by Mr. C.', in *The Scarborough Miscellany*, 1734, p. 4.
106 T. Sheridan, *A Complete Dictionary of the English Language* (London: C. Dilly, 1789), p. 579. On the history of Tomboys see M. A. Abate, *Tomboys: A Literary and Cultural History* (Philadelphia: Temple University Press 2008) and *Journal of Lesbian Studies*, 'Special Issue on Tomboys and Tomboyism', 15:4 (October 2011), pp. 407–11.
107 Blackman, 'Walking Amazons', p. 49.
108 See chapter 1, p. 00.
109 Burney, *Evelina*, pp. 268–9.
110 Burney, *Evelina*, p. 275.
111 Burney, *Evelina*, p. 293.
112 Burney, *Evelina*, p. 343.
113 Colman, *The spleen, or, Islington Spa*, p. 21.
114 Colman, *The spleen, or, Islington Spa*, p. 18.
115 Colman, *The spleen, or, Islington Spa*, p. 18.
116 Foucault, 'Des espaces autres'.

4

Pump room politics and the murky past of spas

Health and control are deeply correlated: prevention and cure request a heightened degree of control over the patient's body and conduct. Various forms of control are applied by parents, partners, friends and physicians who offer advice, comment on doctors' prescriptions, measure progress of both patient and disease, and check their commitment to their treatment. Sickness becomes a social event of sorts, launching a private dynamic of interaction around the patient. Public matters of health are in turn prone to political control. In eighteenth-century spa towns, the sick were monitored and ushered through various places of care and entertainment. Social gatherings required further control from the local authorities who were committed to preserving a good reputation so as to attract more visitors. Social control was not an easy task, as the company of a spa town formed in a day, mixed and conversed intensely for a season, and evaporated as the season ended, leaving the town empty until the next influx.

Spa town sociability was ephemeral and marked by the vulnerable health of its members. Gossip, which was depicted as the main occupation of visitors beyond taking the waters, was emblematic of the kind of uncontrollable forces that such volatile acquaintance could spread, and was therefore the target of much regulatory discourse. Poems, novels and periodicals combine to show that a culture of freedom of speech and entertaining gossip was at odds with the rules and protocols established by the various masters of ceremonies.

Beyond the opposing forces to local policy, spa towns – especially the larger ones – played a role at national level. They attracted enough political actors to become alternative political arenas, with potential international connections. The political colour of spas will be studied in a second section, in parallel with the female politics recently analysed by feminist historians who showed how spa towns facilitated the conversation of women who regularly visited spa towns independently of their husbands and built long-term friendships from one visit to another. As potential hotspots of alternative political gatherings, some spas, most notably Bath, attracted Jacobite sympathies, and for good reason, since Roman Catholics were known to entertain a specific relationship with thaumaturgic waters. Holy wells and miracle springs had been forbidden or destroyed during the Reformation, yet some survived or re-emerged in the form of spas, from Restoration to Regency. Dealing with this murky past could create political controversies, as was the case for St Winifred's Well in Wales. And yet, medical writings and travel literature reveal subtler forms of negotiations and re-appropriations within the Protestant medical cultures of the eighteenth century.

Pump room politics: gossip and power

In Sheridan's *A Trip to Scarborough*, Lord Foppington spells out the minutes of his fashionable routines. He mentions that he reads without thinking, attends concerts without 'having to undergo the fatigue of listening' and loves the Opera above all for its potential for gossip: 'There is my Lady Tattle, my Lady Prate, my Lady Titter, my Lady Sneer, my Lady Giggle, and my Lady Grin – these have boxes in the front and while any favourite air is singing, are the prettiest company in the waurld, stap my vitals!'[1] Foppington's comic enumeration sounds like the allegretto arias of Mozart's operas, where gossip becomes itself an aesthetic performance unfolding in the multiplication of voices and accelerated rhythm of vocal virtuosity. In eighteenth-century literature, gossip, much like its companion, wit, is indeed an aesthetic mode and a comic trope which expresses the fecklessness of fashion and the dangers of unregulated social encounters. In spas, as Lord Foppington suggests, gossip is a necessary ingredient of the small and ephemeral social circles that navigate from pump room to assembly hall. Literature presents gossip as both enjoyable and despicable. Not unlike satire, gossip is a performative conversation sharpening wit's double-edged word, begetting both destruction and cure. Just as libel and slander require monitoring and regulation to protect reputations, so does gossip. Many attributes of middle-sized and larger spa towns – illness, domesticity, ephemeral sociability and regular new visitors – contributed to promote the circulation of gossip as an essential dynamic to the internal politics of the place. Gossip revels in details, as do illness narratives which thrive on unsavoury information about other people's bodies, their infertility, their venereal disease, their returning hypochondria or incurable gout and excessive drinking. In its literary representations, gossip unfolds in the domestic spaces of inns and private lodgings, in the small parties going out for a walk, in the assemblies at the pump room, in the queues for a drink. Unsurprisingly, gossip is depicted as a gendered mode of orality, which is either told by women, or targets them. As such, it acts as a counter-power or a threat to local patriarchal control.

There is more to gossip than meets the ear, however, as the Austenian scholar Patricia Meyer Spacks explains. She charts the function of gossip in letter-writing and literature, focusing on the intimacy provided by the act of gossiping, the pleasure derived from getting new and detailed information, and the common imaginary space shared by a group of gossipers. As she delineates the gossip that 'uses the stuff of scandal', she shifts the common perception of gossip as destructive and uncaring to underline its creative and bonding qualities. Patricia Meyer Spacks quotes from Jane Austen's last completed novel, *Persuasion*, to illustrate the ways in which gossip fosters intimacy, and establishes 'a mode not of domination but of linkage'.[2] Needless to say, this pleasurable gossip happens in Bath.

The gossiping skills under study belong to Nurse Rooke, a character in *Persuasion* already mentioned in relation to the illness narrative of Mrs Smith for her understanding of the multiple aspects of care.[3] Mrs Smith talks to the heroine, Anne Elliott, of her pleasure in listening to Nurse Rooke's comments on other people's lives:

> Call it gossip if you will; but when nurse Rooke has half an hour's leisure to bestow on me, she is sure to have something to relate that is entertaining and profitable, something that makes one know one's species better. One likes to hear what is going on, to be *au fait* as to the newest modes of being trifling and silly. To me, who live so much alone, her conversation I assure you is a treat.[4]

To Meyer Spacks, Nurse Rooke's gossip is a form of 'healing talk', which, in the context of the spa, makes even more sense. In the domestic space of her lodgings, Nurse Rooke's comments on

trifles soothe the angst of solitude for Mrs Smith, who cannot go
to the pump room and partake in a global act of care. Gossip, in
that sense, is a performative act of language to reinforce the bond
between the sharers.

There are, as Meyer Spacks explains, several forms of gossip,
ranging from idle – and abundant – talk to slander and scandal-
ous rumours, yet they always involve the experience of being the
privileged recipient of private information. Gossip is often connected
to drinking: tea, wine or, in this particular context, spa waters.
'How goes Scandal at the *Wells* today?' young Reynard asks a
group of women coming back from their morning drink in the
play *Tunbridge-Walks* (1703); 'What fine Lady had an Intrigue last
night, which the rest out of Envy has reported?'[5] The bold Hillaria,
who had just greeted his approach with the remark 'here come the
He-things', replies 'Rather, Sir, what intrigues have your Vanities
boasted of, which neither of your Persons, nor Accomplishments,
had force to gain you?'[6] Hillaria reverses the gendered vision of
gossip, as she points out how the competitive boasting of young men
about their recent female conquests is as much a form of gossip – let
alone more destructive and vile – as the collaborative sharing of
secrets by women. Gossip, in this case, is an object of homosocial
interaction despised by the other gender.

Although literature predominantly represents gossip as a feminine
pastime appreciated by male fops and beaux only, it occasionally
celebrates other forms of gossip that imply heterosocial interaction.
In the 1733 *Scarborough Miscellany*, a poem entitled 'On the Elegant
Entertainement and Mix'd Company at the Ordinaries' depicts the
modes of relaxed pub talk at lunch, after 'each Morn at the Wells
we've our draught done repeating'.[7] The poem insists on the social
mixing of pub-goers, who share the custom of mingling spa water
and wine:

> Then soon as from Table the Dinner re-passes,
> The bottle goes round, and we toast in full Glasses.
> According to custom whose word is a Law,
> The first Glass you take, you dilute it with Spaw:
> Then we club for the Wine, and to finish the Jest,
> Each fair Nymph pays her quota as free as the rest.
> We soon grow acquainted, familiar and hearty,
> And lose in *good Humours* the *ill ones* of the Party.

> No intricate whisper, no Prude affectation,
> We drink, and we prattle in free Conversation.[8]

In this idyllic representation, gossip, like drinking, acts as a social leveller, erasing both distinctions of gender and class.[9] Toasting games usually implied multiple customs of poems, challenges, witty compliments or gossipy innuendoes that made this kind of drinking even more of a social act.[10] The poet contrasts 'free conversation' with the potentially harmful 'intricate whisper' and idle talk which are depicted here as a form of healing for the assembly of sick people. In fact, the whole poem starts on treatment and ends on diversions ('a walk or the play'), which represent a form of care for ill humours.

The letter on watering places published in *The Guardian* in 1713 also connects gossip and ill humours, as if the desire for gossip was deeply ingrained in physical discomfort. In the character of Nestor Ironside, gossip takes the metaphorical shape of sickness and contagion. Ironside associates gossip and female letter-writing from watering places: 'I have had Rheams of Letters from *Bath*, *Epsom*, *Tunbridge*, and St *Wenefride's* Well; wherein I could observe that a Concern for Honour and Virtue proceeded from the want of Health, Beauty, or fine Petticoats'.[11] Needless to say, the narrator revels in the gossipy letters, and finds that illness begets ill-will: 'A Lady, who subscribes herself *Eudosia*, writes a bitter Invective against *Chloe* the celebrated Dancer, but I have learned, that she herself is lame of the Rheumatism. Another, who hath been a Prude, ever since she had the SmallPox, is very bitter against the Coquets, and their indecent Airs.'[12] In his fantasy of female denunciation, Ironside ascribes the cause of all their sourness to the bitter humours stemming from the social experience of deformed bodies gathered in one place, and acting upon each other as jealous censors, begetting much pain and gall. He takes the role of a male physician, curing the root of all gossip with his own satirical quill:

> I shall make it my Business, in this Paper, to cool and assuage those malignant Humours of Scandal which run throughout the Body of Men and Women there assembled; and, after the manner of those famous Waters, I will endeavour to wipe away all foul Aspersions, to restore Bloom and Vigour to decayed Reputations, and set injured Characters upon their Legs again.[13]

Satire acts like the miracle waters of St Winifred about to be discussed in this chapter, which are rarely mentioned in such-like enumerations and might have been added to the list to insist on the superstitions of mineral water users. It restores the order of the social body and renders justice to the victims of gossip and idle talk by directing well-crafted published words at the gossip-mongers.

The social dynamics of gossip in watering places are sources of power and counter-power that were thought to belong to women. In contrast to Ironside's letter to *The Guardian*, women were often represented as gossip masters who played the reputation of visitors thanks to tried methods of collecting stories and secrets. When Hillaria, the impetuous and witty woman character in *Tunbridge-Walks*, is asked by her brother how she insinuates herself into the world, she promptly answers: 'As most women that live by their Wits do; I prais ev'ry Body to their Face, and mimick every Body behind their backs, so that all court my Favour, because they are afraid of being Abus'd'.[14] She further explains her constant mockery as a strategy of self-defence: 'By keeping a World of Company, appearing in all publick Places, and giving myself a liberty of Railing I have acquired the character of a Judge'.[15] Hillaria draws a link between wit, mockery and fear, which clearly exposes how gossip begets power. Malignant gossip in turn leads to blackmail, where Hillaria is courted by subjects who cannot afford to refuse her lest she exposes their dirty secrets. She thus revels in a position apparently well suited to the town of Tunbridge Wells in 1703, when the play was published: 'Well, this *Tunbridge* is the Joy of my life: such Treating, Dancing, Serenading, Ragglins and Scandal, I cou'd die here'.[16] Baker chose his location carefully as the whole town of Tunbridge Wells – and most specifically the Walks – is emblematic of gossip in the first half of the eighteenth century. One specific reason is the influential character of Bell Causey, a woman who raised subscriptions for events, ushered people along the Walks or in the rooms, and welcomed new visitors, informing them of the programme for the season.

Although Bell Causey is regularly mentioned in the contemporary literature on watering places, little is known of her character. She presided over ceremonies in Tunbridge from the 1720s until her death in 1734. She was not an appointed master of ceremonies, as

Rachael Johnson explains. 'Her role was to manage rather than to lead society', she writes:

> Causey had no authority or standing in polite society and so could not mould the visiting company in the way Nash was attempting at Bath. Instead her role, apparently self-appointed, was organisational and opportunistic, drawing on the increasing need to manage the company's entertainments but also exploiting the lack of a governing authority (such as the Bath corporation) that held the power to make an official appointment.[17]

Johnson quotes a late eighteenth-century guide to Tunbridge Wells which portrays Causey retrospectively as a large woman who raised subscriptions and managed to rally new company to assembly rooms and entertainments provided during the season.[18] Earlier literature on watering places seems to agree with this retrospective portrait, and draws a direct link between Causey's power in Tunbridge and her skilful manipulation of gossip. The 1722 *Tunbrigialia* opens on a poem entitled 'On B— C':

> Bright Nymphs o' the train
> That adorn *Tunbridge* Plain,
> And continue our Season so long;
> Beware, e'er too late,
> And avoid your sad Fate,
> Which depends on *B*—'s flattering tongue.[19]

The poem, which starts a series of derogatory lampoons targeting female visitors, contributes to an atmosphere of fear, placing reputation as the most precious asset a woman can safeguard during the season. Bell's methods are exposed to the reader in a cautionary poem which has her start her manipulation by following a step-by-step ritual of preliminary conversation aimed at gathering gossip:

> When the Tea-Pot comes out
> And her *Nants* flows about,
> Then she cants, to prepare you the better;
> But her View and Design
> Is to take you all in,
> With, My Dear, O my Dear, here's a Letter![20]

Gossip, Markman Ellis argues, is organised around the equipage of the tea-table, which is idealised, in contemporary literature, as 'a safe place for heterosocial discussion about matters of significance'.[21] In this case, the tea-table is a manipulative safe space, in which brandy ('Nants') and careless gossip ('cant') are cleverly controlled to untie the tongues of the assembly. 'Tea-table conversation was habitually represented as gossip and scandal', Ellis further argues, relying on the work of sociologists for whom the function of gossip is to maintain moral values and cohesion.[22] The representation of Bell Causey in control of gossip is a depiction of her power which goes beyond the blackmailing strategies of Hillaria. As she has power over what is said and thought of others, she is in direct control of the moral and social values of the restricted circle of Tunbridge visitors.

Another portrait of her, similar to this view, was published seven years after her death and included in one of the *Pamelianas*, the shortened and rewritten chapbook versions of Samuel Richardson's *Pamela*, which tended to exalt the titillating scenes and add more peripeteia to the celebrated sentimental novel.[23] In the rewriting of the second volume, in which Pamela is married and accompanies Lady Davers, her sister-in-law, on a trip to Tunbridge Wells, Bell Causey appears as the saviour of an embarrassing situation:

> When People upon the Walks come to hear of Lady *Davers's* being robbed, both she and Pamela are plagued with so many impertinent questions, and formal condolences from the Ladies, that they were glad to get into *Bell's* Long Room to Cards to avoid the fatigue of answering all the idle People that stock'd about them: and Bell sitting with her arms on Kimbo, at her Door, kept Centry, and told the story to every Body, to save my lady the Trouble of repeating it a Thousand times over.[24]

Bell is ironically represented as the guardian of gossip in town, her physical position and the 'Centry' that she keeps being a way of monitoring the flow of curious questions and idle talk. She thus channels the internal politics of public spaces – the wells and the long room – acting as the perfect master of ceremonies whose function historians and contemporary guide-writers were reluctant to acknowledge because she was not appointed as such. Her ambivalence, and authoritarian and abusive power are other traits that Bell Causey shares with masters of ceremonies. The poem just mentioned calls her a 'Monster well-known for Fineness and Art in Intrigue' and suggests that she is a go-between at best, a Madam at worst:

> Full many a Maid
> Has she lur'd by her Trade
> And broke many a Conjugal League.[25]

Unsurprisingly, Bell Causey's trade is sexualised, and the brothel is never far from the tea-table, subduing young women through the mere power of joining in the murky waters of common cant.

Bell Causey's successor in Tunbridge Wells, Beau Nash, seems at first to differ radically in his moral views. As the famous master of ceremonies of Bath from 1701 to 1761, whose model inspired other spa towns to do the same – Bath being, as always, leader in spa town cultures – Beau Nash entertained a solid reputation for balancing out wit and politeness. He was officially appointed master of ceremonies in Tunbridge Wells after the death of Bell Causey. He kept his function in both towns until his own death in 1761, at age eighty-seven. His persona, like Bell's, was satirised and celebrated in local ephemeral literature. They ruled in opposite ways: rather than promoting gossip to maintain himself in power, Nash endeavoured to censor gossip to reinforce his moral authority. One year after Nash's death, the physician, novelist and playwright Oliver Goldsmith published his biography as he was staying in Bath and got access to his papers.[26] Goldsmith examines the ways in which Nash's soft power was executed through quiet diplomacy, conversation and wit, regulation at the gambling table and the management of reputations. *The life of Richard Nash* reads like a progress, as Goldsmith traces the political ascension of the master of ceremonies within the spa: 'In order to proceed in every thing like a king, he gave his subjects a law, and the following rules were accordingly put in the pump-room'.[27] Most notably, he records Nash's policy against gossip, which he calls, like Nash, 'scandal and lies': 'He endeavoured to render scandal odious, by marking it as the result of envy and folly united. Not even Solon could have enacted a wised law in such a society as *Bath*.'[28] Greek ruler Solon's laws were remembered as a reaction to the moral decay of Athens, so that Goldsmith hints at the social decay of the spa town in the early eighteenth century and further illustrates it in a derogatory overview of the water-drinkers. He subsequently lists the rules of protocol Beau Nash posted in the pump room where all new 'worthy' visitors were welcomed on arrival:

10. That all whisperers of lies and scandals be taken for their authors.
11. That all repeaters of such lies, and scandal be shun'd by all company; – except such as have been guilty of the same crime.[29]

The political strategy implemented to regulate gossip is thus to make the spreader of false news accountable for his act of sharing it. To Goldsmith, the main reasons for such quick penetration of scandal in the social circles of spa towns lie in sickness, levity and boredom. His vision of the population of spa towns (he mostly has Bath in mind, but also Tunbridge) is no better than a society of sick dunces:

> The gay, the heedless, and the idle, which mostly compose the group of water-drinkers, seldom are at the pains of talking upon universal topics, which require comprehensive thought, or abstract reasoning. The adventures of the little circle of their own acquaintance, or of some names of quality and fashion, make up their whole conversation.[30]

In one sentence, Goldsmith draws a sketch of the ignorant society, driven by irrelevant details and matter-of-fact observations with no notion of intellectual conversation. And yet, his own biography is rife with details, as John Eglin, the author of the most recent biography of Beau Nash, explains: 'Goldsmith, who took Nash at his word too often, manufactured anecdotes, or borrowed them from other sources'.[31] Yet Eglin does not denigrate Goldsmith's writings altogether, judging that despite such creative accounts, 'his interpretive instincts, however, were good'.[32]

The life of Richard Nash reads indeed like a collection of anecdotes, a major form pervading the literary genres involved in spreading knowledge in the eighteenth century, from medical treatises to periodicals and biographies. Goldsmith's perspective on Beau Nash, however, is not hagiographical. He makes several forays into the ambivalence of the character, and most notably into his complex relationship with gambling and money which I will explore in the next chapter. Yet what clearly fascinates Goldsmith, who never knew Nash directly, is the master of ceremonies' ability to regulate manners through conversation and immediate action. As a playwright and novelist, Goldsmith tries to catch Nash in action in a set of lively anecdotes which thrive within the theatrical setting of the spa. I would like to dwell on one anecdote set in Tunbridge, rather than Bath, which is representative of Goldsmith's method of staging Nash *in media res*:

> Nothing offended him more, than a young fellow's pretending to receive favours from ladies he probably never saw; nothing pleased him so much, as seeing such a piece of deliberate mischief punished. Mr. *Nash* and one of his friends, being newly arrived at *Tunbridge* from *Bath*, were one day on the walks, and seeing a young fellow of fortune, with whom they had some slight acquaintance, joined him. After the usual chat and news of the day was over, Mr. *Nash* asked him, how long he had been at the wells, and what company was there? The other replied, he had been at *Tunbridge* for a month; but as for company, he could find as good at a *Tyburn* ball. Not a soul was to be seen, except a parcel of gamesters and whores, who would grant the last favour, for a single stake at the Pharaoh bank. 'Look you there, continued he, that Goddess of midnight, so fine, at t'other end of the walks, by Jove, she was mine this morning for half a guinea. And she there, who brings up the rear with powder'd hair and dirty ruffles, she's pretty enough, but cheap, perfectly cheap; why, my boys, to my own knowledge, you may have her for a crown, and a dish of chocolate into the bargain. Last *Wednesday* night we were happy.' Hold there, sir, cried the gentleman; as for your having the first lady, it is possible it may be true, and I intend to ask her about it, for she is my sister; but as to your lying with the other last *Wednesday*, I am sure you are a lying rascal – she is my wife, and we came here but last night. The Buck vainly asked pardon; the gentleman was going to give him proper chastisement; when Mr. *Nash* interposed in his behalf, and obtained his pardon, upon condition that he quitted *Tunbridge* immediately.[33]

This anecdote is reminiscent of the farcical poem 'The Unfortunate Blow' I quoted in the previous chapter and might well have been borrowed from similar anecdotical verse. It is a good example of gendered gossip exacerbating masculine sexualities which Hillaria calls 'boasting'. The gossip at stake relies on men watching women stepping out on the Walks and objectifying them ('pretty enough but cheap, perfectly cheap'). The setting of the Walks is more dynamic than the assembly in the pump room or the audience in a theatre

and allows for a better view of each visitor as they walk past the
observer. The chivalrous defence of women in this mishap is quite
theatrical, showing nonetheless no alternative for women but to be
sisters and wives, or whores. Nash is represented as a peacemaker,
preventing further aggression and preserving the place from brawl
and duel, which he had already done in Bath by forbidding gentlemen
from wearing a sword.[34]

   In the first half of the eighteenth century, masters of ceremonies
started to be officially appointed by the corporations of major spa
towns such as Bath, Tunbridge, Scarborough and Cheltenham.
They held different titles, and they supervised various perimeters:
some managed assembly rooms only, like Vipont in Hampstead in
the 1730s; others supervised both the wells and the rooms, like
Richard Dickinson ('Dickie Dickinson') who was Governor of the
Wells in Scarborough until 1738; while yet others held a function
modelled after Beau Nash, or Simeon Moreau who was master of
ceremonies at Cheltenham Spa, and whose presence could apparently
be sensed all over town. They were committed to the contradictory
objectives of gathering visitors for entertaining parties and regulating
the manners of the assemblies. Naturally, the internal politics of the
spa town revolved around them, as the various local institutions had
a direct interest in their action, while the social politics of a season
gave visitors little time to know everyone and everything, making
them quite dependent on the master of ceremonies's expertise. This
probably explains why their power and authority were under such
scrutiny. A broadside poem on Dickie Dickinson revolves around his
disability,[35] comparing the master of ceremonies to two antagonistic
French figures. On the one hand, his authority is said to be similar
to the absolutism of 'Lewis Grand' (Louis XIV). On the other hand,
Dickinson's writings give him the status of 'Scarron', a well-known
seventeenth-century French satirical writer who was also disabled
and wrote a long epistle in verse on Bourbon l'Archambault, a major
spa town in seventeenth-century France.[36] Scarron was married to
Madame de Maintenon, who is herself compared to Dickinson's
mistress Peggy, and was later Louis XIV's favourite.

> The Sea itself does twice a day
> Advance and Homage to me pay;
> Yet some infer (like Sons of Wh—res)
> *Neptune*, grown jealous of our Pow'rs
> Turns Me and *Peggy* out Doors.[37]

The poem follows up with Apollo's interjection on his wonderful creation in the body of the Governor, and connects Dickinson's disability with his sway over the spa town:

> I'll make him *Sov'reign* of the *Spaw*
> To keep the squirting Tribe in awe,
> The loosest shall obey his Law.[38]

It concludes on the beauties of the mind of the Governor, as Dickinson was the author of several literary pamphlets, and he is represented at his writing table in Hans Hysing's engraving which circulated in several reproductions with the concluding words: 'France may glory in her late *Scarron*, While England has a Living *Dickinson*' (Figure 4.1).[39]

Most masters of ceremonies were regularly celebrated and ridiculed in literature for their awkward relationship to power. Samuel Derrick, for example, who succeeded James Collet in Bath and Tunbridge who had stayed only two years after Nash's death in 1761, is laughed at in Smollett's *Humphry Clinker* (1771). The scene starts as Tabitha Bramble, Matthew's sister, walks into the assembly room with her dog:

> Chowder no sooner made his appearance in the Room, than the Master of the Ceremonies, incensed at his presumption, ran up to drive him away, and threatened him with his foot; but the other seemed to despise his authority, and displaying a formidable case of long, white, sharp teeth, kept the puny monarch at bay.[40]

Like Dickinson, Derrick is mocked for his awkward physical appearance – he was said to be much smaller and less imposing than his predecessor, hence the title of 'puny monarch'. The confrontation with the dog strips him entirely of his dignity as he runs from the barking and biting little dog, who proudly takes control.[41] The fight degenerates further as Tabitha's dog is 'kicked in the jaws' by the very Baronet his mistress was trying to impress. The scene ends in a general brawl, with Derrick running after Tabitha to remind her 'upon the rules and regulations of the place'.[42]

If we compare the two representations of rules and regulation, it appears as if internal politics were person-dependent rather than the result of a common adherence to democratic rules of civility. The leadership of masters of ceremonies and their relationships to civility and entertainment were culturally modelled on monarchical power with a propension to autocracy. Against this top-down,

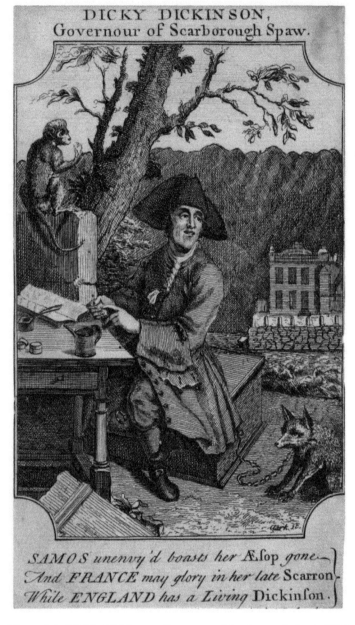

Figure 4.1 'Dickie Dickinson, Governor of Scarborough Spa', 1725

conventional approach of civility, some expressed a nostalgic attachment to earlier forms of a self-regulated society which allowed for
the free conversation originally praised in the 1733 poem 'On the
Elegant Entertainement and Mix'd Company at the Ordinaries',
quoted at the opening of this section.[43] Such nostalgia can also be
found in a later form of soft satire, as Sim writes to his friend in
Mavor's *The Cheltenham guide*:

> Without form we were gay – good humour went around,
>> And mirth and contentment society crown'd;
>>> Till lately an Ape in the shape of a Beau
>> With the outlandish name of Monsieur M——u,
>>> Has officially come at the balls to preside,
>>> To preserve *etiquette* and pay homage to pride.
> · Some use there may be in the creature, 'tis true,
>> Their way to the Temples the ladies to shew;
>>> But I still lament, that forms should efface
>>> The native politeness and ease of this place!
>> Perhaps you may call me low-liv'd and ill-bred,
>>> But, *sans* form, I am truly,
>>>> Yours.[44]

Mavor, who dedicated himself to pedagogical novels, cannot be taxed
with lacking morals. His work has none of the satirical pungency
of the model it is claiming to follow, Anstey's *New Bath Guide*.
Yet he uses the (much assuaged) character of the young Oxonian
student Sim B—N—R—D to criticise the continence imposed upon
the company by the new top-down protocol imported from Bath.
Simeon Moreau, the master of ceremonies under criticism, was elected
by the Cheltenham committee to preside over both assembly rooms
from 1784 to 1801, and he imported many regulations from Bath.[45]
He wrote a guide to Cheltenham Spa, and seems to have adapted
rather quickly many of the rules in effect at Bath. As a spa town,
Cheltenham was praised for its modest rusticity, which was contrasted
with the busy urbanity of Tunbridge, Bristol and Bath. The 'native
politeness' is the expression of an idealised society in a pastoral,
amiable environment that needs no authoritative ruler to thrive.

At local level, spa towns raise some of the political questions at
stake for the whole nation. What should be the degree of involvement of the police? Can society be self-regulated? Is the democratic
appointment of a ruler better than letting the most authoritarian

figures rise to power? Should the news be allowed to circulate freely, with the collateral damage of slander and gossip, or should they be channelled and controlled with adequate censorship? Like the experimental island staged in Marivaux's play *La Dispute*, spa towns appealed to the political imagination because they were self-contained in space and time – each season was an opportunity to start anew.[46] Visitors, governing bodies and the space itself were scrutinised by contemporaries as feedback on how the system of the town as a whole responded to competing political principles – whether concerning national spirit, the social role of women or the regulation of manners.

Healing the nation

Because they attracted visitors from various regions, and sometimes from the continent or the colonies, spas served as veritable spyglasses to observe the nation. Watering places enabled social and political gatherings outside of London and were sometimes presented as the summer house of government. Yet official governors were not the only visitors with political interests. Spa towns rallied influential people with dissenting opinions and were represented as such in some pamphlets and poems. Some women also envisioned spa towns as places to express their concerns and experiences in the alternative modes of social life that were not as readily accessible to them otherwise. Finally, the expanding British Empire gave spas a double function that worked towards its globalised organisation: the model was reproduced in the colonies which abounded in mineral waters, while in Britain waters were advertised as a cure for 'exotic' diseases.

At national level, spa towns were sometimes caricatured as the summer quarters of Parliament. As Hannah Greig explains, they were not the only places to follow a seasonal pattern.[47] The social life of the *Beau Monde*, which can roughly be defined as a restricted circle of aristocrats who held a seat in one of the parliamentary houses, was structured by the parliamentary season in London during which elite landed gentry would stay in their newly constructed houses in the West End.[48] Spa towns found a place within the larger map of national seasonal migrations. Calendars of the social seasons of spa towns varied and overlapped, but some of them, like Bath and Tunbridge Wells, were juxtaposed to enable visitors to make the most of the various seasons. Although the landed aristocracy usually went back to their country houses when the parliamentary sessions were over, many members of the London gentry planned to leave the city for the summer months, and regularly resorted to a spa town, especially when a member of their family was sick. Tunbridge, Epsom and the ring of smaller spas around London were favoured during the winter and spring while the summer allowed for more distant destinations such as Buxton, Harrogate, Cheltenham and Scarborough. Once they arrived in a spa town, remarkable visitors were announced by the ringing of the bells. Sometimes, their names could be called at the balls. They partly recreated some of the circles they frequented in London. A poem from the 1734 *Scarborough Miscellany* gives a panorama of the society gathered in the long room as a political assembly from London:

> Without Regret I leave the Town and Court,
> For Shades, where the Polite and Gay resort.
>
> Think not that softer Joys alone delight, –
> Here Senators harangue, and Sages write,
> Whilst Raptur'd I attend the Patriot's Themes,
> The *Long-Room* like *St. Stephen's Chapel* seems.
> Here, W—t—y Zealous in his Country's Cause,
> There, florid *Walsingham* the Audience draws.[49]

Although it is tempting to read the name of William Pulteney, Robert Walpole's opponent, under the letters W—t—y, the use of dashes does not quite fit the name. Walsingham, on the other hand, was the pen name of William Arnall, a pamphlet- and periodical-writer at Walpole's service, whose fierce prose was always a ready defence of the ministry.[50] The comparison between Vipont's long room and St Stephen's Chapel brings the political hypercentre into the distant periphery, as Scarborough, more than two hundred miles away through uncouth roads, was hard to access from London. Was this phenomenon, as has been argued among spa historians, a mark of the 'artificial life of society leaders playing at rusticity, and that but for a few months in summer'?[51] Surely, contemporary accounts of spa society are addressed to visitors much more than they are to local people, and give the impression that the 'company' is entirely made up of external visitors, as Ronald Cooley argues in his article on Tunbridge Wells.[52] As a result, spas were perceived as peripheral political centres in which new alliances could be explored and unofficial conversations pursued. Miscellanies probably overplayed their own roles as political pamphlets and satirical spa literature wove its way into the political debates of the time. Towards the end of the century, for example, Burnby's *Summer Amusement*, published in 1782, contained a poem entitled 'on the enlargement of John Wilkes', which praised the release of the radical politician. It is followed by another enthusiastic poem, 'To John Sawbridge, esq., one of the representatives in Parliament for the City of London'.[53] John Sawbridge was a fervent advocate of Wilke's radical ideas, which John Burnby, who had written *An Address to the People of England; on the Increase of Their Poor Rates*, was undoubtedly supporting.[54] Burnby, whose writings have a strong Kentish identity, used spa towns as a platform to enter national political debates.[55]

Pump room politics were also influenced by the dynamics of patronage. The role played by noble and royal patronage in the construction of spa tows has been widely studied and analysed by Phyllis Hembry.[56] Securing a patron was a way for a spa town to expand its clientele, receive coverage in periodicals and pamphlets, and manufacture objects of commerce related to said patron. Although Hembry insists on the Stuart patronage of spa towns during the Elizabethan and Jacobite period, the practice was still very much alive throughout the whole century, as shown by the royal visit of George III to Cheltenham in the summer of 1788. The king had been ill, and his court came on the advice of his physician George Baker for five weeks in July and August, calling national attention to the rural spa town. A comment from the *Morning Post* illustrates the craze that ensued, a craze which, of course, was partially created by the article itself, which lists all the fashionable objects of summer 1788: 'The Cheltenham cap – the Cheltenham bonnet – the Cheltenham buttons – the Cheltenham buckles – all the fashions are completely Cheltenhamised'.[57] As the waters were expected to heal the king's body, the author of the article in the *Morning Post* suggests that a paraphernalia of patriotic objects celebrated the Cheltenham waters for their potential healing of the nation.

Several caricatures of George III drinking at the pump circulated in London. One of them pictures the king eagerly opening his mouth under the flow of water (Figure 4.2). His servants are pumping the

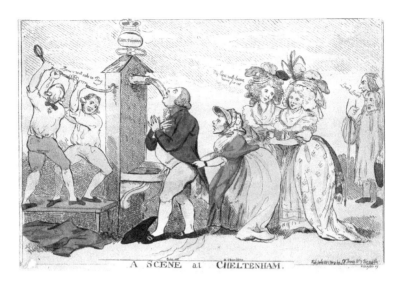

Figure 4.2 'A Scene at Cheltenham', 1788

water; his daughters, Charlotte and Augusta Sophia, complain that 'Papa will leave none for us', a possible allusion to the problems of water shortage encountered in many spa towns, Cheltenham especially, which is echoed by the interjection of the two men who have taken their coats off to pump the water vigorously: 'Zoons a will suke en Dry'.[58] His wife, Queen Charlotte, is pulling him by the jacket to interrupt his excessive drinking. The peasants in the background stand gaping, suggesting that even they are unused to drinking this amount of purging waters, in spite of a common belief among spa-goers that the poor drank excessive quantities, unaware of the consequences.[59] The king's enthusiastic gulping down of the waters as well as the position of his arms and head falling backwards denote absolute trust and dedication to his water treatment. His red, white and blue habit matches the colours of the nation whose future is at stake within the body of the king.

Such visits could give a spa town its political colour, perhaps beyond its own wishes, as was the case for Bath at the end of the seventeenth century. Mary of Modena visited the spa town in the summer of 1687, hoping that the waters would cure her barrenness – they were prescribed to her daughter-in-law, Princess Anne, for the same reason. Mary of Modena's delivery of a healthy infant son in June 1688 was attributed to the beneficial effects of the waters. The town was then imbued with long-lasting Jacobite sympathies, especially after the warming pan scandal of 1688 revolving around the legitimacy of the heir to the English crown.[60] Parliament asked for an inquiry to be made, hearings were organised, and a servant testified that her queen had become pregnant after a visit to Bath.[61] The richly decorated dome and cross erected within the cross bath in September 1688 in celebration of its effects on the queen, therefore, had heavy political implications (Figure 4.3). The monument was financed by the Earl of Melfort, close advisor to James II, newly converted to Catholicism. By celebrating the effects of the waters, the Melfort monument reasserted the authenticity of the queen's pregnancy, and God's action on the queen's body through the natural effects of the waters, which, as John Eglin remarks, 'had not purged the distinctly popish odour of the miraculous'.[62] Although the inheritance of the Roman Catholic tradition of holy waters in the English Protestant world is a complex question which I will try to disentangle in the next section, it is undeniable that the Melfort monument was an ostentatious sign of Jacobitism that the Bath corporation would gradually seek to erase. It was eventually removed in the 1780s as it embarrassed the corporation, its members having wished to distance themselves from any Jacobite sympathies since the first days of the Glorious Revolution.[63] That Bath would be the hosting place of dissenting political groups was in line with a representation of spas inherited from Renaissance writings. From the beginning of the early modern period, European spas were thought to be a favoured spot to meet and plan alliances, or prepare coups. In his article on politics and balneology in sixteenth-century France, for example, Xavier Le Person explains that spas are both a real and imagined space for political plotting and quiet diplomacy.[64] According to him, it was acceptable within a European court to leave quickly for health reasons to seek a water treatment rather than wait for permission to leave court for personal reasons, which put spa towns on the top list of destinations that could justify a quick departure – a good pretext for hiding other political agendas.

Whether for political, medical or leisure purposes, international visitors came to visit major English spas, and their visits were commented upon in the writings of the times, which tended to insist

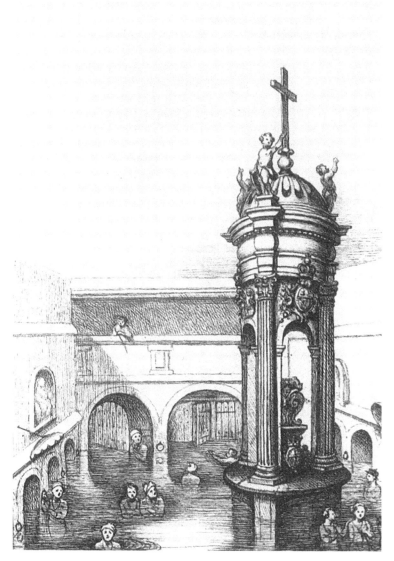

Figure 4.3 John Fayram, The Melfort monument in the cross bath, 1739

– not always positively — on the cultural diversity of spa towns. Elizabeth Montagu, for example, regrets the international and multi-confessional crowd present at Tunbridge Wells in 1745:

> We cannot complain of want of numbers, for all nations and sects contribute to make up complement of people. Here are Hungarians, Italians, French, Portuguese, Irish and Scotch. Then we have a great many Jews, with worse countenance than their friend Pontius Pilate, in a bad tapestry hanging. In opposition to these non-believers, we have the very believing Roman Catholics; and to contrast with these ceremonious religionists, we have the quaint puritans, and rigid Presbyterians. I never saw a worse collection of human creatures in all my life. My comfort is, that as there are not many of them I ever saw before, I flatter myself there are few of them I shall ever see again.[65]

Montagu has a knack for describing crowds, as in her 1740 letter from Bath in which she calls the company 'an assembly of disorders'. In this letter, she also distances herself from the rest of the company at Tunbridge, using denominations and national identities to disembody the other visitors and turn their presence into an assembly of religion and politics. The juxtaposition of religious groups and national characters creates a hotchpotch that can only be transient, yet seems a concentrate of the urban composition of the English nation. As Linda Colley explains, visiting the countryside could be reassuring for those who were anxious over the internationalisation of Britain and eager to entertain the idea of an authentic Englishness: 'patrician tourists enjoyed the comforting illusion that they had travelled back in time, when their world was still safe'.[66] Representing the inaccessible countryside, she argues, contrasted with 'the well-established watering-places and spas, which had long been taken up by the bourgeoisie', displaying the cosmopolitan qualities of international cities.[67]

In the same vein, the variety of food and entertainments provided at the spa were mocked in hackneyed conservative satire, which saw spas as places of importation of foreign taste: Italian singers, French food and all the elements of 'false grandeur' displayed in spa towns reek of continental origin. A scathing nationalist poem published in 1777 entitled 'Modern Refinement' targeted Bath and the Hotwells (Bristol) by opposing the roast beef of Old England and the meagre banquets of the spa town:

> some vile French Cook supplies the frugal board
> With here a snail, and there some hash'd-up Toad.[68]

Such discourse partakes of a more general attack on the foreign taste corrupting urban life, consumption and high-manners. It considers the major spa towns as porous points of contact through which permeated the taste for foreign goods, foreign manners and foreign culture. In 'Modern Refinement', for example, Squire Dilettanti gives weekly concerts and serves no food.[69] It would be wrong, however, to consider that foreigners were systematically presented as a threat. In a poem entitled 'The Humours of Brighthelmstone', written by Jane West in 1788, the poet stages Brighton as a neutral or 'diplomatic' space between the English and the French:

> The French from Dieppe in great numbers come hither
> Shake hands with John Bull, and deal *friendly* together.[70]

West, whose famous didactic novels and cautionary tales were most probably known to the readers of this poem, preferred to see spas as an opportunity for quiet diplomacy and the soft mending of old political feuds, a subject she also defended in other writings on private and family relationships. Her political views on the role of spas are therefore rooted in the belief in the virtues of social and international mingling. At the opposite end of Montagu's annoyance with social and national mixité, West depicts Brighton as an ideal space for relaxed encounters and tolerance:

> Here English and French* noble visitors mingle,
> The old and the young, and the married and single.[71]

She provides further context in the following footnote: '*The Duke of Chartres (now Duke of Orleans), the Duke de Fitz James, and the Marquis de Constans, visited Brighton in the year 1785; as also did the Princess de Lamballe'.[72] The poem was published five years after the peace of Paris was signed, and five years before another war broke out between England and France. Jane West cleverly transforms Brighton into a diplomatic hotspot, while most readers would have known that the Duke of Orléans, the future Philippe Égalité, was an enthusiastic anglophile who had found temporary quarters in London. Clearly, the poem is on the side of the French aristocracy ('noble visitors'), whose powers are about to be shattered by the French Revolution. West depicts Brighton as a haven of hospitality on the other side of the channel, a potential refuge for French aristocrats in search of new alliances. In all its polite under-tones, the poem reinforces the contrast between the utopian world of Brighton and other spa towns and seaside resorts, as 'Bright-helmstone' surpasses, says the poet, 'the pleasures of Margate and old Tunbridge Wells'.[73]

The term 'alliance' best describes another kind of political aspect of spa towns – women's relationships, their common activities, their shared experiences and their epistolary conversations. In her book *Female Alliances*, Amanda Herbert shows how early modern women, by fostering family bonds and friendships, worked at a micro level to strengthen the social structures on which the British Empire was being built. In her chapter on spas, 'Hot spring sociability', she charts the various ways in which women bonded and exchanged practices. Herbert focuses on confectionary as one of the common activities of women, who worked at making sweets, fruit pastes and medicinal lozenges, spending time together in conversation, negotiating with transpacific commercial dealers, and exchanging goods and recipes.[74] In many ways, the multiple networking activities of women in spa towns can be seen as another form of 'healing the nation', as it is now widely acknowledged that patients depended on the ways in which women invested the various forms of care within their networks, as well as on their access to medical knowledge and their multiple handiworks related to the medical trade. In an earlier article entitled 'Gender and the spa', Herbert shows the connection between female sociability in spa towns and the general sociability of care, as women provided for each other and each other's friends and families 'by visiting and taking the waters in tandem, by exchang-ing medical advice and providing childcare, and by sharing the physiological experiences of illness and of emotional care for others'.[75] Although no public danger, no direct threat of plotting or revolution-ary mobs were at stake, women clearly nurtured modes of sociability that nourished their existence quite independently of the patriarchal public spheres, a sociability which could prove resourceful and fostered a sense of same-sex companionship. To Alison Hurley, spa towns were even more charged with potentially subversive female alliances, as they were central to the correspondence of bluestocking intellectuals. They worked as an imaginary space around which their intellectual exchanges gravitated. 'Spa towns provided these women with a locus, at once imagined and real, upon which to elaborate a distinctive style of correspondence', she writes, showing how Elizabeth Montagu and her correspondents led epistolary 'spa conversations' in which a playful yet caring tone enabled them to 'address themselves more directly to the world in which they lived'.[76]

Like most social, political and medical phenomena in England at the time, the development of mineral waters had multiple ramifications in the growing Empire. Within the British Isles, Welsh, Scottish and Irish spas flourished in parallel with English spas, sometimes mirroring them, sometimes clearly demarking themselves through specific cultural traits. In the next section of this chapter, I will deal with the Roman Catholic inheritance of holy wells which was a strong component of some of the most popular Welsh and Irish wells, even when their waters had been analysed and validated as mineral waters by local physicians. In Ireland, as James Kelly explained, there were many holy wells still visited throughout the century on the days of their patron saint, yet wealthier visitors, in the first part of the eighteenth century, chose to go to England, Belgium or France and visit the spa towns there.[77] The Dublin-based Quaker doctor John Rutty, like Thomas Short in Yorkshire, promoted the Irish spa towns which were developing, such as Ballyspellan in county Kilkenny, Templeogue in county Dublin and Swanlinbar in county Cavan, in his 1757 *Methodical Synopsis of Mineral Waters*. His controversy with the Irish Protestant doctor Charles Lucas, who was then in exile in England, contributed to render Irish spas more visible. In Scotland, Moffat was probably the most visible of all spa towns, but it was certainly not the only one. As Alastair Durie explains, spa towns developed in parallel with seaside resorts, which promoted the medical benefits of sea-bathing. Some spas, like Peterhead in Aberdeenshire, offered both mineral waters and sea water. Salt water treatment, Durie writes, received '*general* endorsement of science and medicine'.[78] Scotland's role in the development of medicinal sea-bathing needs to be explored further, as it did not offer the same leisurely activities as those found in the southern parts of England. Similarly, John Andrews identifies several seaside towns in Wales in his 1797 map of mineral waters, and several spas developed on ancient holy wells, like St Winifred in Flintshire or St Justinian in Pembrokeshire. Traces of ancient thermal baths testify to a long-lasting bathing culture in Wales, as Robert Sanders argues in his *Complete English Traveller* (1771) when he narrates how a gardener of Caergwrle in Flintshire was digging to find the ruins of an ancient Roman bath.[79]

Far beyond the provinces, watering places were also developing in the colonies at White Sulphur or Bath in Virginia, at Saratoga Springs in Connecticut, at Ballston Spa in the state of New York, at Berkeley Springs and Harrogate in Pennsylvania, to name but a few.[80] As Thomas Chambers explains, the urban development of the spas started in the late eighteenth century, and they tended to be set in a rather 'rustic' environment with little accommodation and entertainment provided to visitors. Chambers argues that 'only by equalling the European spas would American springs earn the cultural legitimacy that the elite demanded', and thus 'Federalist groups continued to look to England for cultural models', even when they were advised to develop their own American identity.[81] Yet Vaughn Scribner shows that the watering places in early America also developed in areas already known and used by Native American tribes, many of whom 'centered their cultural identities around water immersion' and entertained a 'mystical relationship with water'.[82] Such practices were known to the colonial doctors who, in turn, reported the fact to their counterparts in England. This was then turned into a general discourse on the natural healing practices of the natives that justified the use of mineral waters as a universal and ancestral practice. Thomas Short, who was otherwise well versed in chemical analysis, interspersed his scientific discourse with these early and general anthropological observations: 'We may add to waters penetrating the skin, that as hurtful things applied outwardly, convey into the body something of their own duality, so must things of a healing nature convey something salutary into the body; for which reason the wild Americans, Asiatics, Africans and savage islanders in all those places, have the highest opinion of bathing, both cold and warm', he writes, looking for universal principles that would justify his Yorkshire-based obsession with mineral waters.[83]

Short's analytical practices were familiar to the physician Benjamin Rush, who turned to the waters in the Philadelphia region and analysed them with similar methods.[84] About the mineral waters at Harrogate, he writes that 'It is proper in all those Colics, which arise from mere weakness of the bowels, and particularly in that species, which is accompanied with an overflowing of the bile, a disease this to which the inhabitants of the warm climates are most subject'.[85] He advertised the mineral waters of Philadelphia as a proper cure for typical Western diseases such as hysteria, gout and palsy, and insisted on their helpful preservation of Western bodies which they assisted in their struggles with the diseases contracted in the colonies, such as the obstinate diarrhoea which affected 'Sailors from long voyages, or from warm climates'.[86] E. T. Jennings maps the ways in which mineral water resorts were used as places of adaptation to warmer climates, as well as to heal the colonisers' bodies on their return to the metropole.[87] Although the book deals with the French context, Jennings's reflexion on the relationship between the anxiety of becoming sick in warm climates and the reconstruction of mineral waters in the French colonies as a sort of medical and social quarantine which re-enacted modes of nostalgic continental sociability, is a good starting point to analyse the use of mineral waters in British colonies:

> If altitude and water cures came to be seen as essential to detoxify, recalibrate, or otherwise heal the constitutions, organs, even the blood composition of French people who had spent time in 'hot climes,' then said climes must indeed have been considered highly noxious. Nowhere is the anxiety over colonial settlement and over the inherent toxicity of the tropics more apparent than in the interminable debates over human acclimatization, which weighed considerably on modes of European behavior in the colonies.[88]

A similar reasoning justified the development of Jamaican spas, especially the Bath waters near St Thomas, which had been developed since 1695 and found to be 'a powerful remedy in the cure of the dry belly-ache and some other prevailing diseases of the climate', as Thomas Dancer argues at the beginning of his chemical inquiry of the said waters in 1784.[89]

Similar reasonings could be found in England when mineral waters cured patients suffering from 'exotic' diseases. A narrative reported by the Westphalian doctor Diederick Wessel Linden in 1748 about Shadwell Spa reports the case of a young servant – a '*Black Boy* belonging to his Grace, the Duke of *Cleveland*'[90] – suffering from the yaws, a skin disease forming ulcers on the upper body and spreading in the whole system, which Linden identified as 'Distemper happily unknown to these our Climates, being peculiar to that of *Negroes*, or *African* Nations; But, as this Distemper is of a putrid Nature, so as to rot the human Flesh insensibly, and without the affected Part feeling any Pain, also without any inflammation or Fever, preceding or accompanying it'.[91] The detailed account of the young man's disease resembles the earlier narratives of miraculous cures presented in the second chapter of this book:

> All his Head was crusted over with large Scabs, his Shoulders and Neck interspersed with ugly hard Swellings, and other Parts of his Body broke out in putrid Ulcers. Such was his Condition, when their Grace of *Cleveland*, from their innate Tenderness and Humanity, suffered no Means to be spared, for the Recovery of this their Servant; for the Space of eight Months, he had the Advice and assistance of many eminent Gentlemen of the Profession, in which Space, he was thrice salivated to no Purpose, or perceivable Melioration whatever: But, at length, he being sent by their Graces Order, to the *Shadwell Spaw*; the Under-steward of that noble Family, and a Surgeon under whose Care he had been for some Time, brought him thither, where he both drank and bathed every Day, first drinking a Pint of this Water in the Morning, upon an empty Stomach, and then, some Hours after, he went into a prepared warm Bath of this Water, in which he remained an Hour and upwards. And with this Method alone, this black Servant became cured in eighteen Days Time.[92]

The servant, who seems to have been the object of much speculative and painful medical treatment at the hands of the physicians, is brought to the spa by a medical man. The London mineral water manages to cure a distemper which, in this case, had attacked the body of a young African man, or of African descent, carrying a distemper coming from warmer climates. The water treatment is at odds with the useless and cruel salivation – a mercury-based treatment – of 'gentlemen of the profession'. They seem to be the recourse of people of common-sense. The patient is brought by a surgeon – not a physician – and an under-steward, whom the reader might suppose to be close to the patient, all under the 'innate tenderness and humanity' of his master. The flattering term, commonly used for seeking patronage, reasserts the ownership of the duke while partaking of a sentimental representation of good management of his servants.[93] The patient's case is therefore used as a medical and moral example that is mediated by the natural healing of the virtuous spa.

Dealing with the past: holy wells

The virtuousness of the waters and their miraculous cures is an ambivalent aspect of the healing waters which is deeply ingrained in the religious and political history of the British Isles. This ambivalence lives on to this day. In 2020, several Facebook groups track the ancient holy wells of Great Britain and Ireland. Their members take pictures of the holy wells and, most often, of their ancient location, often covered by ferns or buried underneath an industrial warehouse. They are well informed, in every sense of the term, on the history and original locations, and highly trained in cultural hiking. They collectively chart the map of medieval holy wells in the countries. Group members come from diverse backgrounds: some have an interest in history, some believe in the ever-lasting properties of healing waters, some are environmentally minded.[94] They all share a sense of citizen science, and collaborate to university-led crowdsourcing initiatives such as the 'Well well well!' event in the 2020 festival of archaeology in Northern Ireland.[95] All seem to agree on the fact that Britain was severed from its heritage of holy wells during the Reformation. The dissolution of monasteries (1536–41) was linked with a series of bans and destructions of sacred places, and of the thaumaturgic waters of holy wells and fountains related to the intercession of a saint. The memory of these wells, however, has persisted in British culture until the twenty-first century, and many eighteenth-century writings mention their existence and persistence. As they were dealing with Catholic inheritance, the various narratives surrounding the (re)discoveries of holy wells had political implications. Medical authors mention them as part of an earlier form of superstitious cures, Anglican authors condemn them, travellers express some curiosity at their exoticism. As I will now show, several spas in eighteenth-century British culture were associated with Roman Catholicism, and its representation was ambivalent and contradictory.

Resurgences of the murky past could happen in one's own house, sometimes for the better. Among the many narratives of spa discoveries, the story of Sadler's Wells (also called the Newfound Wells at Islington) by Thomas Guidott is a sample of domestic archaeology:

> M. Sadler, being made Surveyor of the Highways and having good
> Gravel in his own Garden, employed two men to dig there, and when

they had dug, pretty deep, one of them found his Pickax strike upon
something that was very hard, whereupon he indeavoured to break
it, but could not; whereupon thinking with himself that it might
peradventure be some Treasure hid there, he uncovered it very carefully,
and found it to be a Broad Hat Stone; which having loosened and
lifted up, he saw it was supported by four Oaken Posts, and had
under it a large Well of Stone Arched over, and curiously carved; and
having viewed it, he called his fellow Labourer to see it likewise, and
asked him whether they should fetch Mr. Sadler, and shew it him?
Who having no kindness for *Sadler* said, no; he should not know of
it, but as they had found it, so they would stop it up again, and take
no notice of it; which he that found it consented to at first, but after
a little time he found himself (whether out of Curiosity or some other
reason, I shall not determine) strongly inclined to tell *Sadler* of the
Well; which he did one Sabbath Day in the Evening.[96]

Thomas Guidott was a physician whose literary skills had been
largely trained by the writing of several treatises and biographies,
interspersed with satirical poems. He stages the discovery of the spa
with theatrical effects. The labourer's digging 'pretty deep' and the
allusion to a treasure hidden in the garden are relevant within the
economic context of the Restoration, as finding mineral waters near
London could be the promise of a steady income. Within this rather
short pamphlet of four pages, Guidott dedicates several lines to
insist on the labourer's refusal to tell Sadler, which is both puzzling
and interesting within the context of an early scientific discovery.
The work of contractors must have been put off by any archaeological
discovery, which explains why the labourer uses his sudden power
to get back at Sadler, hindering the potential economic progress of
his employer as it curbs his own: it shows that Thomas Guidott
was aware of the ways in which economic and personal interest
interfered with scientific opportunities. The labourer's offer to cover
up the treasure and remain silent is also emblematic of the obscurant-
ism at work, probably tainted with a cultural bias against the Catholic
heritage of holy wells, which should be kept under ground.

Sadler, as we know, made the most of his well. He opened a
theatre and a beer garden, and commercialised the waters. Guidott
shows his sense of business by describing his prompt reaction:

Sadler upon this went down to see the Well and observing the Curiosity
of the Stone Work, that was about it, and fancying within himself

that it was a Medicinal Water, formerly had in great esteem, but by some accident or other lost, he took some of it in a Bottle, and carried it to an Eminent physician, telling him how the Well was found out, and desiring his Judgement of the Water.[97]

The physician tells Sadler that the waters are mineral indeed, and that he should start by brewing beer with them.[98] Guidott explicitly traces the origin of the waters to a well 'before the Reformation, very much famed for several extraordinary Cures performed thereby, and was thereupon accounted sacred, and called *Holy-Well*'.[99] He then reminds the reader of the Roman Catholic parishes and abbeys charting the city of London: 'The Priests belonging to the Priory of *Clerken-well* using to attend there, made the People believe that the vertues of the Waters proceeded from the efficacy of their Prayers'.[100] The well disappeared, Guidott argues, because of the great historical rupture in England: 'But upon the Reformation the Well was stopt up, upon supposition that the frequenting it was altogether Superstitious, and so by degrees it grew out of remembrance, and was wholly lost until found out'.[101] His emphasis on memory, which coincides with the burying of the well, shows that memory of the waters, their identity within the history of a neighbourhood, and their serendipitous reappearance, were several elements that belonged to a historical narrative that Guidott trusted and passed on.

For some contemporaries, the persisting existence of holy waters was part of a superstitious paraphernalia of Roman Catholicism that was to be strictly condemned, mocked and rationalised into other explanations. In its most extreme satirical forms, the Catholicism and Jacobitism surrounding the history of thaumaturgic waters led to accusations of plotting and poisoning. Sadler's Wells, for example, is violently mocked in a broadside sheet published in 1684 and previously studied in this book, *An Exclamation from Tunbridge and Epsom against the Newfound Wells at Islington*. This diatribe accounts for the wells' healing property by accusing the 'Papist' of poisoning the wells, 'as chronicles tells us, the Jews did of old'.[102] It revels in a hotchpotch of popular accusations of plotting and poisonous remedies, blatantly asserting that 'all their operations proceeds from *Jesuits Powder* or *phanatical Quicksilver*'.[103] Clearly, Roman Catholicism here is just another element in a long list of social ills attributed to Sadler's Wells.

In some sites such as Glastonbury, charges of Roman Catholicism were more serious, as they had more grounds. Phyllis Hembry's account of the Glastonbury waters and their transient success in the middle of the eighteenth century shows how they are built on Roman Catholic culture, from the way they were discovered – Matthew Chancellor was directed to the waters in a dream – to their management – the bath house run by Anne Galloway was 'closed on Catholic Fast Days'.[104] Surely, the ruins of Glastonbury abbey nearby, which attracted many visitors to the Somerset town, must have contributed to the promotion of the miraculous healing powers of these waters, with Roman Catholic undertows. A song published in 1751 mocking the 'Popish inventions' of the Glastonbury waters starts indeed with the legend of the holy thorn, which flourishes at Christmas and Easter:

> I'll sing you a song to the tune of down derry,
> Concerning the waters of fam'd *Glastonbury*;
> Where *Arimathy Joseph* of old fix'd his staff,
> A story some credit, while other folks laugh.
> > *Derry down &c.*

> From this, says tradition, there sprang up a thorn,
> That constantly blossoms each *Christmas-day* morn;
> Which as firmly some credulous people believe,
> As the serpent seduc'd our old grandmother *Eve*.
> > *Derry down &c.*

> But this spring was found out by a man in a dream,
> Who was bid by an angel go drink of the stream
> Seven Sundays successive; what e'er he endur'd,
> If faith was not wanting, he'd surely be cured.[105]

The song inscribes the healing waters within the local Roman Catholic tradition, fashioning it as a powerful legend with the seductive, serpent-like manipulative powers of popish narratives. Credulity and belief are at the centre of the song, which correlates the thaumaturgic waters with the faith of the patient.

The debate over the Glastonbury waters soon took a political and medical turn.[106] Several periodicals took part in the controversy, and among them a letter from the *London Daily Advertiser* argues that waters tested through amateur methods of chemistry (they simply evaporated the water) should be deemed no different from common water.[107] The author of the letter calls for further chemical analysis of the waters, 'that people may be undeceived and not flock thither in multitudes, from the most distant places, with great expense, and loss of life to many'.[108] No direct accusation of Catholicism is to be found in the article, yet the terms of the letter express a clear anxiety over what resembles a Roman Catholic pilgrimage generating uncontrollable crowd movements. Beyond attacks on credulity, the political anxiety over popular Catholic beliefs tainted with Jacobite culture is implicitly presented as a threat by the amateur chemist. An answer to this letter from the *London Daily Advertiser*, published in the same issue of *The Gentleman's Magazine*, takes up the medical thread and leaves aside all religious hints, accusing the previous author of being a 'pipkin chemist'. He insists that 'facts are stubborn things', as he claims to have been cured of a distemper himself.[109] By moving the dispute onto medical grounds, the author of the *London Daily Advertiser* can give some credit to the waters without claiming any affiliation with the Roman Catholic Church. His concern is to oppose facts to superstition, and professionalism to amateurism. A similar economy of proof was adopted by J. Davies in his pamphlet published that same year, *A Short Description of the Waters at Glastonbury*. On the cover page, he claims to be 'a disinterested Clergyman, not at all obliged to the inhabitants, nor in the least concerned in the Interest of that Town'.[110] Not a physician himself, Davies displays all the marks of a reliable witness and collects a series of cases, some of them confirmed by affidavits, to cram his argument with facts and avoid any discussion on the religious inheritance of the waters – while his own status as a clergyman is sufficient to counter potential suspicions of Roman Catholicism.[111] The disclaimer on the front page is a way of addressing what Alexandra Walsham calls 'the latent conflict between profit and piety that crystallized around healing springs'.[112]

Clergymen played a leading role in the debates surrounding the inheritance of holy waters. As they condemned or rationalised the healing virtues of holy wells into the acceptable boundaries of the Anglican Church, they made a local political statement on the social dynamics at stake around sacred spaces and sanctuaries. In 1727, for example, the Church of Ireland dean, John Richardson wrote a diatribe against the resurgence of pilgrimages which is a good example of how miraculous waters were condemned by the Anglican Church. As he describes the healing waters of St Patrick's Well in Lough Derg in Ireland, he hammers that 'because some have been healed of their Diseases by drinking of the Waters of St. *Patrick*'s Well, it doth not follow that St. *Patrick* wrought the Cure'.[113] Richardson, who had previously authored a pamphlet entitled *A Short History of the Attempts that have been Made to Convert the Popish Natives of Ireland* (1712), was part of the Anglo-Irish elite seeking to convert the Catholic peasantry. He claimed to have made more effort than his Anglican peers at meeting the natives halfway, as he learned Gaelic and believed it should be one of the languages in which priests should preach. In *The Great Folly, Superstition, and Idolatry, of Pilgrimages in Ireland*, he partly rationalises superstitious rituals and beliefs among Catholics, and reframes them within Protestant beliefs: 'For Protestants, who hold it unlawful to invocate Saints, have received as much Benefit by the Use of these Wells, as Papists, whereof many Instances might be given: And therefore, I do not see, how any Papist can be assured, that it was done by St *Patrick*, or through his Intercession'.[114]

Richardson also describes the pilgrims as uncouth natives 'who run bare foot and bare-Head, with their beads in one hand a stick like a † in the other'.[115] He gives many details of the ritualised gestures of the peasants whose barbarous bodies clearly fascinated and disgusted him at the same time.[116] Unsurprisingly, he attempts to rationalise miracles of holy waters in the county of Meath by mentioning their minerality: 'When Pilgrims come within Sight of the Well, they walk bare Head and bare Foot up to it, and drink plentifully of the Water, which is purging, and impregnated with some Mineral'.[117] The pilgrims' Roman Catholic beliefs in saints are also set in a wider frame of Irish mythology which, according to Richardson, coexists with Catholic rituals. He thus implies that Roman Catholics came from lower illiterate classes, prompt to believe any mythological narrative, be it of Christian or pagan origin. He narrates the edifying tale of Conan, a giant who threw away a worm in a nearby lake and came back to be swallowed up by the worm, which had grown in monstrous disproportion, eating men and cattle alike. Conan simply cut off the head of the monster from its insides: 'The Monster immediately died, and Conan having cut off his head, threw it upon the shore, where the stones were coloured red with

Blood, that gushed out of it (as the Natives believe:) whereas it is obvious to observe that it is a Mineral Spring flowing over them, that gives them this Colour'.[118] The redness of the pebbles was no miracle, produced neither by the head of a holy saint, nor that of a vulgar monstrous worm decapitated by a giant: it was merely the trace of a chalybeate spring nearby.

Within the medical world, similar attacks were made upon the belief in Roman Catholic saints either to clear the mineral waters of any aftertaste of holiness, or to bring some suspicion on mineral waters in general, and the way they operated. Tobias Smollett, for example, in his treatise on the waters of Bath, expresses little trust in the healing properties of minerals:

> I have known the most sordid and inveterate *scrophulous* and *scorbutic* ulcers cured by the *aspersion* of common Well-water, which to the taste and smell, exhibited no sign of mineral impregnation; but, at first, derived its reputation from the superstition of the people, by whom, in times of ignorance, it had been dedicated to one of the legendary saints on the Roman calendar'.[119]

The force of belief, however, and the power of the imagination, are recurrent themes in eighteenth-century medicine to account for miraculous cures.[120] Some historians of medicine have seen this rationalisation as a wider attempt to secularise healing practices. According to them, the multiplying treatises on mineral waters were striving to medicalise the holy waters. In his article on chemistry and the legitimisation of spas, Christopher Hamlin observes a shift in the strategies of legitimisation after 1537, as wells were destroyed and saints banned:

> During the Reformation attempts were made, often successfully, to stamp out the association of waters with saints and sometimes to close the springs themselves. Sometimes these attempts were founded in appeals to hard-headed rationality: those who used and believed in the springs had been duped by con men who saw an easy profit; it would be a public service to root out such superstitious gullibility by demonstrating that the waters were no different from any others.[121]

The new legitimisation processes, he argues, were now focused on the analyses of waters, and the collection of cures witnessed by the local people.

To the literary scholar Daniel Cottom, the double inheritance of Catholic and pagan beliefs such as Conan's monster triggered new strategies of medicalisation, and potential suspicions of Jacobitism in some spa towns: 'One consequence of the English Reformation was a more or less concerted effort to strip these holy wells of their religious associations and, not incidentally, of their suspected role as gathering places for recusants and schemers against the Protestant succession'.[122] The medical historian Daphne Oren-Magidor gives a more nuanced interpretation of the medicalisation of holy wells. As she details the various cures for infertility in early modern England, she pays particular attention to the ways in which medicine and religion interacted: 'Spa towns were not always popular among upper-class women. Immediately after the Reformation, water cures actually fell out of favour, because they were associated with specific saints and with Catholic rituals.'[123] Even though she explains that the holy waters were 'recast in medical terminology', she refrains from concluding that spas were entirely cast out of the religious sphere. On the contrary, spas were 'understood within a religious framework that saw the spas as God's particular divine gift to England and would work, like all medicine, through God's will'.[124] This statement is in line with the analyses of the religious historian Alexandra Walsham on early modern sacred spaces and the memory of Catholicism: 'The rampant secularism that was a feature of health resorts centred on medicinal waters cannot be ignored', she writes, 'but nor should we fall into the trap of assuming that it was inherently incompatible with devotion and piety'.[125]

A good example of such Protestant rhetoric can be found very early on within the chronological scope of this book, in the two sermons preached at Tunbridge Wells during the Restoration by Anthony Walker, published in 1685 under the title *Fax Fonte Accensa, Fire out of Water: or, an Endeavour to kindle Devotion, from the Consideration of the Fountains God hath made*. Walker was a clergyman in Fyfield, Essex, and came regularly to Tunbridge Wells to accompany his wife, Elizabeth Walker, whose medical knowledge as a druggist and practitioner of medicine must have influenced Anthony in his perception of the medicinal use of waters.[126] His sermons enjoin readers to recognise that the works of God are at the origin of the blessed waters, and patients should engage in their physical healing with a spiritual conversion of the heart. In deep strains of religious lyricism, Walker starts one of the meditations of his sermon on the mineral waters as a sign of an abundance of blessings given freely to all:

> These waters have a Voice, and joyn the *Chorus*, which ecchoing the call of the Spirit, and the Bride (the Church on Earth, and God from Heaven) invites us to come and take the Waters of Life freely. The Perennity of their Streams, the free access that, from the Prince to the Peasant, all have to them; their equal Helpfulness to rich and poor, to bad and good; and many more like Properties, are all instructive.[127]

The waters of life invite the sick to meditate on the waters of eternal life, and on the alliance between God and humanity through the intercession of the Church at large – not through the specific interces-sion of a Saint who would answer individual prayers. Theological imagery of the relationship between God and his Church on earth replaces the hagiological accounts of extraordinary events associated with the waters. In Walker, waters are indeed miraculous, yet they are as part of a wider context in which any natural healing plant or matter is considered as a blessing of God and a wonder. He focuses on the minerality of the waters and their taste as the physical sensation of God's grace: 'O Lord my God, thy Goodness is the rich Mineral, through which our Springs to glide! 'tis this which gives them, both their Tincture and their Taste, renders them whole-some, makes them healthful.'[128] The emotional burst of gratitude is a devotional trait that partakes of a religious culture of grace-giving in front of the abundance of natural blessings, some of which, like the waters, or many other natural drugs, were also acknowledged as valid medical cures. As Alexandra Walsham reminds us, there is no linear 'narrative of the onward march of secularization'.[129] She insists on the role played by Protestantism in the remediation of holy waters in early modern British culture:

> The transition from sacred springs to spas was seen in terms of the triumph of scientific rationalism over blind superstition, and Protestant-ism was typically accorded the role of an able and enthusiastic midwife in this process. But it is important to stress that contemporary percep-tion of healing baths and wells remained firmly locked within a framework of pious assumptions.[130]

Some spas bore their Roman Catholic inheritance more ostenta-tiously than others. Bath and its Melfort monument or Buxton,

whose waters were originally dedicated to St Anne and were
famously taken by Mary Stuart not long before her death, were
regularly acknowledged for their Catholic tradition. They could
not rival, however, the popular outreach of St Winifred's Well in
Wales as a Roman Catholic sanctuary. Contemporary guidebooks
and periodicals testified that numerous pilgrims continued to flock
to the well throughout the eighteenth century, and the Catholic
sanctuary kept its strong religious identity in coexistence with the
Church of England. There are many variations on the name of St
Winifred (Wenifrede, Wenefrede, etc.), yet they all refer to the same
virgin martyr from the seventh century who lived in Holywell and
was held as a saint in the Roman Catholic Church. Later, legendary
accounts of her life report that she was pursued by a man named
Caradog, who made several attempts at ravishing her, and, being
rebutted by her refusal and her steady commitment to become a
nun, decapitated her. Her head rolled down the hill, giving birth to
a spring, and was gathered by her hermit uncle, Beuno.[131] He put
the head back on Winifred's body and invoked godly punishment
upon Caradog, who fell dead. Just like the waters in Lough Derg
in Ireland, the pebbles at the bottom of the well were said to be
coloured as if stained with blood.

The well is mentioned all through the century, as shown by a
late eighteenth-century broadside sheet printed in Liverpool, narrating
the life of the saint and her struggle with 'the Heathen Prince, named
Cardoc'.[132] In the second column, it blends medical prescription
with the rhetoric of religious healing and salvation: 'it heals those
troubled with the Leprosy and many other Diseases, restores the
Lame to the Use of their Limbs, as well as Sight to the Blind; and
strengthens such as are recovered of the Small Pox'.[133] In the header
of the broadside, a picture of St Winifred shows her in a nun's habit,
with a trace on her neck and the well in the background, on top of
which stands the figure of Cardoc ominously raising his sword over
his head (Figure 4.4).

St Winifred became a symbol of popish idolatry for eager adepts
of Protestant theology such as the Welsh convert Myles Davies, a
former Roman Catholic priest converted to the Church of England,
and later controversial biographer, who dedicates his *Recantation*
to the Bishop of St Asaph 'in whose neighbourhood stands that
famous Popish Idol, call'd St *Winefred*'s Well, which must be own'd

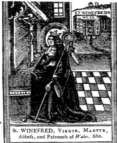

A Description of St. *Winefred's* at *Holy-Well* in *Flintfhire*, produces, every Minute, One Hundred Tons of Water; and many Distempers, and dinary Manner, all fuch Pox, or any other fevere

St. *Winefred's* North *Wales*; which Night and Day, One Hundred BATHING therein cures ftrengthens, in an extraordinary as have had the Small-Pox, or any other fevere Diforders.

LIVERPOOL: Printed by Wm.

St. WINEFRED, Virgin, Martyr, Abbefs, and Patronefs of *Wales*. 660.

Nevett, in *Caftle-ftreet*, 1784.

The firft Rife of St. *Winefred's* Well is by fome accounted a Miracle, and related as follows:

Figure 4.4 'A Description of St. Winefred's at Holy-Well in Flintshire', 1784

by all that has the least Tincture of Ecclesiastical History, to be one of the most groundless Fables that can be found amongst all those Myriades of impossible, for the most part; as well as improbable Popish Legends'.[134] He goes on to note that the hagiographers did not mention St Winifred's story, which makes it even more folkloric, as they 'pick and rake up all that they could hear of far and near, of all sorts and sizes', blaming the murky dealings of Roman Catholic propaganda at the bottom of the well.[135]

The success of St Winifred's Well occasioned several disputes, one of which is mentioned in a 1713 edition of Richard Steele's *The Guardian* in a letter penned by a character who was particularly sensitive to the subject of water, and whom we have met in every chapter of this book – Nestor Ironside:

> Last year a Papist (or to please Mr. Examiner, a Roman Catholic), published the life of St Wenefrede, for the use of those devout pilgrims who go in great numbers to offer up their prayers to her at her well. This gave occasion to the worthy prelate, in whose diocese that well is, to make some observations upon it; and in order to undeceive so many poor deluded people, to show how little reason, and how small authority there is, not only to believe any of the miracles attributed to St Wenefrede, but even to believe there ever was such a person in the world.[136]

The 'worthy prelate' is William Fleetwood, Bishop of Asaph, who published his comments on the life of St Winifred in 1713, in an attempt to reintegrate the use of the waters within Protestant culture. In his introduction, he clearly delineates two religious behaviours at odds with each other:

> The Papist come to St *Wenefrede*'s Well for Help, and so do the Protestants; the Papist expect some Help from *Wenefrede*, the Protestants none; if the Papist receive any Help, they impute it to the Merits and Intercession of St *Wenefrede*, and are thankful to God and her; if the Protestants find any Benefit there, they thank God, and mind not *Wenefrede*, but impute it to God's blessing and the cold Waters.[137]

As Bishop of Asaph, Fleetwood strategically integrates the Protestant sick with the pilgrims potentially healed by the waters, extending the powers of the waters beyond the community of Roman Catholics. Although he is distancing the Protestant faith from any direct intercession of the saint, he allows a certain degree of divine action through the waters, which are not entirely destitute of their holiness. This careful rhetoric – quite distinct from the earlier diatribes on popish credulity – is a trend within eighteenth-century Anglican thought. As Walsham explains, it negotiates with the permanence of folkloric practices, the prayer to saints and other ritualistic behaviours: 'With Bob Scribner, we may perhaps describe this as a species of Protestant "magic": not as a survival of "popish" (let alone pre-Christian) belief so much as an example of the pragmatism that made people willing to experiment with any technique that might help them cope with their adversities'.[138]

Such middle ground is found in the writings of the naturalist and traveller Thomas Pennant, who was born and raised in Flintshire, near Holywell, and who describes his native region in *The History of the Parishes of Whiteford, and Holywell*. Of Saint Winifred's Well he writes: 'There are two different opinions about the origin of this stream. One party makes it miraculous. The other asserts it to be owing only to natural causes' without determining who should have the final word.[139] As for the cures performed at the well, he follows Fleetwood's account of non-discriminatory waters: 'This saint is equally propitious to Protestant and Catholics; for among the offerings are to be found these grateful testimonies from the patients of each religion'.[140] The testimonies are described by another traveller, Henry Penruddocke Wyndham, who was Pennant's contemporary and wrote a *Gentleman's Tour through Monmouthshire and Wales*. Wyndham remarks 'the numerous trophies of hand-barrows, crutches, &c. which adorn the roof; and which have been left at different times by pious patients, whose faith contributed undoubtedly not a little, towards making them whole'.[141] These crutches, left as ex-votos around the well, and sometimes in the trees leading to the area, were the material traces of the belief of sick people who probably had little access to print culture. I would like to investigate further into the material history of these crutches, which could be read, perhaps, as signs of hope, or as the significant token of an individual pilgrimage, as most crutches were engraved with the name of their owner.[142]

Just as Protestant strategies of integration tried to process miracle cures in their belief system, medical discourse was not always constructed on the radical denial of miracle cures. Holy wells could thus be the object of intellectual compromise. In 1748, Diederick Wessel Linden, the Westphalian doctor who compared the chalybeate waters of Britain and Europe, gave an account of the legend of St Winifred which resembles the religious broadside in every point, without inserting any commentary on Catholic superstition. He then goes on to describe the moss that grows around the wells:

> On the Sides of the Wood, and stones of the Bason, there grows green Moss, which has a grateful fragrant Smell, and is vulgarly called St *Winifred's Hair*, which makes likewise Part of the above traditional Miracle. This moss is frequently applied to the ulcerated Wounds, with signal Success, in the Way of contracting, cohering, and healing them. Which inherent sanative faculty cannot be better accounted for than this Moss drawing or collecting from the Water a more than ordinary Portion of the *Spiritus Rector*, by some called, *Spiritus Mundi*, or *Spiritus universalis*, by which is to be understood that vegetating Power imbibed by the Air, which maintains and furnishes the Principles of Growth and Life to the whole Vegetable and Animal Kingdoms.[143]

Linden's account of the effect of the moss gives a spiritual dimension to the material transformations of the water, which seem to retain traces of alchemical reasoning in search of a universal principle in all elements. Considering Linden's interest in chemistry, and his thorough knowledge of German medicine, the notion of a 'spiritus rector' comes from the early eighteenth-century vitalist ideas that sought to reassert the existence of a universal organising principle at work in living organisms. And yet, this 'spiritus' is here being transferred from the elements to the living moss. Within the controversial religious context of St Winifred, the Latin term itself easily blends a Christian rhetoric on miracles, apt to reconcile Protestants and Catholics on a common agreement over the healing virtues of the well.[144] St Winifred's Well and its waters have survived to this day, which is quite rare for British healing waters. It was touted 'the Lourdes of Wales' in the twentieth century, which surely denotes the profound attachment to Roman Catholic miracles, yet fails to acknowledge the long-standing medieval persistence of Catholic beliefs in Protestant grounds as well as the mediation of such beliefs in religion, science and touristic discourse since the Reformation.

Spa towns were woven into the political construction of the nation, most specifically in the imaginary construction of politics. As a self-contained space, they were often seen as a blank page on which political utopias and dystopias could be projected. The reaction of a whole social system to new rules could be observed, and spa towns could be seen as a sample of the whole nation. Yet, spas also occupied another function with the political dynamics of the nation beyond that of an observatory. Like harbours or metropolises, yet smaller and perhaps less frightening, they were a point of contact between Britain and the continent, Britain and its colonies, and, at national level, between town and country. As such, they were an important meeting point for cultural interaction that was not strictly related to business, like London, Liverpool or Dover, yet remained an area of possible political encounters. For some, they became a rallying point – albeit more imaginary than real – for dissenting or unwelcome opinions. The persistence of Roman Catholic traditions and pagan beliefs attached to healing waters was emblematic of the political charge of spas, as an object of anxiety or praise or a starting point for more integrating strategies in contemporary literature.

Notes

1 Richard Brinsley Sheridan, *A Trip to Scarborough: A Comedy* (Dublin: R. Marchbank, 1781), p. 19.
2 P. Meyer Spacks, *Gossip* (New York: Knopf, 1985), p. 9.
3 See chapter 1, p. 47.
4 Austen, *Persuasion*, p. 126.

5 Baker, *Tunbridge-Walks*, p. 20.
6 Baker, *Tunbridge-Walks*, p. 20.
7 'On the Elegant Entertainement and Mix'd Company at the Ordinaries', in *The Scarborough Miscellany*, 1733, p. 32.
8 *The Scarborough Miscellany*, 1733, p. 32.
9 The poem insists on social mixing: 'Without rude Distinction all Huddle together / Young, old, handsome, ugly, there's no chusing whether', *The Scarborough Miscellany*, 1733, p. 32.
10 Several studies on the history of toasting have shown the ambivalence of the practice, traditionally built on consensus yet was sometimes seen as an opportunity to assert dissenting political opinions, as Ian Newman explains. Newman, 'The anti-social convivialist: toasting and resistance to sociability', in V. Capdeville and A. Kerhervé (eds), *British Sociability in the Long Eighteenth Century* (Woodbridge: The Boydell Press, 2019), pp. 219–36. On drinking and conviviality, see M. Hailwood, *Alehouses and Good Fellowship in Early Modern England* (Woodbridge: The Boydell Press, 2014).
11 *The Guardian*, 174, p. 500.
12 *The Guardian*, 174, p. 500.
13 *The Guardian*, 174, p. 501.
14 Baker, *Tunbridge-Walks*, p. 15.
15 Baker, *Tunbridge-Walks*, p. 15.
16 Baker, *Tunbridge-Walks*, p. 14.
17 Johnson, 'Spas and seaside resorts in Kent', p. 124.
18 Johnson, 'Spas and seaside resorts in Kent', p. 124; *The Tunbridge Wells Guide* (Tunbridge Wells: J. Sprange, 1780), pp. 286–7.
19 'On B— C—', in *Tunbrigialia, or the Tunbrige Miscellany for the year 1722* (London: A. Moore, 1722), p. 5.
20 'On B— C—', p. 5.
21 M. Ellis, 'The tea-table, women and gossip in early eighteenth-century Britain', in Capdeville and Kerhervé (eds), *British Sociability*, p. 72.
22 Ellis, 'The tea-table, women and gossip', p. 82.
23 On *Pamelianas*, see P. Sabor and T. Keymer (eds), *The Pamela Controversy: Criticisms and Adaptations of Samuel Richardson's Pamela, 1740–1750* (London: Pickering & Chatto, 2001).
24 From 'A piratical adaptation of Richardson's original, author unknown', *The Life of Pamela* (London: C. Whitefield, 1741), p. 390.
25 'On B— C—', p. 5.
26 Goldsmith, *The life of Richard Nash*.
27 Goldsmith, *The life of Richard Nash*, p. 99.
28 Goldsmith, *The life of Richard Nash*, p. 97.

29　Goldsmith, *The life of Richard Nash*, p. 33. This rule is also mentioned by Glover in 'Polite society and the rural resort', p. 72, and the rules are historicised and analysed by John Eglin in his biography of Richard Nash (Eglin, *The Imaginary Autocrat*, pp. 63–4).

30　'But it is too likely, that we mention those, we wish to depress them, in order to render ourselves more conspicuous; scandal must therefore have fixed her throne at Bath preferable to any other part of the kingdom'. Goldsmith, *The life of Richard Nash*, p. 99–100.

31　Eglin, *The Imaginary Autocrat*, p. 19.

32　Goldsmith, *The life of Richard Nash*, p. 19.

33　Goldsmith, *The life of Richard Nash*, p. 98.

34　'It must be acknowledged, that he always took pains to prevent the ruin of the youth of both sexes, and had so guarded against duelling, that he would not permit a sword to be worn in Bath.' Goldsmith, *The life of Richard Nash*, p. 230.

35　The British Museum website specifies that Dickinson was suffering from 'Acromegaly, "a disease characterized by hypertrophy and enlargement of the extremities"' (OED); yet this term was not available to Dickinson nor his contemporaries, and this retrospective diagnosis does not inform twenty-first- century readers of the ways in which this chronic disease and disability might have been understood and lived.

36　On Scarron see A. Gimaret, 'Scarron aux eaux de Bourbon: le burlesque comme thérapeutique', *Littérature et voyages de santé* (Paris: Classiques Garnier, 2017), pp. 221–42.

37　'Richard Dickinson Governor of Scarborough Spaw', 1725.

38　'Richard Dickinson Governor of Scarborough Spaw', 1725.

39　'Richard Dickinson Governor of Scarborough Spaw', 1725.

40　Smollett, *Humphry Clinker*, p. 62.

41　According to Phyllis Hembry, Derrick was also called 'insignificant puppy' (Hembry, *The English Spa*, p. 138), a nickname at which the scene may be hinting.

42　Smollett, *Humphry Clinker*, p. 62.

43　'On the Elegant Entertainement and Mix'd Company at the Ordinaries', p. 32.

44　Mavor, *The Cheltenham guide*, p. 28.

45　Moreau was from Bath, where he had applied for the same post in 1777 but failed to secure it. See Hembry, *The English Spa*, p. 139 on his application to Bath, and p. 188 on his supervision of the assembly rooms at Cheltenham.

46　P. de Marivaux, *La dispute: comédie en prose en 1 acte* (Paris: N.-B. Duchesne, 1758).

47 H. Greig, *The Beau Monde: Fashionable Society in Georgian London* (Oxford: Oxford University Press, 2013), pp. 1–31.

48 H. Greig, 'Uses and meanings of "Beau Monde": a supplementary essay', in Greig, *The Beau Monde*, pp. 257–8.

49 'A view of the Long Room, by Mr. C.', in *The Scarborough Miscellany*, 1734, p. 8.

50 P. Carter, 'Arnall, William [pseud. Francis Walsingham] (d. 1736), political writer', *Oxford Dictionary of National Biography*.

51 Cooley, '"Sexy in a 'Tunbridge Wells' sort of way"', p. 96. Cooley quotes from C. H. Strange, 'The history of Tunbridge Wells', in J. C. M. Given (ed.), *Royal Tunbridge Wells: Past and Present* (Tunbridge Wells: Courier, 1946), pp. 36–71.

52 'This is a theme [short lived, transient populations] echoed in most historical accounts of early modern spas, Accounts that insist on the absence of any permanent population or native character, and present spas as receptacles for the character of the "company" that descended on them each season', Cooley, '"Sexy in a 'Tunbridge Wells' sort of way"', p. 96.

53 Burnby, *Summer Amusement*, pp. 64, 65.

54 J. Burnby, *An Address to the People of England; on the Increase of Their Poor Rates* (London: J. Dodsley, Pall-Mall, 1780).

55 He published a political satirical poem, *The Kentish Cricketers* (Canterbury: Richardson and Urquhart, 1773) as well as J. Burnby, *An Historical Description of the Metropolitical Church of Christ, Canterbury* (Canterbury: Simmons and Kirkby, 1772).

56 Hembry's table on the 'Initial promoters of minor provincial spas, 1660–1815' is organised in five categories: nobility, gentry, medical men, ministers and others. Hembry, *The English Spa*, pp. 361–4.

57 *The Morning Post*, 25 July 1788.

58 'Zounds! He will suck them dry'. Gwen Hart describes the water shortage in Cheltenham in the 1790s: G. Hart, *History of Cheltenham* (Gloucester: Sutton Publishing, 1981), pp. 136–7.

59 See chapter 2, 'Waters as pharmakon', pp. 83–92.

60 Mary of Modena was said to have had a child brought in a warming pan during an orchestrated false delivery, and that her child was not a legitimate heir. See for example J. Mctague, 'Anti-Catholicism, incorrigibility and credulity in the warming-pan scandal of 1688–9', *Journal for Eighteenth-Century Studies*, 36:3 (2013), 433–48.

61 I mention Mary of Modena's water treatment for infertility and the cross erected in the cross bath in another article: Vasset, 'Mineral waters as a treatment for women's barrenness'.

62 Eglin, *The Imaginary Autocrat*, p. 30.

63 Eglin, *The Imaginary Autocrat*, pp. 31–2; Hembry, *The English Spa*, pp. 174–5.

64 X. Le Person, 'Thermalisme et politique à la Renaissance: les stratagèmes en l'absence de temporisation nobiliaire', in Scheid et al. (eds), *Le thermalisme*, pp. 196–213.

65 Elizabeth Montagu, Letters III, 8 (To the Duchess of Portland, 27/?/1745), quoted in Kerhervé, 'Writing letters from Georgian spas', pp. 275–6.

66 L. Colley, *Britons: Forging the Nation, 1707–1837* (New Haven, CT: Yale University Press, 2005), p. 173.

67 Colley, *Britons*, p. 173.

68 The Invalid, *Modern Refinement: A Satire* (Bath: S. Hazard, 1777), p. 8.

69 The Invalid, *Modern Refinement*, p. 14.

70 J. West, *The Humours of Brighthelmstone* (London: Scatcherd and Whitaker, 1788), p. 6.

71 West, *The Humours of Brighthelmstone*, p. 6.

72 West, *The Humours of Brighthelmstone*, p. 11.

73 West, *The Humours of Brighthelmstone*, p. 9.

74 From Harrogate toffees to Pastilles Vichy, European spa towns are often associated with typical confectionaries, and more research needs to be done on the interface between confectionary and medicine.

75 Herbert, 'Gender and the spa', p. 373.

76 Hurley, 'A conversation of their own', p. 2.

77 Kelly, '"Drinking the waters"'.

78 Durie, 'Medicine, health and economic development' p. 198.

79 R. Sanders, *The Complete English Traveller: or, a new Survey and Description of England and Wales* (London: J. Cooke, 1771).

80 See T. Chambers, *Drinking the Waters: Creating an American Leisure Class at Nineteenth-Century Mineral Springs* (Washington, DC: Smithsonian Institution; Combined Academic, 2003); Scribner, '"The happy effects of these waters"'; Lewis, *Ladies and Gentlemen on Display*.

81 Chambers, *Drinking the Waters*, p. 4.

82 Scribner, '"The happy effects of these waters"', p. 427.

83 Short, *A General Treatise on Various Cold Mineral Waters in England*, p. 101.

84 B. Rush, *Experiments and Observations on the Mineral Waters of Philadelphia, Abington, and Bristol, in the Province of Pennsylvania* (Philadelphia: J. Humphreys, 1773).

85 B. Rush, *Directions for the Use of the Mineral Water and Cold Bath, at Harrogate, near Philadelphia* (Philadelphia: Melchior Steiner, 1786), p. 4.

86 Rush, *Directions for the Use of the Mineral Water*, p. 4.

87 Jennings, *Curing the Colonizers*.

88 Jennings, *Curing the Colonizers*, p. 13.

89 T. Dancer, *A Short Dissertation on the Jamaica Bath Waters* (Kingston: D. Douglass & A. Aikman, 1784), p. 48.

90 Linden, *A Treatise on the Origin, Nature and Virtues of Chalybeat Waters*, p. 166.

91 Linden, *A Treatise on the Origin, Nature and Virtues of Chalybeat Waters*, p. 166.

92 Linden, *A Treatise on the Origin, Nature and Virtues of Chalybeat Waters*, pp. 166–7.

93 I am not discussing here the nature of the work they might have been submitted to, only the management of sick servants.

94 'Holy wells of Britain', www.facebook.com/Holy-Wells-of-Britain-173020806222717/ (last consulted 7 July 2020).

95 In this festival, inhabitants were asked to find their local holy well thanks to historical digitised maps of Northern Ireland (https://festival.archaeologyuk.org/events/well-well-well-1593794172 (last consulted 10 March 2021)). I am grateful to Catherine Porter from the University of Limerick for pointing this out.

96 T. Guidott, *A true and exact account of Sadlers Well, or, The new mineral-waters lately found out at Islington* (London: T. Malthus, 1684), p. 2.

97 Guidott, *A true and exact account of Sadlers Well*, p. 2.

98 This advice was taken later to be a misunderstanding of the medicinal potential of waters, but I would argue that it makes sense in the context of this house on the outskirts of London – the type of water used for beer is essential.

99 Guidott, *A true and exact account of Sadlers Well*, p. 1.

100 Guidott, *A true and exact account of Sadlers Well*, p. 1.

101 Guidott, *A true and exact account of Sadlers Well*, p. 1.

102 *An Exclamation from Tunbridge and Epsom*, p. 2.

103 *An Exclamation from Tunbridge and Epsom*, p. 2.

104 Hembry, *The English Spa*, p. 170.

105 *The Gentleman's Magazine*, August 1751, p. 373.

106 Hembry explains that '*The General Evening Post* and *The Gloucester Journal* attacked the Glastonbury project and hinted at a popish plot'. Hembry, *The English Spa*, p. 170.

107 This letter was published again in the *Gentleman's Magazine*, August 1751.

108 'An Examination of the *Glastonbury* Waters', *The Gentleman's Magazine: and historical chronicle*, January 1736–December 1833;

September 1751; 21, p. 416. I am thankful to Will Slauter for pointing out this reference to me.

109 'The following, taken from the London Daily Advertiser, was wrote as an Answer to the above', *The Gentleman's Magazine: and historical chronicle*, January 1736–December 1833; September 1751; 21, p. 416.

110 J. Davies, *A Short Description of the Waters at Glastonbury* (Exon: Andrew Brice, 1751), cover page.

111 Davies, *A Short Description of the Waters at Glastonbury*, p. 24.

112 Walsham, "Reforming the waters," p. 450.

113 J. Richardson, *The Great Folly, Superstition, and Idolatry, of Pilgrimages in Ireland; Especially of that to St. Patrick's Purgatory* (Dublin: J. Hyde, 1727), pp. 84–5.

114 Richardson, *The Great Folly*, p. 85.

115 Richardson, *The Great Folly*, p. 132.

116 Richardson, *The Great Folly*, p. 132.

117 Richardson, *The Great Folly*, p. 65.

118 Richardson, *The Great Folly*, p. 65. The involuntary and yet unnamed 'smiley' is authentic.

119 Smollett, *An Essay on the External Use of Water*, p. 5.

120 Vasset, *Décrire, prescrire, guérir*, pp. 85–101.

121 Hamlin, 'Chemistry, medicine', p. 68.

122 Cottom, 'In the bowels of the novel', p. 159.

123 D. Oren-Magidor, *Infertility in Early Modern England* (Basingstoke: Palgrave Macmillan, 2017), p. 147.

124 Oren-Magidor, *Infertility in Early Modern England*, p. 147.

125 Walsham, "Reforming the waters," p. 454.

126 For more information on Elizabeth Walker as a practitioner of medicine, see K. P. Long, *Gender and Scientific Discourse in Early Modern Culture* (New York: Routledge, 2016), pp. 199–200; L. Whaley, *Women and the Practice of Medical Care in Early Modern Europe, 1400–1800* (Basingstoke: Palgrave Macmillan, 2011), pp. 138–9.

127 A. Walker, *Fax Fonte Accensa, Fire out of Water: or, an Endeavour to kindle Devotion, from the Consideration of the Fountains God hath made* (London: Ranew, 1684), p. 137.

128 Walker, *Fax Fonte Accensa*, p. 136.

129 Walsham, "Reforming the waters," p. 431.

130 Walsham, "Reforming the waters," p. 431.

131 Beuno was also a saint in the Roman Catholic Church, and was credited with several other resuscitations.

132 The propagandising text associated the spring with the resuscitation of the saint, 'That at the very Instant *Winifred* was restored to life this

Spring arose in that very place'. *A Description of St. Winefred's Well, at Holy-Well in Flintshire, North Wales* (Liverpool: Nevett, 1784).

133 *A Description of St. Winefred's Well.* The blind, the lame and the lepers stand among the topoï of the religious sick, all of them being the object of miracles in the gospel. The juxtaposition of the smallpox, a major contemporary epidemic, with religiously charged illnesses, creates a discourse in which religion and medicine are entangled.

134 M. Davies, *The recantation of Mr. Pollet, a Roman priest* (London [?], 1705).

135 Davies, *The recantation of Mr. Pollet.*

136 *The Guardian* 90 (24 June 1713), p. 36.

137 W. Fleetwood, *The Life and Miracles of St. Wenefrede* (London: Buckley, 1713), p. 12.

138 Walsham, "Reforming the waters," p. 462.

139 T. Pennant, *A Tour in Wales* (Dublin: Sleater, 1779), p. 32.

140 Pennant, *A Tour in Wales*, p. 32.

141 H. P. Wyndham, *A Gentleman's Tour through Monmouthshire and Wales, in the Months of June and July* (London: printed for T. Evans, 1794), p. 167.

142 Twenty-first-century visitors to St Winifred's Well will see crutches on display, with dates and names inscribed on them. Some of them are specifically shaped in the form of ancient crutches to be left at the well.

143 Linden, *A Treatise on the Origin, Nature and Virtues of Chalybeat Waters*, p. 127.

144 Further research needs to be undertaken on St Winifred's, including Linden's ambivalence on the well. Linden was based in Llandrindod for a while, and came from Westphalia, which was a Roman Catholic German province. See R. C. B. Oliver, 'Diederick Wessel Linden, M.D.', *National Library of Wales Journal*, 18 (1974), 241–67.

5

Pumping and pouring: watering places and the money business

From Restoration to Regency, around a hundred and thirty new spas were found and built on, albeit frugally, still creating many economic opportunities for local investors. Publications were booming: more than three hundred independent treatises were published on various waters.[1] As Phyllis Hembry explains,

> the success of the Tudor and Stuart spas, several attracting a steady local trade and some outsiders, also led to an upsurge of resort activity; the few of ephemeral existence, like Wellingborough, being exceptions. A vogue for spa-going encouraged speculators to invest into converting a local spring of mineral water into a spa.[2]

Although the phenomenon of spas, as I argued in the first two chapters of this book, cannot be reduced to the commercialisation of leisure and the new craze for touristic consumption, it cannot be denied that the phenomenon expanded throughout the eighteenth century, and that it represented an influx of money to local people, and to new investors who sometimes came from neighbouring cities deliberately to invest in the spa, spurring credit, patronage and advertising to increase their profits. In this closing chapter, and to follow up on the thread of the book, I would like to investigate the contemporary narratives on the murky dealings of spa town money.

Investment, speculation and corruption were part of the picture of the financial business of spas which contemporaries perceived as risky. They potentially constituted a substantial profit but could also result in a dramatically speedy loss – and in that way resembled the gambling craze that accompanied the development of spa towns. Gambling is a good place to start this investigation. Before casinos existed in the spas of continental Europe, gaming practices evolved somewhat organically, and spa towns of all sizes were key to their development.[3] Following up on the eighteenth-century association between speculation, risky investment and gambling, I wish to map out the contemporary imaginary of financial risk-taking in spa towns. Such versatile money culture attracted a variety of sharpers and fortune-hunters. Contemporary narratives insisted on the necessity to recognise the signs of a predator, and to identify sharpers and fortune-hunters in spa towns within a hotchpotch of unknown visitors of undetermined social rank. One of the challenges for spa corporations was to usher the visitors from various social classes into the same space. It was thought that the poor, who would 'come flocking' to take the waters for their health, would have to be kept apart from the *bon ton*, who happened to come for the same reason, so that the reputation of the spa would be maintained. I will explore, at the end of this chapter, the ways in which the juxtaposition of the two was dealt with and represented in contemporary literature.

High stakes

In the creative 1732 issue of *The Scarborough Miscellany*, a familiar reference at this stage, a mock-heroic poem entitled 'The Battle of the Sugar Plums' charts the deeds of an elegant tea party splitting in two over matters of precedence and protocol. The initial tensions quickly spiral into a revolting food battle such as those much later encountered in twentieth-century Christmas pantos. The guests throw sugar plums at each other, while 'custards, tarts and cheesecake speak their rage'.[4] The 'bloodless field' is left in disarray, with various streams of 'jellies, claret, sillabubs and creams', but the poet turns to the new battlefield with more conflict unfolding around the gaming tables:

> One Chance in twenty-four is fairly shown,
> And each believes that Chance will be her own.
> At *Pharo*, or at *Hazzard*, who can view,
> Without a Smile, the strange promiscuous crew,
> Where rakes and bullies mingle with the Fair,
> The fleecing Sharper and the unfleg'd Heir.
> Lords, – who, if Honour's question'd, draw their Swords,
> Yet scorn – to pay their Debts, or keep their Words.

Dull, solemn Coxcombs, Fops, and *Irish* Beaux,
Whose whole Estate is Impudence and Cloaths,
All in the Circle mix, Distinction's lost,
'Twixt Knight o'th' Garter here, and Knight o'th' Post.[5]

The burlesque and playful description of food-fighting is abandoned
for a darker satirical tone once gambling enters the picture, with
gloomier prospects and higher stakes for the gamblers. As the gaze
of the poet sweeps over the tables, all the elements commonly
associated with gambling are evoked. White geese are trying their
luck over-confidently while sharpers of all sorts exploit their gullibility
and empty their purse. The higher ranks (knights of the garter) and
the gentry (solemn coxcombs) are betting amounts they do not have,
and threatening their adversaries with duelling. All the protocol and
respect due to higher social ranks ('Distinction') is forgotten in the
excitement of loss and gain. As Donna T. Andrew reminds us,
gambling was often depicted as an 'aristocratic vice' that could lead
to suicide or duelling – two other such vices in the public opinion
of contemporaries.[6]

The type of gaming performed in the public rooms of spa towns
was much more like the 'gaming of the great' inherited from courtly
entertainment than the street gambling of cups and dice or three-
card-monte found in markets.[7] Eighteenth-century writers usually
traced it back to the French courtly practices which influenced the
English court-in-exile. As the king came back to England, the courtiers
were thought to have imported a whole new set of games, as Oliver
Goldsmith explains in *The life of Richard Nash*:

> A spirit of gaming had been introduced in the licentious age of *Charles*
> II, and had by this time thriven surprisingly. Yet all its devastations
> were confined to *London* alone; To this great mart of every folly,
> sharpers from every country daily arrived, for the winter, but were
> obliged to leave the kingdom at the approach of summer, in order to
> open a new campaign at *Aix*, Spaw, or the *Hague. Bath, Tunbridge,
> Scarborough,* and other places of the same kind here, were then
> frequented only by such as really went for relief.[8]

Goldsmith goes on to show how the court accompanying the royal
visits of Queen Anne spread the new games to the whole resort.
Gambling, to him, was of aristocratic descent.

In 'The Battle of the Sugar Plums', the poet mentions 'Pharo and
Hazzard'. Hazard (or hazzard) was a betting dice game, while faro

(pharao or pharo) was a popular card game that spread throughout Europe – and especially France – from the end of the seventeenth century.[9] Faro and hazard relied entirely upon chance, unlike other card games requiring strategic skills from the players to win their bets, such as whist and quadrille, both four-player games, and ombre, a three-player game. Gaming houses developed all over Europe, under the name Ridotto or Redoute, Maison de Jeux, Vauxhalls and, later in the eighteenth century, casinos, all submitted to changing regulations in the seventeenth and eighteenth centuries. In Britain, two laws were passed in 1739 and 1745 banning public gaming houses managed by professional staff who were in control of the 'banks'. As Donna T. Andrew explains, 'the desire to control or eliminate such places had something to do both with the desire to establish order and control crime, with the wish to protect property in "Mannours, Lands, and Lordships" from being squandered away'.[10] The laws, however, were not very effective in preventing public gambling, and Henry Fielding as magistrate 'was regularly breaking up similar gaming establishments, and attempting, largely unsuccessfully, to fine the proprietors, and more successfully, to destroy their gaming tables'.[11]

Spa satire was a fertile context for medical and bodily metaphors about gambling. It might have been encouraged by the common medical idea that 'recreations' were welcome to entertain the sick and help keep their minds away from their own condition. Of course, they were first and foremost thought of as forms of physical exercise, as the author of a treatise on the waters of the Irish spa town of Ballyspellan, county Kilkenny, explains: 'Bowling, Shooting with Bows and Arrows, or the moderate pursuits of Game proper to the Season, whereby the Lazy motions of the Blood, and other Juices are gently push'd forward by the Compression, the active Muscles give certainly advantageous Exercises', he writes, adding that: 'in Stormy and wet Weather, the Shuttle-Cock, and the Billiard-Table, or in the want of that the Shuffle-Board, will very well answer the Defects of external Recreations'.[12] In the letter on watering places published in *The Guardian* in 1713, Richard Steele sarcastically brings together sporting games and gambling under the pen of Nestor Ironside, also calling it an exercise: 'In such a Place as the *Bath* I might urge, that the Casting of a Dice is indeed the properest Exercise for a faire Creature to assist the Waters; not to mention the Opportunity it gives to display the well-turned Arm, and to scatter to

Advantage the Rays of the Diamond'.[13] In all its ironical pique, Steele does touch upon one of the possible explanations for the surge of gaming in spa towns: other than boredom, the debilitated bodies of the sick were often unable to enjoy any other kind of entertainment, as dancing must have been excluded for many people suffering from rheumatic diseases.

In contemporary literature, the gaming tables had all the characteristics of vice, as Donna T. Andrew argues, including the powerful irresistibility and attraction they exerted on inveterate gamblers. Several poems express the internal struggle with the gambling passion that twenty-first-century readers would be tempted to call 'addiction', and might have been linked to consumption of 'intoxicants' served in the gaming rooms – alcohol, tobacco, tea and coffee. In the 1735 *Bath, Bristol, Tunbridge and Epsom Miscellanies*, for example, two short poems, 'The Interrogatories' and 'The Resolution', are juxtaposed, the first sounding much like the moral catechistic tone of early medical preventative discourse:

> The interrogatories
>
> Tell me Andrea, Goddess kind,
> the worst of passions in mankind,
> And shew me, Justice, if you can,
> The worst of characters in man?
> The Goddess answers 'Lose or win
> Gambling produces every sin
> With rapid strides from bad to worse
> It soon completes the gamester's curse'.[14]

This awkward poetic form – an octave – hinges around the opposing outcomes of gambling. 'Lose or win' both amplifies the desire to invest more money into another round and the deception brought about by escalating problems. Gambling, therefore, only brings on more gambling, with a new wave of problems amplifying each loss. The second poem printed on the same page, 'The Resolution', takes a strategical counterpoint to the attractiveness of gaming:

> Farewell Quadrille, thou sweet deluding game
> Parents of slander, female sex's shame!
> Music in future shall my sense drown
> And cushion dances moonlight evening crown,

> I'll figure in and out with any Lass,
> Tho' men of figure set me down an Ass.[15]

As the author heavily suggests, 'figuring in and out' here means more than dancing. He whimsically elaborates a hierarchy of pleasure where for other 'men of figure', gaming – in this case, strategical gaming like quadrille, which was of a higher standard than faro or hazard – is better than sex. Asses and aces, however, bring about different kinds of trouble. In both poems, no matter how ironical and light, the powerful attraction of gambling is shown to compete with other passions, and to pervade the atmosphere of evening parties with a different kind of murk than the waters visitors bathed in during the day, one boiling with greed, cheating and excitement.

In his biography of Beau Nash, John Eglin also spins the medical metaphor, comparing the cultural anxiety over gambling to the fear of epidemics:

> The increasingly central place of gaming at Bath and other resorts was a key element of their success, but was also more and more a liability over time as gaming came to be viewed as that social pathology of affluent society that gin was for the lower class. Bath's close identifications with gaming was enough liability to necessitate a fundamental redirection in the development of the resort. Like the Hindu deity Shiva, gaming was creator and destroyer, the engine of cataclysmic change felt beyond the circle of resorts. The spas, especially Bath, became the forcing grounds of crucial social reconfigurations.[16]

Through Nash, Eglin talks of Bath and Tunbridge Wells. In this book, as I argued earlier, Bath is considered as a model and counter-model, and the prevalence of gambling in Bath, as well as its management, was clearly a point of reference for other resorts. The ambivalence of its master of ceremonies, Beau Nash, played a key role in the persistence of gaming in Bath in spite of a rising concern for its impact on public opinion and lawmakers. Beau Nash, as we know, was never officially appointed as master of ceremonies, and his biographers all seem to agree in stating that his income came mostly from gambling and from reaping part of Bath's gambling profits. *The Life of Richard Nash*, by Oliver Goldsmith, is largely dedicated to gambling, and gives an informative perspective on late eighteenth-century attitudes towards early eighteenth-century 'gaming', as Goldsmith calls it. He abruptly interrupts his narrative of Nash's eccentricities to address the reader directly: 'But I hear the reader now demand, what finances were to support all this finery, or where the treasures, that gave him such frequent opportunities of displaying his benevolence, or his vanity?'[17] The question leads him to a darker part of the character of Beau Nash: 'by gaming alone at that period, of which I speak, he kept up so very genteel an appearance. When he first figured at *Bath*, there were few laws against this destructive amusement. The gaming-table was a constant resource of despair and indigence, and the frequent ruin of opulent fortunes.'[18] Goldsmith writes in 1762, as gaming is still authorised on the continent, and many English people go to Spa in Belgium to enjoy gambling at the English Club there.

There were 'honest' ways to acquire a steady profit from the gambling tables, such as keeping the bank at faro, or striking deals with addicted gamblers to prevent their ruin. According to Goldsmith, Nash, who was adamant to protect gullible players from sharpers and frauds, regularly intervened when he saw they were in danger. Notwithstanding this vigilance, he never banned sharpers from the room. After all public gaming was banned by the law of 1745, however, the fortune of Beau Nash was undone: 'by this means the public became acquainted with what he had long endeavoured to conceal. They now found that he was himself concerned in the gaming-tables, of which he only seemed the conductor, and that he had shared part of the spoil, though he complained of having been defrauded a just share.'[19] That the most renowned master of ceremonies could be a fraud, in spite of all his regulation of manners and attacks on sharpers, and generally exquisite politeness, was an object of fascination for Goldsmith, similar to that exerted on Defoe and Fielding by the figure of Jonathan Wild and his criminal dealings while he held the position of 'Thief-taker general'.[20] Such characters epitomise the ways in which criminals can infiltrate the very institutions that fight them. The ambivalence of Beau Nash was never as clear and criminal as Wild's, but he nonetheless pretended to regulate the gambling assemblies when he was, in fact, profiting from opaque dealings with the bankers.[21]

The murky waters of gambling were also rife with suicidal threats. Contemporary writings argue that combating gambling was a matter of public health for the nation. Beyond the preservation of the interests of the landed aristocracy, the number of gambling-related suicides raised major concerns. Some heartbreaking stories made the news and circulated in various literary genres. Goldsmith's *Life of Richard Nash* included several such narratives, probably meant to warn readers while satisfying their thirst for narrative tension, in line with the novel-writing strategies of the century. Goldsmith used the effective novelistic trope of inserting a letter within the book at the end of the narrative. He added a sense of Nash's agency in the public discussions over gaming in the title of the letter 'from Mr. *** in Tunbridge, to Lord — in London' that would add yet another gambling story to those already accumulated in the biography as it was 'found among the Papers of Mr. Nash, and prepared by him for the press'.[22] This letter opens on the sad news of yet another suicide at Tunbridge Wells:

> What I foresaw has arrived, poor *Jenners*, after losing all his fortune, has shot himself through the head. His losses to *Bland* were considerable, and his playing soon after with *Spedding* contributed to hasten his ruin. No man was ever more enamour'd of play, or understood it less. At whatever game he ventured his money, he was most usually the dupe, and still foolishly attributed to his bad luck, those misfortunes that entirely proceeded from his want of judgement.[23]

A long, convincing discourse on the fatality of loss at gambling follows. It relies on the initial cautionary tale of Jenners's death to warn against sharpers who mix within the polite society of watering places, enjoining the readers to identify them: 'The great error lies in imagining every fellow with a laced coat to be a gentleman. The address and transient behaviour of a man of breeding are easily acquired, and none are better qualified than gamesters in this respect',[24] the author of the letter writes, implying that the lower classes can imitate their betters through dress and deportment. Mastering education, however, requires skills that are not as easily available to sharpers:

> At first, their complaisance, civility, and apparent honour is pleasing, but upon examination, few of them will be found to have their minds sufficiently stored with any of the more refined accomplishments, which truly characterise the man of breeding. This will commonly serve as criterion to distinguish them, tho' there are other marks which every young gentleman of fortune should be apprized of.[25]

Conversation acts as a test of gentlemanly culture and is presented here as a probing tool for the honesty of your gaming partner, a test that sharpers will most certainly fail.

Another strategy to protect gullible gamblers is actually to strike a deal with sharpers. The letter continues with another cautionary tale from Tunbridge Wells. It relates the parallel downfall of a young gentleman of fortune, J. Hedges, with the prudent management of his wife in the background. 'He knew nothing of gaming, for he seemed to have the least passion for play', yet he was 'unacquainted with his own heart', and got involved at the gaming tables, 'he was soon surrounded with sharpers, who with calmness lay in ambush for his fortune, and coolly took advantage of his passions'.[26] The calmness of sharpers echoes their genteel demeanour, denoting the premeditation of their crime, as well as the mastery of sleight of hand such as 'palming', 'cupping', or 'ace up the sleeve'.[27] As commonly reported in the news, a gambler's ruin was his family's ruin. Hedges's wife, perceiving 'the ruin of her family approaching', warns his brother. She understands that reasoning her husband out of his passion will be in vain: 'she was determined therefore to let him pursue fortune, but previously take measures, to prevent the pursuits being fatal'.[28] By admitting that reasoning and moralising are excluded, Mrs Hedges ascribes a pathological feature to gambling. Passions ranked, after all, among the 'non-naturals' in preventative medical treatises of the time. They were understood as constitutive elements of preventative health which required long-term education and bodily regulation. In the meantime, Hedges marched to his own downfall: 'he lost his estate, his equipage, his wife's jewels, and every other moveable that could be parted with, except a repeating watch'.[29] A scene follows, making the violence of ruin tangible to the reader:

> *Hedges* was at last furious with the continuance of ill success, and pulling out his watch, asked if any person in the company, would set him sixty guineas upon it: the company were silent; he then demanded a fifty; still no answer; he sunk to forty, thirty, twenty; finding the company still without answer, he cried out by G—d it shall never go for less, and dashed it against the floor, at the same time, attempting to dash out his brains against the marble chimney-piece.[30]

The reverse bid that Hedges launches in front of an embarrassed crowd of players echoes the gradual shrinking of his own fortune symbolised by the final destruction of his watch as the countdown to misery is now over. The company takes over and brings him back home to his wife. She shares with him the 'good' news of the death of her uncle, who had bestowed his fortune upon her husband. He answers by confessing his own ruin in the pathetic tone of sentimental tragedies.[31] As he takes 'frantic steps across the room', and after his wife – pricelessly – 'had a little enjoyed his perplexity', letting the excruciating lesson sink in just long enough, she launches into a passionate outburst of affection, and renewed fortune:

> No my dear, cried she, you have lost by a trifle, and you owe nothing, our brother and I have taken care to prevent the effects of your rashness, and are actually the persons, who have won your fortune; we employed proper persons for this purpose, who brought their winnings to me; your money, your equipage, are in my possession, and here I return them to you, from whom they were unjustly taken, I only ask permission to keep my jewels, and to keep you, my greatest jewel, from such dangers in the future.[32]

By owning her husband's fortune, she finally owns control of him through the clever management of the very deceptive qualities of sharpers. As she returns his money in a redemptive sentimental gesture, she also objectifies him with tender masculine name-calling ('my jewel').

This anecdote is at odds with many contemporary representations of gambling women, which focused rather on women's propensity to lose control. Women were generally believed more liable than men to become prey to sharpers, and extremely vulnerable to the fatal consequences of financial ruin.[33] Fanny Braddock's tragic suicide in 1731 certainly made the news and epitomised the fragility of gambling women. She was found dead in her room at John Wood's at Bath, having committed suicide after she considered herself stuck in a deadlock of accumulated gambling debt. Her story 'was several times repeated through the century, both in Britain and abroad', Andrew writes, and it was quite representative of 'the fear and concern that the female gambler seemed to evoke'.[34] Andrew examines the coverage of Braddock's death, and the moralising comments on self-murder. She compares it with the coverage of male suicides for the same reason, concluding that 'female gaming seems disproportionately represented in literature and non-fictional texts, suggesting that it was the focus for powerful social anxieties'.[35] Braddock's

fortune was undone in Bath, which must have confirmed the association her contemporaries made between gambling and watering places.
The 'Battle of the Sugar Plums', for example, which describes the
gambling rooms of Scarborough, mentions the name of Braddock
as a warning against the fate awaiting women playing quadrille:

> See wrangling at *Quadrille*, the anxious Fair:
> What ardent Hope to see the *Spadille* appear?
> Propitious Card! On *thee* the Fair depends:
> For *thee*, neglects her Family and Friends:
> For *thee*, she breaks thro' Nature's strictest Ties;
> For *thee*, she quits Love's softest tender Joys:
> Her Peace she forfeits, and her Rest destroys.
> For *thee*, the fatal Knot poor B–DD–K tied,
> For *thee*, the baneful Drug sad L—RE try'd:
> How dear has Love of *thee*, the Fair-ones cost?
> What Beauty spoil'd, – what Reputation lost![36]

The other name hidden in the poem is Lady Lechmere, the wife
of a prominent Whig politician. She was known to have lost
'furious sums' at Bath,[37] according to her contemporary Lady
Mary Wortley Montagu.[38] Montagu even wrote in 1725 that 'the
melancholy catastrophe of poor Lady Lechmere, is too extraordinary
not to attract the attention of everybody. Having played away her
reputation and fortune, she poisoned herself. This is the effect of
prudence!'[39] As the poem specifies the poisoning was not fatal, but
her 'reputation' was damaged by her suicide attempt. The insistent
anaphora (for *thee*) gives a mock-lyrical tone to the complaint of the
poet, who sexualises quadrille and makes it an object of passionate
love, driving women out of their prudence and quiet, into desperate
suicidal acts.

Tangible links were acknowledged between public gambling and
capital management, as well as metaphorical connections between
gambling and contemporary economical models of investment and
speculation.[40] To John Eglin, games that relied entirely upon chance
were emblematic of early capitalism. He claims that critics reserved
'genuine opprobrium for hazard, basset, faro and other such games
played against a "bank" (the terminology cannot have been acci-
dental), games which powerfully symbolised the most pernicious
aspects of commercial culture'.[41] In the specific context of spas,
which multiplied in the eighteenth century throughout Britain and

attracted new local or external investors hoping to transform villages into profitable resorts, gambling was all the more significant as it brought more money to the newly-built spa towns and attracted more visitors than just the sick. Goldsmith ironically pointed out the magnetic power of gambling prospects:

> To a person, who does not calmly trace things to their source, nothing will appear more strange, than how the healthy could ever consent to follow the sick to those places of spleen and live with those, whose disorders are ever apt to excite a gloom in the spectator. The truth is, the gaming table is probably the salutary font, to which such numbers flocked.[42]

As I argued in my first chapter, the culture of pleasurable pastimes should not make us forget that spas were primarily health resorts.[43]

Nonetheless, as Goldsmith underlines, a sick person would not travel alone: friends and family came along, hoping for some diversion to pass the time, and to form new acquaintances. Roy Porter, whose view of the eighteenth century was much focused on the development of commerce, argued that 'city fathers and individual estate-developers were quick to capitalize upon the opportunities for the creation of a speculative hedonic culture surrounding the spa'.[44] Spas were investment magnets.

Urban speculations

Investing in a spa – in the bathing facilities, in the pump room, in the assembly rooms, in the theatre, and in the urban planning it entailed – was a risky business. The stakes were high, with investors who often expected stupendous returns based primarily on the reputation of the spa town which, in turn, depended on fickle fashion. According to Peter Borsay,

> Watering-places encouraged change and innovation, particularly in the fields of services and property development. They also tended to attract those with surplus capital and who were willing to take a risk, from theatre managers to bankers, since the scope for investment, and the *potential* returns, were high. All this ensured that resorts nurtured an economy, and an economic culture, that was opportunistic and entrepreneurial.[45]

Some visitors were aware of the potential high profits made by the owners of the spa and of the facility rooms. For example, in *The Register of Folly: or, Characters and Incidents at Bath and the Hot-Wells* published in 1773, the author, calling himself 'An Invalid', complains of his want of money on his arrival at the Hotwells and contrasts the generosity of the Bristol waters to the stinginess of their owners:

> How diff'rent it's virtues to WOODALL AND CO.!*
> Each season it causes fresh spirits to flow
> And their pockets replenish, tho' ever so low;
> To them it most truly gives strength to the nerves,
> And the name of *specific* most richly deserves;
> For each idle bibbler is now such a ninny,
> Tho' *pennyless* left, they at least give a guinea,
> And the nymph of the fountain gold quarter-piece,
> While their tradesmen they bilk, and their bosom-friends fleece:
> For debts of *true honour*, and those, *must* be paid,
> But *just* ones: – quite gothic! – mere vulgar-bred trade.[46]

* The Proprietors of the Pump

The company owning the Hotwells is criticised for charging for a good which Nature supplies for free. For 'the 'Invalid', spending money for waters literally means throwing money out (into the fountain) which, like gambling, is a mere act of spending with no return.[47] That easy money and a steady cash flow resulted from the exploitation of natural resources certainly contributed to entertain the idea that spas were highly profitable. In addition, they seemed to put visitors in a spending mood, and the permanence of sickness was a sure guarantee of future incoming patients.

Similar ideas spread in medical treatises. In the middle of the eighteenth century, Charles Lucas, a physician and a Protestant Irish politician who had just fled from Dublin into England, published *An Essay on Waters*. The essay, as I stated earlier, started a long controversy with the Quaker physician John Rutty, who, unlike Lucas, had dedicated his whole career to the study of waters.[48] Lucas, who had started his medical career by denouncing frauds in the preparation of drugs among Irish apothecaries,[49] spotted a major conflict of interest (before the term existed) in the medical treatises of waterdoctors:

most of the voluminous and numerous tracts, and of these the most pompous we have upon mineral waters, have been published by men living and practicing upon the spot, not always competent judges of the subject, but always interested in the fame of the particular water, which was their idol, the Diana of the Ephesians, and always interested in letting the world know, by a book or pamphlet, calculated for the purpose, where the mouth of the oracle, the Priest of the mysteries was to be consulted: Such a man's evidence must therefore be deemed as doubtful, concerning the efficacy of his favourite water, as that of any other priest touching the miracles of the shrine, by which he gets his daily bread.[50]

As Adam Mason has shown, this controversial rhetoric targeted the Bath corporation, and Lucas's treatise was an important turning point in the 'sulphur controversy' around the Bath waters.[51] Beyond the discussion on the methods for detecting sulphur in mineral waters, however, Lucas's bitter attack on the water doctors is rooted in a long history of anti-Catholic writings which he had published in Ireland.[52] Doctors and priests, he argues, have high stakes in the shrines that bring money to their purse, and supposed relief to the sick. As he evokes the temple of Diana, one of the seven wonders of the ancient world, Lucas suggests that priests and water doctors encourage miraculous narratives to spread, so that pilgrimages and early spa tourism bring them a steady income. Such a discourse, as I have shown in my second chapter, has had an important legacy on later historiography. It is part of a wider condemnation of quackery which was a classic trope among medical writings at the time. Nevertheless, Lucas's comparison between ancient priests of Ephesus, Roman Catholic priests and water doctors is a comment on the hubris of the investors in spas worth exploring.

Profits made from investments in spa towns could turn overnight, as was the case for many eighteenth-century businesses. In *A Tour of the Whole Island of Great Britain*, Defoe gives the example of Barnet Wells, in Hertfordshire:

The Mineral Waters, or Barnet Wells, are a little beyond this house, on the declivity of a hill; they were formerly in great request, being very much approved by physicians; but of late, they began to decline, and are now almost forgotten: Other waters at Islington, and at Hampstead having grown popular in their stead.[53]

The decline of Barnet Wells could be explained by the high competition with other spas in the proximity of London. It was located on the road to Tunbridge Wells, yet the Barnet waters were certainly muddier than the chalybeate waters of Tunbridge.[54] The Somersham waters in Huntingdonshire are another example of such rapid decline. A network of medical scholars and wealthy patrons, as Phyllis Hembry explains, tried to pump up the reputation of the Somersham waters, yet the spa never attained the degree of celebrity it was expected to.[55] Daniel Layard, a medical doctor who tried to rescue the waters from oblivion, launched a rehabilitation programme in 1763. According to him, the waters had partly suffered from a malicious account of their toxicity:

> Some having injudiciously drank the SOMERSHAM Water while they laboured under a fit of the Stone or Gravel, which proved fatal to them; a report was spread that this Water was productive of the Stone; all that could be said in defence of the Water by the Physicians, upon the strictest examination, was to no purpose.[56]

Like gossip, slander cannot be fought easily and all the investors in the Somersham spa saw their profits dwindle down to nought: 'the torrent of prejudice could not be stemmed; the spring became totally neglected, and so few persons continued the use of the Water, that the attendant's profit being very small, the house fell to ruin; and lest it should become a harbour for loose people, the materials were all removed'.[57] Several early eighteenth-century examples of disaffected spas showed that the atmosphere could rapidly deteriorate, and spa corporations were on the watch for signs of corruption, prostitution and criminal dealings.[58]

In spite of this risk, or perhaps because of it, spa towns are a good place to gather material for a cultural history of ambition. William Casey King shows how the idea of ambition evolved from vice to virtue, and shifted in the early modern period to become a spur quickening the pace of colonisation.[59] In the history of medicine and urbanisation, spa towns represented an attractive potential for rapid urban development and, as Borsay writes, '*potential* high returns'. Spa towns, however, satisfied ambition in many other ways by fostering the hope of bettering one's social status through extended networks, new friends or even a fortunate marriage. Katharine Glover's study of the Scottish town of Moffat, sixty miles south of Glasgow, is a good example of the determination of local investors.

She describes the coordinated efforts of two ambitious men: John Hope, Earl of Hopetoun, who overtook the management of the estate from his incapacitated uncle and worked on 'a visual representation of the town as a refined and unified space'; and James Hunter, a physician who 'took the lease of the farms around the well' and undertook legislative processes to launch the construction of an assembly room.[60] 'Print culture', Glover says, 'played a crucial role in the promotion of a polite reputation'.[61] Several local authors played on the pastoral image of the Scottish lowlands to differentiate Moffat from other spa towns at national level, reassuring local genteel visitors on the politeness of its entertainments. Glover also maps the multiple private efforts of Robert Adam to use Moffat early in his career for the improvement of his family network. He was the son of the successful architect William Adam and brother to his partner architect James Adam, later called 'the sovereign architect of Great Britain'. Robert Adam 'encouraged his unmarried sisters back home in Edinburgh to take advantage of any opportunity for social elevation',[62] Glover writes, and to make the most of the social occasions procured by the three weeks they spent in the summer at Moffat drinking the waters: 'It was at Moffat, Robert believed, that Peggy Adam could hope to gain access to the sort of society that would help to rub off the edges of what he saw as her informality'.[63] Glover further analyses how Adam constructed his social ambitions through spa sociability, by shaping his sister's manners as he thought she had 'nursed up a foolish Shyness & Modesty'.[64] She thus shows the intricacy of personal, intimate ambition with bolder strategies of urban development that crystallised around watering places.

More endearing, perhaps, than the real-life personality of Robert Adam, the character of Mr Parker in Austen's (unfinished) *Sanditon* shows similar energy in embarking his family on his ambitious project, which aims at turning the little sea village of Sanditon into a major health resort. Early in the narrative, Austen describes Parker's investment in the city and his obsession with profit-making:

> Sanditon was a second wife and four Children to him, hardly less dear, and certainly more engrossing. – He could talk of it forever. – It had indeed the highest claims; – not only those of Birthplace, Property and Home; it was his Mine, his Lottery, his Speculation and his Hobby Horse; his Occupation, his Hope and his Futurity.[65]

Although she uses 'lottery' rather than other games of chance, Austen's description of Parker's speculation is reminiscent of a gambler's obsession with his game:

> A very few years ago, it had been a quiet Village of no pretensions, but some natural advantages in its position and some accidental circumstances having suggested to himself, and the other principal Land Holder, the probability of its' becoming a profitable Speculation, they had engaged in it, and planned and built, and praised and puffed, and raised it to something of young Renown – and Mr. Parker could now think of very little besides.[66]

Mr Parker's speculating efforts are inscribed in Austen's prose, like the heartbeat of the narrative. Incidentally, in the 2019 TV adaptation of the novel, the project rises, falls and rises again, a plausible plot if one thinks, as I do, that Parker's love affair with urban planning is, in fact, the real love story of the narrative.[67] There was some debate about the ending of the series, as the heroine does not marry, which many have considered an unorthodox adaptation of Austen's signature plot lines and obligatory happy endings, only complete with one or more marriages.[68] If orthodoxy and 'faithfulness' were in fact an aesthetic objective of the series, it could be argued that Sidney Parker's final rescue of his brother's investment in Sanditon is the cathartic outcome of the central narrative.[69] In Austen's novel, the early set-up certainly makes the reader feel the high stakes of Parker's enterprise, and the disproportion between his description of Sanditon and the reality of the village as ironically depicted by Austen.

One of the effects of Parker's obsession is that it turns every visitor into a financial venture – a prospective client or patron – with the hope of high returns. His discussion with Lady Denham, the principal investor of his urban scheme, as they review the list of future visitors coming to Sanditon, testifies of this diffuse fortune-hunting: '"Very good, very good," said her Ladyship. – A West Indy Family and a school. That sounds well. That will bring Money." – "No people spend more freely, I beleive [sic], than West Indians," observed Mr. Parker.'[70] The influx of money coming from the colonies is seen as the life-saving nourishment of the resort. And yet as a local – of the thrifty kind, to say the least – Lady Denham worries over how the wealthy newcomers would influence the price of goods:

'because they have full Purses they fancy themselves equal, may be, to your old Country Families. But then, they who scatter their Money so freely never think of whether they may not be doing mischeif [sic] by raising the price of Things. – And I have heard that's very much the case with your West-injines. And if they come among us to raise the price of our necessaries of life, we shall not much thank them, Mr. Parker.'[71]

The way Lady Denham's fear of inflation contradicts her desire for new money reflects the growing ambivalence towards colonial money at the turn of the century. Yet Parker reassures her with an encouraging narrative of a trickle-down economy, which he hopes the whole village may benefit from:

'My dear Madam, they can only raise the price of consumable Articles by such an extraordinary Demand for them and such a diffusion of Money among us as must do us more Good than harm. – Our Butchers and Bakers and Traders in general cannot get rich without bringing Prosperity to *us*. – If *they* do not gain, our rents must be insecure – and in proportion to their profit must be ours eventually in the increased value of our Houses.'[72]

Such a view was not isolated either. In her satirical 'Letter on Watering Places', published two decades earlier, Anna Laetitia Barbauld had depicted a series of relationships that were entirely based on money. In the letter, the narrator is appalled by the reverse of aristocratic values: 'Here the continual fluctuation of money takes away all regard to character', he complains. 'As to the settled inhabitants of the place, all who do not get by us view us with dislike, because we raise the price of provisions; and those who do – which, in one way or other, comprehends all the lower class'.[73] This statement in the name of the local poor mirrors Lady Denham's concerns. They project similar anxieties over the confrontation of old and new money, rich and poor, locals and visitors caught in structural contradictions which permeated the culture of watering places.

Rich and poor

It was a common trope of spa discovery narratives that whenever a new mineral spring was found, the poor came flocking, while most spa-owners aimed to attract the rich. When Diederick Wessel Linden wrote in 1752 about the discovery of a London spring called 'Shadwell Spa', for example, he pointed out the irony of the situation: 'its Medicinal efficiency was much sooner known by the Poor, and lower Sort of People, than by the Proprietor himself; and it was upon the Account of the extraordinary Resort of such sick and afflicted Persons, that the Proprietor inclosed this Well, and also erected a Pump and Bathing-house'.[74] Linden's account highlights the tension between users and owners, raising an implicit question about the ownership of water. There was no clear rule regarding ownership: in most cases, the waters rose on the grounds of a private owner, who either gave access to them, or built a well to start charging for the water. In Cheltenham, according to Simeon Moreau, who dedicated a portion of his guide to the history of the place, the spa was accessible to drinkers in the early eighteenth century, just after it was discovered:

> The ground was originally the property of Mr Higgs, of Charlton Kings; but not knowing of a medicinal spring being on the spot, he sold it with the adjoining lands in 1716, to Mr. Mason, who discovered the spring, which for some time after its discovery was open, and the people of the town and neighbourhood drank of it.[75]

And yet, like Shadwell, soon enough it was closed by its owner, who had the waters analysed: 'In the year of 1718 it was railed in, locked up, and a little shed thrown over it'.[76] Further exploitation of the wells was organised by Mr Mason's heirs, and the spa started to develop on a more commercial basis.

Sometimes, right of way was negotiated; at other times the spas were found on the commons, in which case, rights of common prevailed, as the rules and regulation of Somersham Spa stipulated. These rules were clearly geared towards the distribution of rich and poor visitors, the regulation of cash flow and the monitoring of crowds of visitors:

> That the house of attendance at the SPA, be from five o'clock in the morning till seven, for the poor; and from seven till twelve at noon for other persons. That no gratuity be taken by any servant, or servants, from any poor person; the servant in default to be immediately discharged. A certificate of the person being a proper object of charity, signed by the Minister of the Parish, or by some reputable person in

that parish, is to be given to the servant. – Every person claiming, and having a right of Common on SOMERSHAM Heath, to have the water *gratis* for their own use, on giving to the servant their names and places of abode.[77]

The rights of common are thus integrated in a wider system of privatisation, which shows the complex status of water in the eighteenth century. Clearly, the proprietors of the Somersham Spa had the right to charge for the use of water, yet they needed to provide for parishioners who had a poor certificate. The country was still under the regulation of the Old Poor Law, and some of the poor were directed by their local authority to take the waters, which required a certificate for the sick to avoid being charged for vagrancy and sent back to their parishes. Water ownership also had to yield to the supremacy of rights of commons. This shows the composite status of mineral waters within a village, and the ways in which their exploitation was negotiated with the current laws and the local people. Some local craftsmen or lodgers saw an interest in the commercial development of spas, others considered that it might be a threat to the economy of the village.

Waters had to be managed properly, and they could resist profit-making logics. One of the issues was flow: not every spa could rely on a steady flow like St Winifred's Well, which was known to fill its basin of 'two hundred and forty tons' in less than two minutes.[78] In fact, Cheltenham was quite the opposite, and the scarcity of the waters put the economy of the spa at risk. Towards the end of the century, Joseph Smith wrote to the Royal College of Surgeons, complaining of the lack of proper regulation at the pump: 'A third cause of the scarcity is, that many accustom themselves to send in the morning for the waters; and though a pint is sufficient for the generality of drinkers, a quart is the smallest quantity that is ever carried away; and more frequently two or three quarts'.[79] This blocked the way for other users, and contradicted the medical advice to drink water directly at the pump, to prevent the volatile spirits from evaporating. It was made even worse, Smith argued, by servants who, 'notwithstanding they may have no occasion for the waters, often choose to drink them as their betters do'.[80] Waters could hardly be sold as any other good, as they were, after all, freely bestowed on men by nature. Their curing properties were seen, for religious and secular reasons, as natural medicine for all. Regulating access to the waters therefore required that some use be maintained for several social classes, including the poor: specific hours, separate basins or specific springs could be made more accessible to lower social classes. Daniel Defoe even claimed that while 'the nobility and gentry go to Tunbridge, the merchants and rich citizens to Epsome, so the common people go chiefly to Dullwich and Stretham'.[81] In Streatham, he finds that 'throngs' of people were visiting the spa, typically associating the poor with potentially dangerous crowds: 'because it lies near London, that they can walk to it in the morning, and return at night; which abundance do; that is to say, especially of a Sunday, or on holidays, which makes the better sort also decline the place; the crowd on those days being both unruly and unmannerly'.[82]

Some spa towns had had a long experience of providing for the poor. Their corporations set up early charity schemes by applying a local tax to visitors, which was redistributed among the lodgings, baths and costs of care for the visiting poor. This was the case of Buxton in the 1770s, as Mike Langham describes it: 'A collection was taken of all those who stayed in hotels and lodging houses and a subscription book kept' to support sixteen patients chosen and vetted by the local gentry. 'The patient received six shillings for board and lodging together with medicines and water treatment for a maximum period of five weeks'.[83] Similar organisation could be found in towns like Scarborough and Harrogate. In the same vein, Anne Borsay's study of the General Infirmary in Bath is a fascinating account of the ways in which the bodies of the sick poor were handled by institutional regulations: 'In common with other institutions, Bath infirmary allowed patients "to go to their respective places of worship on Sunday, and return directly" although the rules also forbade them to "loiter about the city or go to ale house on pain of expulsion"'.[84] From the opening of the Infirmary in 1731, the town corporation partly delegated to this charity the care and control of the sick poor, which also helped to prevent any vagrancy in the streets of Bath, leaving the town in a peaceful utopian atmosphere.

Failure to find a solution to monitor the incoming sick poor, contemporaries argued, might result in financial difficulties for a spa. Glastonbury was a well-known example of such economic and social failure. It was managed by Mrs Galloway, who could not afford to invest enough to maintain the spa structure in good shape, which would have improved the frequentation of the place. The rest of the town was growing weary of the influx of the poorer sort coming to take the Glastonbury waters – charges of popism, as we saw earlier, came into play, as they did in Buxton and Holywell. In 1751, the Reverend of Plympton complained about the situation, on which he claimed to have neutral views, as he lived in Plympton, which was far enough from Glastonbury:

> I am likewise in Hopes that the Poor that resort hither will soon be put under proper Regulations, that such as are charitably inclined, like yourself, may not be too much importuned and imposed upon by *Mumpers* and such sturdy Beggars as are no probably Objects of Cure, to the great Detriment of others that are real Objects of *Cure* and *Compassion*.[85]

Several attempts were made to rescue the waters from ruin, and Phyllis Hembry explains how an initial scheme of rehabilitation for the spa was set up:

> An injection of capital was necessary, and the remedy proposed in the *Bath Journal* was an annual subscription of one guinea for the use of the rooms, drinking, bathing and attendance. Paupers could be subsidized by a two-guinea subscription from the better-off, carrying the right to send one poor person to take the waters with lodgings and maintenance for seven weeks.[86]

Yet this failed to succeed, and by 1781 'the pump-room had become a shop'.[87]

Regular appeals were made to the charity of visitors with what we would now call 'fundraising events'. As parishes were the local centres of charity and welfare in the confessional state of Britain, charity events were often coordinated with church events: religious feasts, preaching and local gatherings. In the 1730 *Tunbrigialia*, a poem was published with the title 'To *Dr. Lynch*, on his Excellent Sermon preach'd at Tunbridge Wells, Aug. 23, 1730, for the support of the Charity Children, where there was a great Audience, but little given, considering their fortunes'.[88] The poem most probably refers to John Lynch, who was then Dean of Canterbury, and regularly visited the neighbouring counties:[89]

> In vain you shew a happy Nation
> The Gospel's glorious Dispensation

> And plead from thence, to bring up Youth,
> To early Piety and Truth;
> To unattentive ears you preach
> Calamities alone can't teach.

> A neighbouring island boasts a flood,
> Famous for petrifying Wood;
> A greater Change, as Story tells,
> Is plainly wrought by *Tunbridge Wells*,
> Their dire Effects both Sexes feel,
> The Waters turn their Hearts to Steel.[90]

The 'petrifying wood' comically conveys the minerality of waters, together with the term 'steel', which evokes the high concentration of the chalybeate waters of Tunbridge.[91] The effect of the poem is intensified by an epigram printed on the following page, which compares the sums given, which 'wou'd make one think this People poor', with the great amounts of money bet at the 'Hazard-table' by the same:

> *Britons*! 'tis little for your Glory
> That such as hand you down in Story,
> Should of your Wealth their notions frame,
> Not as you *give*, but as you *Game*.[92]

By juxtaposing it with the gaping needs of poor relief, the epigram stresses the idea that gambling is a sign of excessive and wasteful wealth. The representations of watering places in literature enhanced the social gap between the happy few and the poor masses. They revolved around the waters' attractive potentials for rich and poor alike, and revelled in stereotypical portraits of characters from each extremity of the social ladder. As the poor came 'flocking' to drink the waters, the rich came to enjoy public entertainments such as concerts, gaming parties, balls and races, which, should they leave town, threatened to degenerate into gatherings of ill repute.

In Tunbridge, gaming was not the only performance of wealth that might have contrasted with the poorer sort. The central spot of sociability, as we recall, was the 'Walks', paved and built upon at the end of the seventeenth century. The long lines of shops and colonnades along the Walks which were soon called the 'Pantiles' (named by the shape of the tiles on the pavement) were the perfect setting for the performance of shopping. Shopping was gradually becoming a leisure activity for the better sort. Jon Stobart, in his comparison between the luxury trade in spa towns and market towns, insists on the widening importance of shopping, both as a means of acquiring the material trappings of polite society and as a leisure activity in its own right. This socio-cultural function made shopping an important part of the daily routines of the leisured, and the shops themselves became essential in the landscape of leisure towns.[93]

In fact, Stobart concludes that although the luxury goods were more abundantly sold in market towns, they tended to be more advertised, and more easily available, in spa towns.[94] Luxury shopping entertained a cultural function within the town, both enhancing its reputation and serving the sociability of the wealthy or, perhaps even more so, of the would-be wealthy.

Because it was supposed to appeal to the *Beau Monde*, shopping was pictured as an aspiration of the middling sort, as Anna Laetitia Barbauld's comic 'Letter on Watering Places' cunningly suggests. It is allegedly written by a country gentleman, 'Henry Homelove', whose name is self-explanatory, and who remains puzzled (and cranky) in front of the new fashions displayed in the spa town:[95]

> In the country I had been accustomed to do good for the poor; there are charities here too; – we have joined in a subscription for a crazy poetess, a raffle for the support of a sharper, who passes under the title of a German county, and a benefit-play for a *gentleman* on board the hulks. Unfortunately, to balance these various expenses, this place, which happens to be a great resort of smugglers, affords daily opportunities of making *bargains*. We drink spoiled teas, under the idea of their being cheap; and the little room we have is made less by the reception of cargoes of India taffetas, shawl muslin, and real chintzes.[96]

Unsurprisingly, the 'chintzes' were soon caught by custom-house officers and the material, thought to be obtained in contraband, came in reality from 'the home-bred manufacture of Spitalfields'.[97] Henry Homelove's depiction of the desperate attempts of the women of the middling sort at taking part in the consumption culture of their betters is seen as another gamble, bringing displeasure and unexpected losses. Again, the commerce and sociability of spa towns appear as a deforming mirror for the monetary value of things. A few years before Barbauld's letter was published, the author of *Modern Refinement:*

A Satire, who calls himself 'The Invalid' and claims (very plausibly) to have written *The Register of Folly* mentioned earlier, adopts a much angrier tone than the soft complaints of Henry Homelove. He unveils the strategies used at Bath and Bristol Hotwells to give the illusion of abundance in the pump room buffets, and the ways of setting the table 'that Plenty's *Shadow* may appear'.[98] One of the techniques mocked by the Invalid is to serve water instead of wine at buffets, for alleged medical reasons:

> A large decanter of spring-water's plac'd,
> (for since Codogan [sic.] water's all the taste)
> Full in your view – to tell you, tho' there's wine,
> No liquor's half so wholesome, half so fine![99]

In his treatise on gout published six years earlier, Cadogan had indeed warned against the abuse of alcohol, and invited gouty patients to adopt a strict diet and increase their exercise – readers in Bath and Bristol would therefore easily understand the reference as the treatise had been published more than ten times since.[100] From failed contraband to false grandeur, the performance of wealth in spa towns was regularly depicted as a stucco paste which matched the disproportionate ambitions of their proprietors, ready to crumble at the first signs of crisis.

The readiest example of the discrepancy between what watering places claimed to be and the experience they offered lay in the housing stock available to visitors. Complaining about the dodgy lodgings was one of the most respected conventions among the manifold genres of spa writings throughout the eighteenth century. Letters, poems, essays and novels all dedicated a few lines to the dreadful lodgings on offer: their scarcity, their filthiness, their disagreeable landladies and their outrageous prices. It is, of course, one of the items of the list ticked off in the list of complaints from 'A Letter from *Tunbridge* to a friend in *London*': 'Lodgings are here so dear and so scarce, that a Beau is sometimes glad of a Barn, and a Lady of Honour to lie in a Garret: The Horses being commonly put to Grass, for the Servants to lie in the Stable'.[101] Lodgings are thus turned into a social leveller, rather than a sign of social distinction. The narrator of this letter also mentions parasites in a small comic narrative that links stock-keeping and inn-keeping, a very probable association in many rural areas where new spas had been erected:

My Landlord was a Farmer, and his very Out-houses were so full, that having shear'd some Sheep, he abated me Half-a-crown a Week, to let the Wool lie in my Bed-chamber; by which means a Tick one Night had bury'd himself so far in my Belly, that I was forc'd next morning to borrow a Shoe-maker's Pincers to pluck the blood-thirsty Vermin out of his Nest by the Arse.[102]

The tick, it seems, found a better lodging than the narrator.

A satirical poem on Scarborough published in the 1735 *Bath, Bristol, Tunbridge and Epsom Miscellany* also complains of the parasite-laden bed. To ennoble his subject, the anonymous writer juxtaposes private complaints and national pride:

> O Scarb'rough, say, how comes thy Pow'r so great,
>   Thus to attract the Wealthy and the Great!
> What Pleasure can in unceil'd Rooms be found,
> Where buggy Beds with Fleas and Lice abound?
> *Egyptian* Plagues! what Man of common Sense
> Can with thy wild, thy rustic Scenes dispense?[103]

Readers must have easily jumped to the conclusion that the wealthy and the great were another kind of parasite, corrupting the country like an 'Egyptian plague', be it gnats or flies or locusts. The materiality of the buggy beds, however, brings the town corporation back to what it should promote internally: decent accommodation for visitors, which was seen as a major hindrance to the reputation of spa towns and to the development of what we now call early tourism. Similarly, the anonymous 'countryman' author of *A Journey to Llandrindod Wells*, who is otherwise rather enthusiastic about his travels, complains about ghastly lodgings nearby: 'We were introduced in a little nasty Room, by as nasty an old Woman, and were almost suffocated with Smoke'.[104] He explains the irrationality of hastily designed cottages around the wells, which appear to the twenty-first-century reader as early forms of ephemeral touristic constructions.

Towards the end of the century, dirty lodgings and want of beds still fuelled many a satirical comment on spa towns, including Barbauld's above-mentioned 'Letter on Watering Places', in which the narrator depicts his disappointment on arrival: 'the place was so full, that when we arrived, late at night, and tired with our journey, all the beds at the inn were taken up, and an easy-chair and a carpet were all the accommodations we could obtain for our repose'.[105] Once he finds lodgings, thousands of little frustrating details depict the estranging physical experience of displaced domesticity: 'we are continually lamenting that we are obliged to buy things of which we have such plenty at home', he writes, the greatest irony lying in the physical results of living thus: 'the rooms we at present inhabit are so pervious to the breeze, that in spite of all the ingenious expedients of listing doors, pasting paper on the inside of cupboards, laying sand-bags, puttying crevices, and condemning closet-doors; it has given me a severe touch of my old rheumatism'.[106] Just like the poet in Scarborough, the poor maintenance of private domestic spaces brings to the fore the absurdity of taking the waters when the rest of the experience is not coordinated with the central medical purpose of spa towns. In all its sombre irony, Barbauld's letter highlights a recurrent problem in health systems: therapeutics undone by lack of a wider approach.

Throughout the century, the idea that the wealthy, the prosperous and the poor classes mingled in dangerous proximity persisted: 'The Sons and Daughters of Fortune thrive here so mightily, it is hard to know the Lady from the Jilt, or the Lord from the Sharper; all higglede pigglede mix among one another', writes the narrator of 'A Letter from *Tunbridge* to a friend in *London*'.[107] Similar imagery can be found in the 1733 poem 'On the Elegant Entertainment and Mix'd Company at the Ordinaries', although this time, social mingling doesn't seem to bring any sign of anxious need for differentiation:

> I can dine with a Lord, or his Grace for my Shilling;
> Where Ladies and Beas mingl'd all in a Row,
> At the same pretty Sport make a Raree fine Show.
> Without rude Distinction, all huddle together,
> Young, old, handsome, ugly, there's no chusin whether.[108]

As Katharine Glover mentions, however, it denotes a 'loosening of social hierarchy' which was 'characteristic of spa sociability permitting hopes of new social contacts among the ranks of the gentry and aristocracy who frequented the resort'.[109] And yet, the social moral of the poem – it is distinction that is rude, not the lack thereof – is rare enough to be mentioned. Anxious criticism was more common in the second part of the century, such as Jerry Melford's famous remark in *Humphry Clinker* on 'the farce of life' displayed in the pump rooms at Bath, which he describes as 'a monstrous jumble of heterogeneous principles; a vile mob of noise and impertinence, without decency or subordination'.[110] At the end of the century, the poem 'Ducks and pease', published in *Trifles from Harrogate*, is built upon a comic anecdote narrating the story of a usurpation of rank. A couple enter an inn in which nothing is left to eat except two roasted ducks ordered by a 'gentleman' already seated in the upper rooms, who cannot be prevailed upon to share his meal with the newly arrived couple. Upon learning that the said gentleman comes from Newcastle upon Tyne, however, and hearing that he sings and dances alone in his room, the couple are soon able to identify him as their previous servant, and they impose upon his supper. 'Lord Joseph', who has reinvented himself thanks to the guise of a 'gold-lac'd hat', has to comply, and social order is restored:

> Joseph obey'd, and up she came
> The Landlord thought it a pleasant game
> So down he went, and told the story
> Not over much to Joseph's Glory
> The waiters laugh'd, to find it so
> For toll de roll, it was plain Joe.[111]

That servants should pretend to be their masters and vice-versa is a well-known feature of comedy. That Harrogate should be the place Joe picks to try his luck at the upper rooms as gentlemen do, as well as the presence of such a plot within the Harrogate miscellanies, is a sign that it was generally accepted that a spa town could be a place of false pretence.

Ironical anxiety prevailed over the possibilities that such social mingling might offer, especially to fortune-hunters.[112] Similar to the 'Ducks and pease' plot, 'The Bath Fortune-Hunter: Or, the Biter Bit', which targets the Irish, tells the story of Brian, 'sprung from kingly Race':

> His Country left, and took his Place
> At *Bath*, among the best, where he
> Claim'd a Superiority:
> A small Estate he had, 'tis true,
> His cloaths embroider'd were, and new,
> Thither a *Fortune-hunting* came,
> In Hopes to allure some *English* Dame.[113]

Brian, it turns out, is unable to read the social conventions of the town. Just like new gamblers are unable to spot the sharpers in a game and have to be taught, he is blinded by his hopes, unable to recognise a 'plain, downright, common Whore' who passes for an English Dame, as he believes she has 'store of Pelf'. Unlike the transvestite characters of the 'Beau-Female, or the Female Beau', who end in mutual embrace,[114] Brian flees after his marriage, leaving Moll 'in dismal Plight'. Plotlines like this pervade spa comedies and the marriage market is as attractive to fortune-hunters as the gaming rooms are to gamblers. In Baker's 1703 play *Tunbridge-Walks*, Hillaria is also desperate to marry a good fortune. She decides to 'Make Love to Mr. Maiden', a character who is clearly presented to have no desire for women other than to dress up as one. He avoids her after she launches heavily into vain attempts to seduce him by talking wigs, turns to the audience and declares: 'She's mighty fond methinks, she may be a Cheat for ought I know; for so many rakish Women come down to *Tunbridge*, to make their fortunes among us Men of Estates, that if a Body ha'n't great care one may be stole – How shall I get away from her?'[115] Baker's play thus cynically presents Tunbridge as a meeting room for the marriage business. The trope is still vivid at the end of the century: in O'Keeffe's play *The Irish Mimic; Or Blunders at Brighton*, two suitors fight over a woman until one of them cries out to his rival: 'Hark'ye, you old raven! Your hovering about for legacies is notorious, thro' almost every public place in England; you have been hooted out of the rooms at Bath, drove from the pantiles at Tunbridge, and, by heaven, I'll have you beat off the Steine at Brighton'.[116] Travelling from one fashionable spa to another, the fortune-hunter, like a gambler, moves to a new spot where he cannot be recognised. In the murky waters of social mingling, marrying for money, satire said, was indeed a risky business.

In the early capitalism that was staged in many areas of spa towns, from gambling and shopping to architectural investments, financial profits were represented as the result of risk-taking. Risk was in fact a common trait to the various discourses on spa towns: patients were risking their lives with the water treatment if it was not properly administered, visitors were risking their reputation by mingling with the mixed societies of spa towns, and players risked their fortunes in the endless escalation of gambling parties. Such representations made watering places the theatre of capitalistic culture, from the early speculating mock-doctors like D'Oyley in Colman's *The spleen, or, Islington Spa* to the compulsive investors like Parker in Austen's *Sanditon*. These representations stood in contrast to the discourse on the waters as a natural remedy, freely bestowed by the earth, a common good that locals should be able to enjoy for free.

Notes

1 A complete and updated bibliography of medical primary sources of eighteenth-century British spas can be found at https://thermal1719. hypotheses.org/ (not yet uploaded on 8 April 2021).
2 Hembry, *The English Spa*, p. 112.
3 D. G. Schwartz has written a general history of gambling. His chapter 'Seeking the cure: spa gambling defines Europe' gives a good overview of the structures devoted to gambling in spas, the kinds of games that were played, and the main affairs surrounding them, in D. G. Schwartz, *Roll the Bones: The History of Gambling* (London: Gotham Books, 2006), pp. 185–215.
4 'The Battle of the Sugar Plums', in *The Scarborough Miscellany*, 1732, p. 15.
5 'The Battle of the Sugar Plums' in *The Scarborough Miscellany*, 1732, pp. 13–14.
6 D. T. Andrew, *Aristocratic Vice: The Attack on Duelling, Suicide, Adultery, and Gambling in Eighteenth-Century England* (New Haven, CT: Yale University Press, 2013).
7 Three-card-monte is also called 'Find the Lady'.
8 Goldsmith, *The life of Richard Nash*, p. 201.
9 On the development of *Pharaon* in France see Schwartz, *Roll the Bones*, p. 101; J.-L. Harouel, 'De François Ier au pari en ligne, histoire du jeu en France', *Pouvoirs*, 139:4 (2011), 5–14. Faro required that someone took the bank, distributed gains and took away the losses. The cards were laid out in a U-shape on the table, and the gamblers would bet if a card was winning or losing. They would be paid or ripped of their bet by the banker each time he drew a losing or a winning card from the deck.
10 Andrew, *Aristocratic Vice*, p. 182.
11 Andrew, *Aristocratic Vice*, p. 182.
12 J. Burges, *An Essay on the Waters and Air of Ballispellan. With Their Various Properties and Uses* (Dublin: W. Wilmot, 1725), p. 32.

13 *The Guardian* 174, p. 503.
14 Burnby, *Summer Amusement*, p. 18.
15 Burnby, *Summer Amusement*, p. 19.
16 Eglin, *The Imaginary Autocrat*, p. 123.
17 Goldsmith, *The life of Richard Nash*, p. 50.
18 Goldsmith, *The life of Richard Nash*, p. 50.
19 Goldsmith, *The life of Richard Nash*, p. 61.
20 D. Defoe and R. Holmes, *Defoe on Sheppard and Wild* (London: Harper Perennial, 2004); H. Fielding, *The Life of Mr Jonathan Wild the Great* ([1734]; London: Hesperus, 2004).
21 On the private arrangement he made with the proprietors of the gaming tables, see Eglin, *The Imaginary Autocrat*, pp. 214–15.
22 Goldsmith, *The life of Richard Nash*, p. 201.
23 Goldsmith, *The life of Richard Nash*, p. 201.
24 Goldsmith, *The life of Richard Nash*, p. 209.
25 Goldsmith, *The life of Richard Nash*, p. 209.
26 Goldsmith, *The life of Richard Nash*, pp. 212–16.
27 See Eglin, *The Imaginary Autocrat*, pp. 128–9.
28 Goldsmith, *The life of Richard Nash*, p. 213.
29 Goldsmith, *The life of Richard Nash*, p. 214.
30 Goldsmith, *The life of Richard Nash*, p. 215.
31 Goldsmith, *The life of Richard Nash*, p. 215.
32 Goldsmith, *The life of Richard Nash*, pp. 215–16.
33 'First, eighteenth-century commentators gave a three-part answer to the question of female vulnerability to such vicious behavior, arguing that in part this was due to their lack of public occupations, in part to their mis-education, and in part to their greater nervous susceptibility. Women were particularly warned to beware "how they suffer this passion [for play] to steal upon them." For, since women had no ordinary paying jobs, they could employ their talents at cards.' Andrew, *Aristocratic Vice*, p. 200.
34 Andrew, *Aristocratic Vice*, p. 197.
35 Andrew, *Aristocratic Vice*, p. 199.
36 'The Battle of the Sugar Plums' in *The Scarborough Miscellany*, 1732, p. 15.
37 'The descreet and sober Lady Lechmere has lost such Furious sums at the Bath that 'tis question'd whether all the sweetness that the Waters can put into my Lord's blood can make him endure it, particularly £700 at one sitting, which is aggravated with many astonishing Circumstances'. Lady Mary Wortley Montagu (1725), quoted in Kerhervé, 'Writing letters from Georgian spas', p. 280.
38 She is not to be confounded with Elizabeth Montagu, the bluestocking letter-writer, who is also mentioned in this book. Lady Mary Wortley

Montagu was the wife of Ambassador Montagu, also a letter-writer, who first observed inoculating practices in Turkey.

39 Wortley Montagu, *Letters and Works*, p. 492.
40 A good example of such connections is the political tensions escalating around the ridottos of Spa in the Belgian province of Liège, eventually triggering the Liège revolution. See D. Droixhe, *Une histoire des Lumières au pays de Liège: livre, idées, société* (Liège: Editions de l'ULG, 2007), pp. 189–91; Schwartz, *Roll the Bones*, pp. 187–9. Spa was a major destination for English gamblers and health-seekers.
41 Eglin, *The Imaginary Autocrat*, p. 124.
42 Goldsmith, *The life of Richard Nash*, p. 22.
43 Porter, 'Introduction', p. ix.
44 Porter, 'Introduction', p. ix.
45 Borsay, 'Health and leisure resorts', p. 792.
46 The Invalid, *The Register of Folly*, p. 57.
47 The society of Merchant Venturers owning the Hotwells pump, however, had enjoyed a ninety-year lease from the town, as Phyllis Hembry explains. Hembry, *The English Spa*, p. 97.
48 Rutty's *Methodical Synopsis of Mineral Waters* has already been studied in chapters 1 and 2.
49 S. Mullaney, 'Charles Lucas and medical legislation in eighteenth century Ireland', *Irish Journal of Medical Science*, 184:3 (2015), 555–6.
50 Lucas, *An Essay on Waters*, p. 126.
51 Mason, 'The "Political Knight Errant" at Bath', pp. 67–83.
52 On Lucas's role as a politician see S. Murphy, 'Charles Lucas, Catholicism and Nationalism', *Eighteenth-Century Ireland / Iris an Dá Chultúr*, 8 (1993), 83–102.
53 D. Defoe, *A Tour through the Whole Island of Great Britain* ([1724–26]; London: Penguin Books, 1986), p. 339.
54 See Curl, *Spas, Wells, and Pleasure-Gardens*, p. 167.
55 Hembry, *The English Spa*, pp. 164–6.
56 D. P. Layard, *An Account of the Somersham Water: In the County of Huntingdon* (London: S. N., 1767), p. 11.
57 Layard, *An Account of the Somersham Water*, p. 11.
58 For example, Lambeth Wells were closed in 1755: a dancing licence was refused because of the frequentation of the assembly rooms (Hembry, *The English Spa*, p. 102).
59 W. C. King, *Ambition: A History* (New Haven, CT: Yale University Press, 2013).
60 Glover, 'Polite society and the rural resort', p. 67.
61 Glover, 'Polite society and the rural resort', p. 67.
62 Glover, 'Polite society and the rural resort', p. 69.
63 Glover, 'Polite society and the rural resort', p. 69.

64 Glover, 'Polite society and the rural resort', p. 69.

65 Austen, *Sanditon*, p. 327.

66 Austen, *Sanditon*, pp. 328–9.

67 *Sanditon* (Red Planet Pictures, Independent Television (ITV), Masterpiece Theatre, 2019).

68 See for example the article in the *Washington Post*, 'Sanditon, finale: fans expect a happy ending', *Washington Post*, 27 February 2020.

69 As Hudelet explains, the criterion of faithfulness does not help evaluate the cinematic rewriting of an adaptation. A. Hudelet, D. Monaghan and J. Wiltshire, *The Cinematic Jane Austen* (London: McFarland, 2009).

70 Austen, *Sanditon*, p. 350.

71 Austen, *Sanditon*, p. 350.

72 Austen, *Sanditon*, pp. 350–51.

73 A. L. Barbauld, 'Letter on Watering Places', in *The Annual Register, or, a View of the History, Politics, and Literature for the Year 1796* (London: T. Burton, 1800). The letter was originally published in *The Monthly* in 1791, see W. McCarthy, *Anna Letitia Barbauld: Voice of the Enlightenment* (Baltimore, MD: Johns Hopkins University Press, 2008), pp. 374–5.

74 Linden, *A Treatise on the Origin, Nature, and Virtues of Chalybeat Waters*, p. 143.

75 S. Moreau, *A Tour to Cheltenham Spa* (Bath: R. Cruttwell, London, 1783), p. 36.

76 Moreau, *A Tour to Cheltenham Spa*, p. 36.

77 Layard, *An Account of the Somersham Water*, p. 23. According to my own article on money in *The Physics of Language*, p. 123, five shillings could be the equivalent of a day's wages for an assistant periwig-maker or for a carpenter by the end of the eighteenth century (C. Emsley et al., 'London history – currency, coinage and the cost of living', *Old Bailey Proceedings Online* (www.oldbaileyonline.org, version 7.0, last consulted 28 July 2020)).

78 According to the broadside sheet studied earlier, the experiment took place on 12 July 1731, in the presence of several important witnesses, showing that 'the Spring rises more than one hundred ton every minute'. *A Description of St. Winefred's Well*, p. 1.

79 Smith, *Observations on the Use and Abuse of the Cheltenham Waters*, p. 12.

80 Smith, *Observations on the Use and Abuse of the Cheltenham Waters*, p. 12.

81 Defoe, *A Tour*, p. 166.

82 Defoe, *A Tour*, p. 166.

83 M. Langham, *Buxton: A People's History* (Lancaster: Carnegie, 2001), p. 112.

84 Borsay, '"Persons of honour and reputation"', p. 290.

85 Davies, *A Short Description of the Waters at Glastonbury*, p. 10.

86 Hembry, *The English Spa*, p. 171.

87 Hembry, *The English Spa*, p. 171. Hembry also explains that another attempt at reviving the spa was made in 1794, but it had become a private dwelling thirty years later.

88 *Tunbrigialia, or the Tunbrige Miscellany for the year 1730* (London: A. Moore, 1730).

89 As we have seen earlier with John Burnby's works (chapter 4), there were regular associations between Tunbridge Wells and Canterbury.

90 *Tunbrigialia, or the Tunbrige Miscellany for the year 1730*, p. 5.

91 Many petrifying wells were known at the time in England, yet this particular example might refer to the submerged forests – or trunks or stumps – regularly uncovered at low tide that can be found on the coasts of Britain and in the Channel Islands.

92 *The Tunbridge and Bath Miscellany for the Year 1730*, p. 4.

93 Stobart, 'In search of a leisure hierarchy', p. 20.

94 'New trends in consumption were set and new consumer goods *show-cased* in London and the spas, but most people obtained their luxuries, decencies and necessities closer to home'. Stobart, 'In search of a leisure hierarchy', p. 20.

95 Barbauld's letter, published ten years after *Humphry Clinker*, gives voice to a narrator that resembles in many points the main character from Smollett's novel, Matthew Bramble.

96 Barbauld, 'Letter on Watering Places', p. 302.

97 Barbauld, 'Letter on Watering Places', p. 302.

98 The Invalid, *Modern Refinement*, p. 10.

99 The Invalid, *Modern Refinement*, p. 10.

100 Cadogan, *A Dissertation on the Gout*.

101 'A Letter from *Tunbridge*', pp. 5–6.

102 'A Letter from *Tunbridge*', p. 6. On the history of parasites in relation with lodgings and tourism see P. D. Mitchell (ed.), *Sanitation, Latrines and Intestinal Parasites in Past Populations* (Farnham: Ashgate, 2015) and A. Mączak, *Travel in Early Modern* (Cambridge: Polity Press, 1995).

103 *The Bath, Bristol, Tunbridge and Epsom Miscellany*, p. 30.

104 Countryman, *A journey to Llandrindod Wells, in Radnorshire* (London: Cooper, 1746), p. 27.

105 Barbauld, 'Letter on Watering Places', p. 298.

106 Barbauld, 'Letter on Watering Places', p. 298.

107 'A Letter from *Tunbridge*', p. 2.
108 'On the Elegant Entertainment and Mix'd Company at the Ordinaries', in *The Scarborough Miscellany*, 1733, p. 32.
109 Glover, 'Polite society and the rural resort', p. 70.
110 'I saw a broken-winded Wapping landlady squeeze through a circle of peers, to salute her brandy-merchant, who stood by the window, propped upon crutches; and a paralytic attorney of Shoe-lane, in shuffling up to the bar, kicked the shins of the chancellor of England, while his lordship, in a cut bob, drank a glass of water at the pump'. Smollett, *Humphry Clinker*, p. 49.
111 *Trifles from Harrogate*, p. 17.
112 For example, in the poem on Islington Wells already quoted in chapter 4, the narrator exclaims: 'Whence comes it that the shining Great, / To Titles born, and awful State, / Thus condescend, thus check their Will, / And scud away to *Tunbridge Wells*, / To mix with vulgar Beaux and Belles?' (Lockman, *The Humours of New Tunbridge Wells*, p. 2). Similarly, a poem 'On the Epsom Horse-Races' written in 1735 frets over the crowd gathering at the races: 'A Scoundrel here, pray take it on my Word, / Is a Companion for the greatest Lord [...] / Here the promiscuous and ungovern'd Crew / Crowd to see what is neither strange nor new' (*The Bath, Bristol, Tunbridge and Epsom Miscellany*, p. 29).
113 *The Bath, Bristol, Tunbridge and Epsom Miscellany*, p. 21.
114 See the poem mentioned in chapter 3.
115 Baker, *Tunbridge-Walks*, p. 39.
116 The Steine, in Brighton, was a green arranged for the visitors' promenades. O'Keeffe, *The Irish Mimic*, p. 5.

Conclusion

Just like the persisting stain of chalybeate waters at the bottom of a well, this book deals with recurrent patterns in the discourse on mineral waters in the long eighteenth century. Hence, it is deliberately organised thematically rather than chronologically, emphasising the echoes rather than the differences between the medical and literary representations of the spas of the Restoration and of the late eighteenth century. Because the back-and-forth chronological flow of each chapter, even when each source is contextualised, can prevent the reader from getting a clear vision of the evolution of the history of spas, wells, spa medicine, sociability and economics throughout the century, this conclusion wishes to reshuffle the main concepts of the book around three ideas commonly attributed to the chronological narrative of mineral waters in eighteenth-century Britain: medicalisation, commercialisation and cosmopolitanism.

The classical historical narrative presents the use of waters as gradually medicalised throughout the century: chemistry was on the rise, natural historians reported new spas to the Royal Society, and numerous medical treatises were published, discussing the uses of spa treatment and accounting for its dangers and benefits. It is undeniable that the 1750s and 1760s were decisive in making the information on the great variety of mineral sources in England better known to the medical world and more accessible to a greater audience thanks to the publication of several systematic treatises. Thomas Short, John Rutty and Diederick Wessel Linden, all of them medical doctors, discussed and compared more than 150 spas in Britain, and some on the continent, giving a detailed analysis and topographical account for each spa, with occasional cases or anecdotes. The way the authors quote each other, and discuss and compare their observations, is a good example of medical knowledge in the making, and a potential illustration for a linear history of ideas. In this teleological perspective, the long eighteenth century would have seen the development of the use of mineral waters, paving the way for nineteenth-century hydrotherapy. I have argued in the introduction and the first two chapters, however, that the theoretical frameworks of eighteenth-century water medicine overlap and re-emerge, so that there is no strict linear evolution in the medical approach to mineral waters.

My interest in middle-sized and smaller spas suggests a counter-narrative to medicalisation: in parallel with the systematic studies of the 1750s and 1760s, other types of medical discourses on mineral waters were published and disseminated. Many a spa discovered at the end of the century was written about with a multitude of cases, blending miraculous cures and chemical analysis in a way which is reminiscent of the compilation of extraordinary cases associated with the end of the seventeenth century. Miracles, as Jane Shaw argues, did not disappear in eighteenth-century Britain, and the religious frame for understanding the effects of mineral waters was not diluted by a uniform discourse of medicalisation.[1] I explained in the fourth chapter how holy waters persisted, reappeared and evolved in eighteenth-century Britain. Some of them kept attracting pilgrims and entertained a deep connection with local Catholic politics (mostly in Ireland and Wales). Others, such as stopped wells found in cellars, were the object of post-Reformation tales. Some local urban wells had their waters analysed and advertised by medical doctors and yet held on to their patron saint's name. Finally, although medical treatises on waters did multiply in eighteenth-century Britain, many of them had already been published in previous centuries. The genre started as early as the fourteenth century, as Marylin Nicoud argues, and the scientific discourse on mineral waters did not unfold solely in medical treatises, borrowing from other theoretical frameworks and blending with chemistry, natural history and travel literature.[2] Finally, the development of medical institutions such as the General Infirmary in Bath remained restricted to the major spas, that is to say, less than 5 per cent of the mineral waters available to the sick.[3]

Although the notion of medicalisation should be nuanced, as it is generally accepted among twenty-first-century historians of medicine, the experience of illness remains central to account for the proliferation of spas, springs and wells throughout the long eighteenth century. As I have explained, sick people turned to local wells, which were more systematically reported on maps and discussed in treatises in the 1760s. The sick were alternatively ready to travel a long way to try new mineral waters, or go back to the spas that had procured them enough relief if the waters nearby did not procure similar relief. Mineral waters were part of the *materia medica* of doctors and chemists, as well as the day-to-day remedies that were advised, used and sold outside of the medical world. As such, multiple discourses on mineral waters and their users found their way through print, from literary miscellanies to songs, plays and religious sermons. Whether spiritual, satirical or sentimental, many of these texts addressed the experience of sickness and relief, including sometimes the disappointed hope for relief, and described the networks of care that could be found close to the spas, from the company of family and friends to local assistance provided through various professions or relations.

Spa sociability, which has been the focus of a great majority of cultural studies on spas, was therefore not independent of healthcare and sickness, even as it was thriving in many directions throughout the century. The development of local social dynamics around spas, accompanied by gambling and the development of urban spaces for the consumption of leisure, has traditionally been put forward as a mode of proto-tourism announcing the leisurely sociability of seaside resorts. The key notion recurrently invoked to account for the chronological evolution of spa sociability is the commercialisation of leisure. As I argued in the introduction to this book, although the rise of urban developments in the spas of the first and second categories is undeniable, the commercialisation of leisure fails to account for the diversity of modes of sociability which have been recently unearthed by critics and historians, from 'female alliances' to alternative political centres.

Throughout the book, led by the flow of the 'murky waters' paradigm, I have studied spa sociability through the literary representation of spas. Spas, I argue in chapter 3, were seen as ambivalent places at the crossroads of the opportunity for social improvement and the possibilities of sexual encounters and gender play. I thus shifted the focus of literary criticism from the consumption of leisure and social display to a darker, yet more playful paradigm of spa sociability that enabled social conventions to be probed and poked. Such is, one might argue, simply a function in literature in any given society, yet what seems more specific to eighteenth-century larger spa towns is that coincidence of extreme regulation, as the days were scheduled from drinking in the morning to dancing late afternoon, and ephemerality. In spa towns, the sense of a season was not restricted to the *Beau Monde* Hanna Greig describes in her book on the landed aristocracy who came to London for the political season before going back to their country houses.[4] Added to the vulnerability of sickness, the sense of an intense, ephemeral time was shared by all visitors coming from various social and geographical backgrounds.

Some changes in the social organisation of first- and second-category spa towns can still be outlined throughout the century. As Phyllis Hembry has shown, patronage seemed to diminish gradually throughout the century.[5] Capitalistic ventures burgeoned in spa towns, from small pump rooms and new assembly rooms to the paved alleyways of urban promenades adorned with shopping windows in Tunbridge and Cheltenham. Spa towns were invested in by a multiplicity of local actors and maintained by a crowd of merchants, doctors, lodgers and bath managers. Among the multiplicity of actors, as Rachael Johnson and John Eglin have pointed out, masters of ceremonies became emblematic figures of major spas towards the middle of the century.[6] Poems, plays, prints, periodicals and novels pictured masters of ceremonies as major power figures of local politics, whose influence on visitors and internal town politics could mend manners, launder money, or both.

A chronological account of spa politics and economics in the long eighteenth century would most probably revolve around gambling and investing schemes. In the light of the revolutionary dealings starting with the controversy around the ridottos of the Belgian town of Spa, gambling started to be addressed as a political point of tension and potential health issue after the 1760s. From the 1780 Epsom horse races to the persistence of private gambling after the laws criminalising gambling were passed in 1745, spa towns remained a favourite background for the depiction of gambling parties in periodicals, novels and satire as well as in the preventative literature that warned against the dangers of irretrievable debt. In the fifth chapter, I contend that the centrality of gambling in discourses on spas is part of a wider paradigm on the speculative investments in spa towns most emblematically exposed in Austen's unfinished novel *Sanditon*. As it focuses on the hubris of one visionary urban developer who builds his hopes on unfeasible urban schemes, *Sanditon* reflects on the magnetic power of spa towns and seaside resorts. Austen casts her acute eye on urban grandeur and cosmopolitan cultures in emergent rural towns luring young entrepreneurs with the last bright idea in disproportionate investments. A history of architectural and medical hubris and failure in spa towns could be written in a transhistorical perspective.[7] Investments in water make for narrative tensions around the myth of the commons and the myth of the placebo effect. In the context of a spa town, medical and architectural hubristic schemes are the epitome of capitalistic desires, as Maupassant's novel *Mont Oriol* will stage in the midst of the French water craze of the nineteenth century: making good money out of free resources.[8]

Cosmopolitanism is another overused chronological thread in the linear narrative of eighteenth-century spas. In this approach, early modern spas are considered attractive at national level until the 1750s, when the development of turnpikes and sea routes started to provide means for travellers from the continent to discover British spa towns and enjoy the season as was the fashion in Spa, Baden-Baden and Vichy. This historical narrative focuses on the largest spa towns of Britain competing with Bath yet never quite managing to supersede the queen of watering places. In chronological order of fame from Restoration to Regency, these famous spas towns can be listed as Epsom, Tunbridge Wells, Bristol Hotwells, Scarborough, Harrogate, Cheltenham, Moffat, Malvern and, finally, Brighthelmstone (or Brighton), a seaside resort also offering artificial mineral water. It is only fair to assume, considering the small number of French, German and Italian publications on British waters compared with British publications on continental spas, that the spas of Britain were not visited as much by continental Europeans as the spas of the continent were visited by the British. Yet it would be unfair to conclude that the recurrent representation of spa town cosmopolitanism in British literature is only a fantasised imperialist representation, as further research is needed on the matter. The fourth chapter, on pump room politics, presented how cosmopolitanism is evoked in periodicals and correspondences of the second half of the eighteenth century. Two opposite visions coexist: cosmopolitanism is either depicted as an object of threat and complaint or as a safe space for quiet diplomacy and transnational friendships, a cultural hub through which art, music and European ideas could be disseminated into Britain. On the continent, early modern and modern spa towns are regularly pictured as the laboratories of European culture, the 'cafes of Europe', as the European Historic Thermal Towns Association contends.[9]

Cosmopolitanism is certainly one of the features of self-representation of spa visitors and the spa towns themselves, yet this narrative tends to leave aside the centrality of sickness. What's more, in all its aspiration for foreign diversity, cosmopolitanism fails to embrace the colonial and imperial dimensions of spa towns. Clearly, the development of Irish, Scottish and Welsh spas, mentioned in the fourth chapter, needs to be addressed with the specific political stakes of each national culture, taking into account the environmental frame of each watering place. As Eric Jennings made visible for nineteenth-century France, the colonial politics of spa towns are overshadowed by the cosmopolitanism narrative.[10] In the same vein, Amanda Herbert's groundbreaking historical study of early modern spas as colonial spaces helps to complexify the narrative of spa towns and foreign diversity. As she gives an account of the discovery and appropriation of mineral waters in British colonies as well as in the internal work organisation and social networks of English spas, her book puts in perspective the social dynamics of spa town diversity by bringing to the table questions of race, the role of enslaved people and slave-owners, and the association of medicine and colonialism in early America and Jamaica.[11]

These representations are quite absent from Jane West's poem *The Humours of Brighthelmstone*, in which she depicts the seaside resort as the ideal setting for cosmopolitan encounters. She stages the polite company of French and Italians coming to the seaside resort and passing their time with the English. Published in 1788, this poem illustrates a shift in the idea of a watering place, as Brighton is not primarily a spa but a seaside resort. Around 1790, Margate, Ramsgate, Brighton and Peterhead were rising in fame while the medical discourse promoting fresh air and sea-bathing developed. Bathing machines – hand-driven cabins on wheels – offered those who could afford it the possibility of a refreshing plunge into the sea in all decency. Austen's *Sanditon* also illustrates the rise of the Regency seaside resort, an idea that may have been reinforced by the recent TV adaptation which cleverly combines the politics of leisure, colonialism and economics yet leaves aside the medical politics of sea water treatment.[12] Although there is no denying that seaside resorts did rise in fame at the end of the eighteenth century, partially to the detriment of spa towns, the idea that mineral waters were gradually forsaken in nineteenth-century Britain to give way to sea water is a partial view of the respective role of seaside resorts and spas.

I have argued in the introduction to this book that, in the long eighteenth century, seaside resorts were a type of watering place that was considered a sub-category of spas. They already existed earlier in the century, especially as some spas like Scarborough and Wellingborough allowed sick people to take both mineral waters and sea waters. Sylvia Mcintyre's account of the history of bottled waters confirms that sea water was even bottled and imported inland to be drunk.[13] Long before the end of the eighteenth century, sea water was part of the pharmacopoeia of water doctors, and it was analysed and compared with mineral waters, especially during the trend for cold water bathing of the 1730s. Similarly, interest in spa towns did not dwindle in the nineteenth century as a variety of methods of hydrotherapy treatment developed in several stations like Malvern and Leamington Spa, while small spas were still thriving in remote rural areas. The nineteenth-century water doctor Augustus Granville vividly depicts them in his comprehensive field study, *Spas of England*, published in 1841.

Perhaps one of the difficulties of writing a chronological history of spas is that spa towns are, in many ways, un-chronological. It is, I find, one of the unsettling aspects of Phyllis Hembry's 1991 book, which remains nonetheless a crucial reference for anyone attempting to launch into a study of British spas. As the reader advances in the chapters, the historical narrative seems to repeat itself in spite of the changes in the political and social context she describes.[14] In spa towns, time is not linear but cyclical, seasonal, ephemeral and, as promotional discourse on spas will later claim, extemporal. Going to a spa town meant retrieving oneself from the schedule of urban *and* rural life and accepting the regulations of a local schedule. As I argued above, seasons allowed enjoyment of the social conventions of a restricted community, with the safety of a way out at the end. In a suspended timeframe, the sick would enjoy rest and the benefits of a longer cure, which even contemporary hydrotherapy doctors insisted on, as they noted that treatments were usually effective three weeks into the cure.[15]

Even now, as some spa towns seem to be frozen in the promotional display of heritage culture, spas claim to provide a timeless experience, an idea already present in the 1728 lyrics of a song on the Irish spa at Ballyspellan:[16]

> THRO' all these parts
> Death throws no darts,
> No sexton's here a knelling;
> Come, judge and try,
> You'll never die,
> But live at BALLYSPELLIN.[17]

An answer to the song, regularly attributed to Swift and published in 1728, is more in line with the murky stream of this book. This second song starts where this book ends, bringing the spa down to earthly matters:

> How e'er you bounce,
> I here pronounce
> Your Med'cine is repelling
> Your Water's Mud,
> And Sowrs the Blood,
> When drank at *Ballyspellin*.[18]

Notes

1 J. Shaw, *Miracles in Enlightenment England* (New Haven, CT: Yale University Press, 2006).
2 Nicoud, 'Les médecins italiens'.
3 Borsay, *Medicine and Charity in Georgian Bath*; see the appendix for a map of eighteenth-century British spas by category.
4 Greig, *The Beau Monde*.
5 Hembry, *The English Spa*.
6 Johnson, 'Spas and seaside resorts in Kent'; Eglin, *The Imaginary Autocrat*.

7 For a discussion of Hardin's 'tragedy of the commons', see S. J. B. Cox, 'No tragedy of the commons', *Environmental Ethics*, 7:1 (1985), 49–61; C. Borch and M. Kornberger, *Urban Commons: Rethinking the City* (New York: Routledge, 2015). On the myth of placebo response see A. Harrington (ed.), *The Placebo Effect: An Interdisciplinary Exploration* (Cambridge, MA: Harvard University Press, 1997).

8 G. de Maupassant, *Mont-Oriol* ([1885]; Paris: Gallimard, 2002).

9 The EHTTA is an international society devoted to preserving and promoting the cultural and architectural heritage of grand spa towns, and cosmopolitanism is a key feature of its argument.

10 Jennings, *Curing the Colonizers*.

11 A. Herbert, *Water Works: Faith, Public Health, and Medicine in the British Atlantic* (forthcoming 2022).

12 *Sanditon* (Red Planet Pictures, Independent Television, 2019).

13 Mcintyre, 'The mineral water trade'.

14 Hembry, *The English Spa*.

15 In a roundtable on contemporary French spa medicine (*thermalisme*) which brought together historians, sociologists and medical doctors working in spas, the latter insisted on the importance of the three-week cure. They argued that mineral water treatment was a slow treatment, combining the effect of time with the patient, repetitive application of water and other water-based forms of care. ("La médecine thermale entre cure et care", March, 17, 2021. Institut La Personne en Médecine.)

16 Borsay explains that the Georgian spa town 'provided an opportunity to escape from the pressures of the present, to establish a sense of continuity and therefore of personal and collective identity, and to celebrate several of the defining myths of western culture'. Borsay, *The Image of Georgian Bath*, p. 348.

17 This poem was probably first printed on a broadside, and it was reprinted in a miscellany: *The Flower-Piece* (Dublin: Walthoe, 1731), pp. 36–9. It has regularly been attributed to Sheridan (see, for example, *Works of Swift*, 1801).

18 J. Swift, *An answer to the Ballyspellin Ballad* (Dublin: Faulkner, 1728).

Appendix: Maps of eighteenth-century spas by category and by area

A note on the maps

The following spas have been classified by the categories presented in the introduction ('putting spas on the map, over- and underground') according to their size and use.

The maps result from an inventory drawn from primary and secondary sources, all listed in the bibliography. Here is a selected list of sources: a more detailed data paper will be published elsewhere, with the list of all mineral waters, the location, type of water, sources and dates of use, but the list is too long to be published here.

Selected list of short-titled references for the maps (chronological order)

Primary sources

Allen, B., *Natural History of the Mineral-Waters*, 1711.

Short, T., *Natural, Experimental, and Medicinal History of the Mineral Waters Derbyshire, Lincolnshire, and Yorkshire*, 1734.

Short, T., *An Essay towards a Natural, Experimental, and Medicinal History of the Principle Mineral Waters*, 1740.

Linden, D. W., *A Treatise on the Origin, Nature, and Virtues of Chalybeat Waters*, 1752.

Rutty, J., *A Methodical Synopsis of Mineral Waters*, 1757.

Short, T., *A General Treatise on Various Cold Mineral Waters in England*, 1765.

Monro, D., *A Treatise on Mineral Waters*, 1770.
Andrews, J., *Historical Atlas of England*, 1797.

Secondary sources

Hembry, P., *The English Spa*, 1990.
Walsham, A., 'Reforming the waters', 1999. (I did not record all the spas mentioned in this article as some were no longer active in the eighteenth century.)
Durie, A., 'Medicine, health and economic development', 2003.
Kelly, J., '"Drinking the waters"', 2008.
Curl, J. S., *Spas, Wells and Pleasure-Gardens*, 2010.

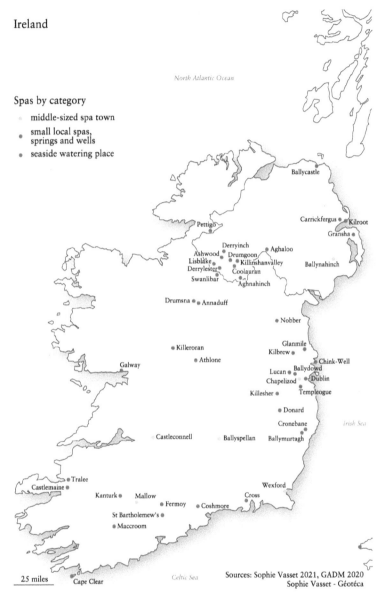

Figure A1 Spas by category in the long eighteenth century – Ireland

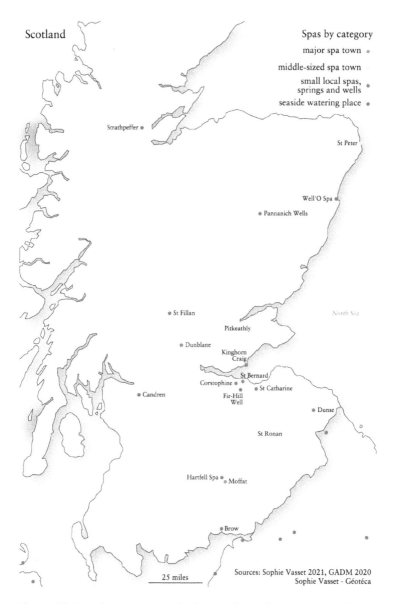

Figure A2 Spas by category in the long eighteenth century – Scotland

Wales

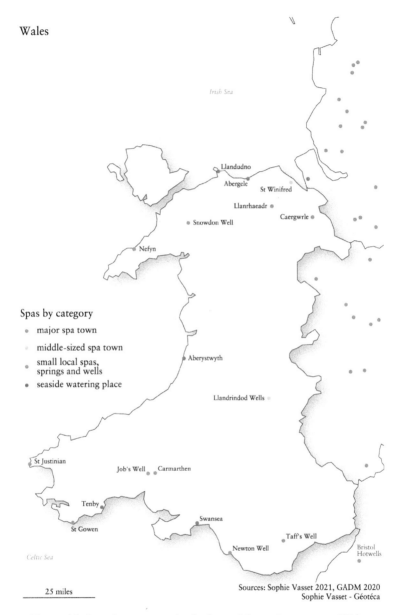

Figure A3 Spas by category in the long eighteenth century – Wales

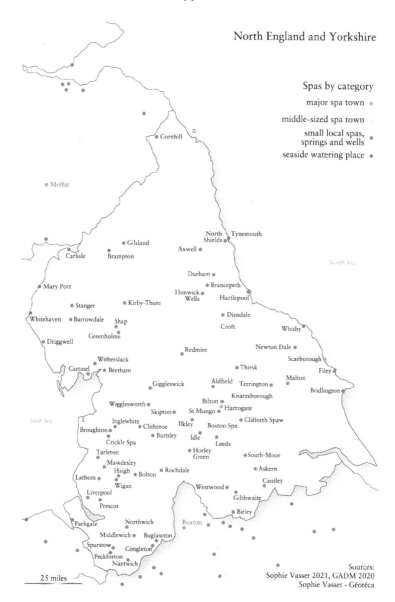

Figure A4 Spas by category in the long eighteenth century – North England and Yorkshire

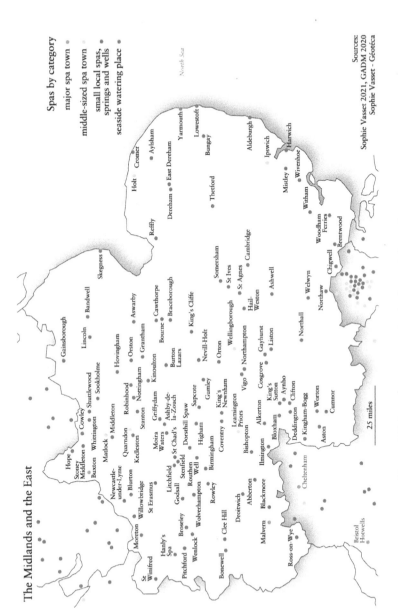

Figure A5 Spas by category in the long eighteenth century – The Midlands and the East

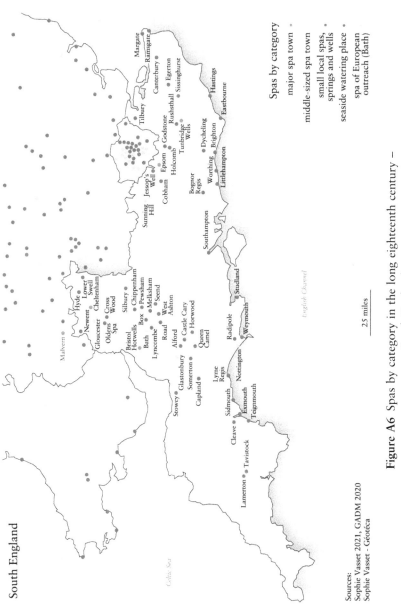

Figure A6 Spas by category in the long eighteenth century – South England

Bibliography

Primary sources

Adair, J. Makittrick, *Medical Cautions, for the Consideration of Invalids; Those Especially Who Resort to Bath: Containing Essays on Fashionable Diseases; Dangerous Effects of Hot and Crowded Rooms; Regimen of Diet, &c. An Enquiry into the Use of Medicine During a Course of Mineral Waters; an Essay on Quacks, Quack Medicines, and Lady Doctors* (Bath: R. Cruttwell, 1786).

Agricola, G., *De Re Metallica: Translated from the First Latin Edition of 1556 / by Herbert Clark Hoover and Lou Henry Hoover* (New York: Dover, 1950).

Allen, B., *The Natural History of the Mineral-Waters of Great-Britain* (London: W. Innys, 1711).

Andrews, J., *Historical Atlas of England: Physical, Political, Astronomical, Civil and Ecclesiastical, Biographical, Naval, Parliamentary, and Geographical; Ancient and Modern; from the Deluge to the Present Time in Which Are Described Its Minerals, Curiosities, Inland Fisheries and Navigation, Commerce, Peerages, Noblemen and Gentlemen's Seats* (London: Smeeton, 1797).

Anon., *A Description of St. Winefred's Well, at Holy-Well in Flintshire, North Wales* (Liverpool: Nevett, 1784).

Anon., *A Gentleman's Tour through Monmouthshire and Wales, in the Months of June and July* (London: T. Evans, 1794).

Anon., 'A Letter from *Tunbridge* to a friend in *London*; being a character of the Wells and the company there', in *A Pacquet from Will's* (London: S. Briscoe, 1705), pp. 159–87.

Anon., *A Morning Ramble or Islington Wells Burlesqued* (London: George Croom, 1684).

Anon., *A Treatise on the Nature, Properties, and Medicinal Uses of the Waters of Pyrmont, Spa, and Seltzers. Also of the Malvern Waters, from Dr. Wall's Observation* (London: W. Owen, 1762).

Anon., 'An Examination of the *Glastonbury* Waters', *The Gentleman's Magazine: and historical chronicle*, January 1736–December 1833; September 1751; 21, p. 416.

Anon., *An Exclamation from Tunbridge and Epsom against the Newfound Wells at Islington* (London: J. How, 1684).

Anon., *Hampstead-Wells* (London, 1706).

Anon., *May-Day: Or, The Original of Garlands. A Poem* (London: J. Roberts, 1720).

Anon., *The Bath, Bristol, Tunbridge and Epsom Miscellany* (London: T. Dormer, 1735).

Anon., *The Diseases of Bath. A Satire* (London: J. Roberts, 1737).

Anon., *The Flower-Piece* (Dublin: Walthoe, 1731).

Anon., *The Grand Mystery, or Art of Meditating over an House of Office, Restor'd and Unveil'd; after the Dublin Edition: Published by the Ingenious Dr. S-Ft* (London: booksellers of London and [Westminster], 1726).

Anon., *The Humours of London, a Choice Collection of Songs* (London: J. Cooke, 1770).

Anon., *The Life of Pamela* (London: C. Whitefield, 1741).

Anon., *The Scarborough Miscellany* (London: J. Roberts, 1732).

Anon., *The Scarborough Miscellany for the Year 1733* (London: J. Wilford, 1734).

Anon., *The Scarborough Miscellany for the Year 1734* (London: J. Wilford, 1734).

Anon., *The Tunbridge and Bath Miscellany for the Year 1714* (London: E. Curll, 1714).

Anon., *The Tunbridge Wells Guide* (Tunbridge Wells: J. Sprange, 1780).

Anon., *Trifles from Harrogate* (Harrogate: Hargrove, 1797).

Anon., *Tunbrigialia, or the Tunbrige Miscellany for the year 1722* (London: A. Moore, 1722).

Anon., *Tunbrigialia, or the Tunbrige Miscellany for the year 1730* (London: A. Moore, 1730).

Anon., *Water poetry: A collection of verses written at several public places, most of them never before printed* (London: G. Pearch, 1771).

Anstey, C., *The New Bath Guide*, ed. A. Cossic (1766; London: Peter Lang, 2010).

Austen, J., *Northanger Abbey* (1817, New York: Norton, 2004).

Austen, J., *Persuasion* (1817; Oxford: Oxford University Press, 2004).

Austen, J., *Sanditon* (Oxford: Oxford University Press, 2019).

Baker, T., *Tunbridge-Walks: Or, the Yeoman of Kent* (London: B. Lintott, 1703).

Baley, W., *A Briefe Discours of Certain Bathes or Medicinall Waters in the Countie of Warwicke Neere Vnto a Village Called Newnam Regis* (London, 1587).

Barbauld, A. L., 'Letter on Watering Places', in *The Annual Register, or, a View of the History, Politics, and Literature for the Year 1796* (London: T. Burton, 1800).

Batt, J., 'Eighteenth-century verse miscellanies', *Literature Compass*, 9:6 (2012), 394–405.

Booth, J., *Epigrams, Ancient and Modern* (London: Booth, 1865).

Bordeu, T. de, *Recherches sur les maladies chroniques, leurs rapports avec les maladies aiguës, leurs périodes, leur nature, et sur la manière dont on les traite aux eaux minérales de Barèges et des autres sources de l'Aquitaine* (Paris: Ruaut, 1775).

Buchan, W., *Cautions Concerning Cold Bathing, and Drinking the Mineral Waters. Being an Additional Chapter to the Ninth Edition of His Domestic Medicine* (London: A. Strahan, 1786).

Burges, J., *An Essay on the Waters and Air of Ballispellan. With Their Various Properties and Uses* (Dublin: W. Wilmot, 1725).

Burnby, J., *An Address to the People of England; on the Increase of Their Poor Rates* (London: J. Dodsley, Pall-Mall, 1780).

Burnby, J., *An Historical Description of the Metropolitical Church of Christ, Canterbury* (Canterbury: Simmons and Kirkby, 1772).

Burnby, J., *Summer Amusement: Or, Miscellaneous Poems: Inscribed to the Frequenters of Margate, Ramsgate, Tunbridge Wells, Brighthelmstone, Southampton, Cheltenham, Weymouth, Scarborough* (London: J. Dodsley, Pall-Mall, 1772).

Burney, F., *Evelina, or the History of a Young Lady's Entrance into the World* (1778; Oxford: Oxford World's Classics, 2002).

Cadogan, W., *A Dissertation on the Gout and All Chronic Diseases, Jointly Considered as Proceeding from the Same Causes; What Those Causes Are; and a Rational and Natural Method of Cure Proposed* (London: T. Bradford, 1771).

Colman, G., *The spleen, or, Islington Spa: a Comick Piece* (London: T. Becket, 1776).

Countryman, *A journey to Llandrindod Wells, in Radnorshire* (London: Cooper, 1746).

Dancer, T., *A Short Dissertation on the Jamaica Bath Waters* (Kingston: D. Douglass & A. Aikman, 1784).

Davies, J., *A Short Description of the Waters at Glastonbury* (Exon: Andrew Brice, 1751).

Davies, M., *The recantation of Mr. Pollet, a Roman priest* (London [?], 1705).

Defoe, D., *A Tour through the Whole Island of Great Britain* ([1724–26]; London: Penguin Books, 1986).

Defoe, D., *The Fortunes and Misfortunes of the Famous Moll Flanders* ([1722]; Oxford: Oxford University Press, 1971).

Defoe, D., and R. Holmes, *Defoe on Sheppard and Wild* (London: Harper Perennial, 2004).

Fielding, H., *The Life of Mr Jonathan Wild the Great* ([1734]; London: Hesperus, 2004).

Fiennes, C., *The Illustrated Journeys of Celia Fiennes 1685–c1712*, ed. C. Morris (London: McDonald, 1982).

Fleetwood, W., *The Life and Miracles of St. Wenefrede* (London: Buckley, 1713).

Floyer, J., *Psychrolousia: Or, the History of Cold Bathing: Both Ancient and Modern* (London: Smith and Walford, 1706).

Floyer, J., *The Ancient Psychrolousia Revived: or, an Essay to Prove Cold Bathing Both Safe and Useful* (London: Walford, 1702).

Fuller, F., *Medicina Gymnastica: Or, a Treatise Concerning the Power of Exercise* (London: Knaplock, 1705).

Goding, G., *Norman's History of Cheltenham* (London: Longman, 1863).

Goldsmith, O., *The life of Richard Nash, of Bath* (London: J. Newbery, 1762).

Grew, N., *Tractatus de Salis Cathartici Amari in Aquis Ebeshamensibus* (London: S. Smith, 1695).

Guidott, T., *A true and exact account of Sadlers Well, or, the new mineral-waters lately found out at Islington* (London: T. Malthus, 1684).

Hippocrates, *Upon Air: Water, and Situation*, ed. F. Clifton (London: J. Watts, 1734).

Hoffmann, F., *New experiments and observations upon mineral waters: directing their farther use for the preservation of health, and the cure of diseases*, trans. P. Shaw (London: J. Osborn, 1731).

J. E., *The Humours of Harrogate* (London: J. Pridden, 1763).

Layard, D. P., *An Account of the Somersham Water: In the County of Huntingdon* (London: S. N., 1767).

Lesage, A.-R., *Histoire de Gil Blas de Santillane* (1715–35; Paris: A. Colin, 2002).

Lesage, A.-R., *The Adventures of Gil Blas of Santillane. A New Translation, by the Author of Roderick Random* (London: Rivington, 1747).

Linden, D. W., *A Medicinal and Experimental History and Analysis of the Hanlys-Spa Saline, Purging, and Chalybeate Waters, near Shrewsbury* (London: John Everingham, 1768).

Linden, D. W., *A Treatise on the Origin, Nature, and Virtues of Chalybeat Waters: and Natural Hot Baths. with a Description of Several Mineral Waters in England and in Germany* (London: T. Osborne, 1752).

Linden, D. W., *A Treatise on the Three Medicinal Mineral Waters at Llandrindod: In Radnorshire, South Wales* (London: J. Everingham, 1756).

Linden, D. W., *Directions for [the Use] of That Extraordinary Mineral-Water, Commonly Called, Berry's Shadwell-Spaw: In Sun-Tavern-Fields, Shadwell, near London. More Especially, in the Several Distempers Wherein It Has Proved by Experience, of the Greatest Efficacy and Success (London: printed for the proprietor; and to be had at the Shadwell-Spaw, in Sun-Tavern-Fields, Shadwell; and F. Jones, Mineral Water Purveyor to His Royal Highness the Duke of Cumberland, in Tavistock-Street, Covent-Garden, 1749).*

Lockman, J., *The Humours of New Tunbridge Wells at Islington: A Lyric Poem* (London: J. Roberts, 1734).

Lucas, C., *An Essay on Waters: In three parts. Treating, I. Of simple waters. II. Of cold, Medicated Waters. III. Of Natural Baths* (London: A. Millar, 1756).

Marcet, A. G., and W. Saunders, *A Chemical Account of the Brighton Chalybeate* (London: Phillips & Fardon, 1805).

Marivaux, P. de, *La dispute: comédie en prose en 1 acte* (Paris: N.-B. Duchesne, 1758).

Mavor, W. Fordyce, *The Cheltenham guide; or, Memoirs of the B-n-r-d family continued: In a series of poetical epistles* (London: Harrison, 1781).

Meighan, C., *A Treatise of the Nature and Powers of Bareges's Baths and Waters* (London, 1742).

Monro, D., *A Treatise on Mineral Waters* (London: G. Nicol, 1770).

Montagu, E. Robinson, *The Letters of Mrs. Elizabeth Montagu: With Some of the Letters of Her Correspondents* (London: Wells and Lilly, 1825).

Montagu, M. Wortley, *The Letters and Works of Lady Mary Wortley Montagu* (Cambridge: Cambridge University Press, 2011).

Moreau, S., *A Tour to Cheltenham Spa* (Bath: R. Cruttwell, 1783).

'News', *The Morning Herald*, 2 August 1785.

Nisbet, W. *A Medical Guide for the Invalid to the Principal Watering Places of Great Britain: Containing a View of the Medicinal Effects of Water* (London: Highly, 1804).

O'Keeffe, J., *The Irish Mimic; Or Blunders at Brighton* (London: T. N. Longman, 1795).

Oliver, W., *A Practical Dissertation on Bath Waters* (Bath: James Leake, 1737).

Oliver, W., *A Practical Essay on the Use and Abuse of Warm Bathing in Gouty Cases* (Bath: Hawes and Co., 1751).

Pennant, T., *A Tour in Wales* (Dublin: Sleater, 1779).

Pierce, R., *Bath Memoirs, or, Observations in Three and Forty Years Practice at the Bath, What Cures Have Been There Wrought (Both by Bathing and Drinking These Waters)* (Bristol: Hammond, 1697).

Rawlins, T., *Tunbridge-Wells: or A days Courtship* (London: H. Rogers, 1678).

Richardson, J., *The Great Folly, Superstition, and Idolatry, of Pilgrimages in Ireland; Especially of that to St. Patrick's Purgatory* (Dublin: J. Hyde, 1727).

Richardson, S., *The History of Sir Charles Grandison* ([1753]; London: Oxford University Press, 1972).

Roberts, P. (ed.), *The Diary of Sir David Hamilton, 1709–14* (Oxford: Clarendon Press, 1975).

Rowzee, L., *The Queenes Vvelles That Is, a Treatise of the Nature and Vertues of Tunbridge Water. Together, with an Enumeration of the Chiefest Diseases* (London: Imprinted by Iohn Dawson, 1632).

Rowzee, L., *Tunbridge Wells* (London: J. Roberts, 1725).

Rush, B., *Directions for the Use of the Mineral Water and Cold Bath, at Harrogate, near Philadelphia* (Philadelphia: Melchior Steiner, 1786).

Rush, B., *Experiments and Observations on the Mineral Waters of Philadelphia, Abington, and Bristol, in the Province of Pennsylvania* (Philadelphia: J. Humphreys, 1773).

Russell, R., *A Dissertation Concerning the Use of Sea Water in Diseases of the Glands* (Oxford: J. Fletcher, 1753).

Rutty, J., *A Methodical Synopsis of Mineral Waters, Comprehending the Most Celebrated Medicinal Waters, Both Cold and Hot, of Great-Britain, Ireland, France, Germany, and Italy, and Several Other Parts of the World* (London: W. Johnston, 1757).

Rutty, J., *An Essay towards a Natural, Experimental and Medicinal History of the Mineral Waters of Ireland* (Dublin, 1757).

Sanders, R., *The Complete English Traveller: or, a new Survey and Description of England and Wales* (London: J. Cooke, 1771).

Shadwell, T., *Epsom-Wells: A comedy* (London: H. Herringman, 1673).

Shaw, P., *An Enquiry into the Contents: Virtues, and Uses, of the Scarborough Spaw-Waters: with The Method of examining any other Mineral-Water* (London: F. Gyles, 1734).

Sheridan, Richard Brinsley, *A Trip to Scarborough: A Comedy* (Dublin: R. Marchbank, 1781).

Short, T., *A General Treatise on Various Cold Mineral Waters in England, but more Particularly on those at Harrogate, Thorp-Arch, Dorst-Hill, Wigglesworth, Nevill-Holt, and Others of the like Nature. With Their Principles, Virtues and Uses* (London: A. Millar, 1765).

Short, T., *An Essay towards a Natural, Experimental, and Medicinal History of the Principle Mineral Waters of Cumberland, Northumberland, Westmoreland, Bishop-prick of Durham, Lancashire, Cheshire, Staffordshire, Shropshire, Worcestershire, Glocestershire, Warwickshire, Northamptonshire, Leicestershire, and Nottinghamshire* (Sheffield: J. Garnet, 1740).

Short, T., *The Contents, Virtues, and Uses of Nevil-Holt Spaw-Water* (London: Corbett, 1749).

Short, T., *The Natural, Experimental and Medicinal History of the Mineral waters of Derbyshire, Lincolnshire, and Yorkshire* (London: F. Gyles, 1734).

Smith, J., *Observations on the Use and Abuse of the Cheltenham Waters* (Cheltenham: Harward, 1786).

Smollett, T., *An Essay on the External Use of Water* (London: M. Cooper, 1752).

Smollett, T., *The Expedition of Humphry Clinker* (1771; Oxford: Oxford World's Classics, 1998).

Swift, J., *An answer to the Ballyspellin Ballad* (Dublin: Faulkner, 1728).

The Bath Chronicle, 17 April 1794.

The Gentleman's Magazine, August 1751.

The Guardian, 90 (24 June 1713).

The Guardian, 174 (30 September 1713).

The Invalid, *Modern Refinement: A Satire* (Bath: S. Hazard, 1777).

The Invalid, *The Register of Folly: Or, Characters and Incidents at Bath and the Hot-Wells, in a Series of Poetical Epistles, by an Invalid* (London: F. Newbery, 1773).

The Morning Post, 25 July 1788.

Walker, A., *Fax Fonte Accensa, Fire out of Water: or, an Endeavour to kindle Devotion, from the Consideration of the Fountains God hath made* (London: Ranew, 1684).

Wall, J., *Experiments and Observations on the Malvern Waters* (1756; Worcester: R. Lewis, 1763).

Wesley, J., *Primitive Physick: or, an Easy and Natural Method of Curing Most Diseases* (London: Thomas Trye, 1747).

West, J., *The Humours of Brighthelmstone* (London: Scatcherd and Whitaker, 1788).

Wilmot, J., *The Complete Poems of John Wilmot, Earl of Rochester* (New Haven, CT: Yale University Press, 1968).

Wyndham, H. P., *A Gentleman's Tour through Monmouthshire and Wales, in the Months of June and July* (London: printed for T. Evans, 1794).

Secondary sources

Abate, M. A., *Tomboys: A Literary and Cultural History* (Philadelphia: Temple University Press, 2008).

Albert, B., *The Turnpike Road System in England: 1663–1840* (Cambridge: Cambridge University Press, 1972).

Anderson, R. G. W., *The Cradle of Chemistry: The Early Years of Chemistry at the University of Edinburgh* (Edinburgh: John Donald, 2015).

Andrew, D. T., *Aristocratic Vice: The Attack on Duelling, Suicide, Adultery, and Gambling in Eighteenth-Century England* (New Haven, CT: Yale University Press, 2013).

Andrews, J., and C. Lawlor, '"An exclusive privilege … to complain": framing fashionable diseases in the long eighteenth century', *Literature and Medicine*, 35:2 (2017), 239–69.

Bachelard, G., *Water and Dreams: An Essay on the Imagination of Matter* (Dallas, TX: Pegasus Foundation, 1983).

Barr, R., S. Kleiman-Lafon and S. Vasset (eds), *Bellies, Bowels and Entrails in the Eighteenth Century* (Manchester: Manchester University Press, 2018).

Benedict, B. M., 'Consumptive communities: commodifying nature in spa society', *The Eighteenth Century*, 36:3 (1995), 203–19.

Berry, S., 'Pleasure gardens in Georgian and Regency seaside resorts: Brighton, 1750–1840', *Garden History*, 28:2 (2000), 222–30.

Blackman, C., 'Walking Amazons: the development of the riding habit in England during the eighteenth century', *Costume*, 35:1 (January 2001), 47–58.

Bogart, D., 'Turnpike trusts, infrastructure investment, and the road transportation revolution in eighteenth-century England', *Journal of Economic History*, 65:2 (2005), 540–43.

Boisseuil, D., and M. Nicoud (eds), *Séjourner au bain: le thermalisme entre médecine et société, XIVe–XVIe siècle* (Lyon: Presses universitaires de Lyon, 2010).

Borsay, P., 'Health and leisure resorts', *The Cambridge Urban History of Britain* (Cambridge: Cambridge University Press, 2000), 775–803.

Borsay, A., *Medicine and Charity in Georgian Bath: A Social History of the General Infirmary, c. 1739–1830* (Aldershot: Ashgate, 1999).

Borsay, A., '"Persons of honour and reputation": the voluntary hospital in an age of corruption', *Medical History*, 35:3 (1991), 281–94.

Borsay, P., *The Image of Georgian Bath, 1700–2000: Towns, Heritage, and History* (Cambridge: Cambridge University Press, 2000).

Borsay, P., 'Town or country? British spas and the urban–rural interface', *Journal of Tourism History*, 4:2 (2012), 155–69.

Bricker, A. B., 'Who was "A. Moore"? The attribution of eighteenth-century publications with false and misleading imprints', *Papers of the Bibliographical Society of America*, 110:2 (June 2016), 181–214.

Brodie, A., 'Scarborough in the 1730s – spa, sea and sex', *Journal of Tourism History*, 4:2 (August 2012), 125–53.

Brown, M., 'Medicine, reform and the "end" of charity in early nineteenth-century England', *English Historical Review*, 124:511 (2009), 1353–88.

Buzon, C. and O. Richard-Pauchet (eds), *Littérature et voyages de santé* (Paris: Classiques Garnier, 2017).

Byrde, P., '"That frightful unbecoming dress": clothes for spa bathing at Bath', *Costume*, 21:1 (1987), 44–56.

Capdeville, V., and A. Kerhervé (eds), *British Sociability in the Long Eighteenth Century* (Woodbridge: The Boydell Press, 2019).

Carey, D., *Money and Political Economy in the Enlightenment* (Oxford: Voltaire Foundation, 2014).

Carey, D., and L. M. Festa, *Postcolonial Enlightenment: Eighteenth-Century Colonialism and Postcolonial Theory* (Oxford: Oxford University Press, 2009).

Castle, T., *Masquerade and Civilisation: The Carnivalesque in Eighteenth-Century English Culture and Fiction* (London: Methuen, 1986).

Chalus, E., 'Elite women, social politics, and the political world of late eighteenth-century England', *Historical Journal*, 43:3 (2000), 669–97.

Chalus, E., *Spaces of Sociability in Fashionable Society* (New York: Routledge, 2019).

Chambers, T., *Drinking the Waters: Creating an American Leisure Class at Nineteenth-Century Mineral Springs* (Washington, DC: Smithsonian Institution; Combined Academic, 2003).

Chiari, S., and S. Cuisinier-Delorme (eds), *Spa Culture and Literature in England, 1500–1800* (Basingstoke: Palgrave Macmillan, 2021).

Cohen, J. J., and L. Duckert, *Elemental Ecocriticism: Thinking with Earth, Air, Water, and Fire* (Minneapolis, MN: University of Minnesota Press, 2015).

Cole, L., 'Of mice and moisture: rats, witches, miasma, and early modern theories of contagion', *Journal for Early Modern Cultural Studies*, 10:2 (2010), 65–84.

Coley, N. G., '"Cures without care": "chymical physicians" and mineral waters in seventeenth-century English medicine', *Medical History*, 23:2 (1979), 191–214.

Coley, N. G., 'Physicians and the chemical analysis of mineral waters in eighteenth-century England', *Medical History*, 26:2 (1982), 123–44.

Coley, N. G., 'The preparation and uses of artificial mineral waters (ca. 1680–1825)', *Ambix*, 31:1 (1984), 32–48.

Colley, L., *Britons: Forging the Nation, 1707–1837* (New Haven, CT: Yale University Press, 2005).

Cooley, R. W., '"Sexy in a 'Tunbridge Wells' sort of way": a study in the literary iconography of place', *Journal for Early Modern Cultural Studies*, 15:1 (2015), 90–118.

Corbin, A., *Le ciel et la mer* (Paris: Bayard, 2005).

Cossic, A., 'Fashionable diseases in Georgian Bath: fiction and the emergence of a British model of spa sociability', *Journal for Eighteenth-Century Studies* 40 (2017), 537–53.

Cossic, A., and P. Galliou (eds), *Spas in Britain and in France in the Eighteenth and Nineteenth Centuries* (Newcastle: Cambridge Scholars Publishing, 2006).

Cottom, D., 'In the bowels of the novel: the exchange of fluids in the Beau Monde', *NOVEL: A Forum on Fiction*, 32:2 (1999), 157–86.

Curl, J. S., 'Spas and pleasure gardens of London, from the seventeenth to the nineteenth centuries', *Garden History*, 7:2 (1979), 27–68.

Curl, J. S., *Spas, Wells, and Pleasure-Gardens of London* (London: Historical, 2010).

Denbigh, K., *A Hundred British Spas: A Pictorial History* (London: Spa, 1981).

Derrida, J., 'La pharmacie de Platon', *La Dissémination* (Paris: Seuil, 1972).

Dhraief, B., E. Négrel and J. Ruimi (eds), *Théâtre et charlatans dans l'Europe moderne* (Paris: Presses Sorbonne Nouvelle, 2018).

Dickie, S., *Cruelty and Laughter: Forgotten Comic Literature and the Unsentimental Eighteenth Century* (Chicago: University of Chicago Press, 2011).

Doron, C.-O., 'The experience of "risk": genealogy and transformations', in A. Burgess, A. Alemanno and J. Zinn (eds), *Routledge Handbook of Risk Studies* (New York: Routledge, 2016), pp. 35–44.

Droixhe, D., *Une histoire des Lumières au pays de Liège: livres, idées, société* (Liège: Editions de l'ULG, 2007).

Durie, A., 'Medicine, health and economic development: promoting spa and seaside resorts in Scotland c. 1750–1830', *Medical History*, 47:2 (2003), 195–216.

Eglin, J., *The Imaginary Autocrat: Beau Nash and the Invention of Bath* (London: Profile Books, 2005).

Evans, J., *Aphrodisiacs, Fertility and Medicine in Early Modern England* (Woodbridge: The Boydell Press, 2014).

Fawcett, T., 'Spa medicine: patients, practitioners and treatments in Stuart and Georgian Bath', www.spamedicine.talktalk.net/main.htm (accessed 25 February 2020).

Fennetaux, A., and B. Burman, *The Pocket: A Hidden History of Women's Lives, 1660–1900* (New Haven, CT: Yale University Press, 2019).

Fissell, M. E., 'Introduction: women, health, and healing in early modern Europe', *Bulletin of the History of Medicine*, 82:1 (2008), 1–17.

Flynn, C. H., *The Body in Swift and Defoe* (Cambridge: Cambridge University Press, 1990).

Forman Cody, L., '"No cure, no money", or the invisible hand of quackery: the language of commerce, credit, and cash in eighteenth-century British medical advertisements', *Studies in Eighteenth-Century Culture*, 28 (1999), 103–30.

Foucault, M., 'Des espaces autres', *Empan*, 54:2 (2004), 12–19.

Foucault, M., 'Of other spaces', trans. J. Miskowiec, *Diacritics*, 16:1 (1986), 22–7.

Gallagher, N., *Itch, Clap, Pox: Venereal Disease in the Eighteenth-Century Imagination* (New Haven, CT: Yale University Press, 2018).

Gentilcore, D., *Medical Charlatanism in Early Modern Italy* (Oxford: Oxford University Press, 2006).

Glover, K., 'Polite society and the rural resort: the meanings of Moffat Spa in the eighteenth century', *Journal for Eighteenth-Century Studies*, 34:1 (2011), 65–80.

Granville, A. B., *Spas of England and Principal Sea-Bathing Places* (Bath: Adams & Dart, 1971).

Greig, H., *The Beau Monde: Fashionable Society in Georgian London* (Oxford: Oxford University Press, 2013).

Gronim, S. S., 'Imagining inoculation: smallpox, the body, and social relations of healing in the eighteenth century', *Bulletin of the History of Medicine*, 80:2 (2006), 247–68.

Guerrini, A., '"A club of little villains": rhetoric, professional identity and medical pamphlet wars', in M. Mulvey Roberts and R. Porter (eds), *Literature and Medicine during the Eighteenth Century* (New York: Routledge, 1993), pp. 226–44.

Habermas, J., *The Structural Transformation of the Public Sphere: An Inquiry into a Category of Bourgeois Society* (1963; Cambridge, MA: MIT Press, 1989).

Hailwood, M., *Alehouses and Good Fellowship in Early Modern England* (Woodbridge: The Boydell Press, 2014).

Hamlin, C., 'Chemistry, medicine, and the legitimization of English spas, 1740–1840', *Medical History Supplement*, 10 (1990), 67–81.

Harcup, J. W., *The Malvern Water Cure: Or Victims for Weeks in Wet Sheets* (Malvern: Winsor Fox Photos, 1992).

Harley, D., 'A sword in a madman's hand: professional opposition to popular consumption in the waters literature of southern England and the Midlands, 1570–1870', *Medical History Supplement*, 10 (1990), 48–55.

Harouel, J.-L., 'De François Ier au pari en ligne, histoire du jeu en France', *Pouvoirs*, 139:4 (2011), 5–14.

Hart, G., *History of Cheltenham* (Gloucester: Sutton Publishing, 1981).

Haslam, F., *From Hogarth to Rowlandson: Medicine in Art in Eighteenth-Century Britain* (Liverpool: Liverpool University Press, 1996).

Hembry, P., M. Cowie and E. E. Cowie, *British Spas from 1815 to the Present: A Social History* (London: Athlone Press, 1997).

Hembry, P. M., *The English Spa, 1560–1815: A Social History* (London: Athlone Press, 1990).

Herbert, A. E., *Female Alliances: Gender, Identity, and Friendship in Early Modern Britain* (New Haven, CT: Yale University Press, 2014).

Herbert, A. E., 'Gender and the spa: space, sociability and self at British health spas, 1640–1714', *Journal of Social History*, 43:2 (2009), 361–83.

Hudelet, H., D. Monaghan and J. Wiltshire, *The Cinematic Jane Austen* (London: McFarland, 2009).

Hurley, A. E., 'A conversation of their own: watering-place correspondence among the Bluestockings', *Eighteenth-Century Studies*, 40:1 (2006), 1–21.

Jarrassé, D., *Deux mille ans de thermalisme* (Clermont-Ferrand: Presses Blaise Pascal, 1996).

Jennings, E. T., *Curing the Colonizers: Hydrotherapy, Climatology, and French Colonial Spas* (Durham, NC: Duke University Press, 2006).

Johnson, R., 'The Venus of Margate: fashion and disease at the seaside', *Journal for Eighteenth-Century Studies*, 40:4 (2017), 587–602.

Johnson, R. M., 'Spas and seaside resorts in Kent, 1660–1820' (PhD Thesis, University of Leeds, 2013).

Katritzky, M. A., *Women, Medicine and Theatre, 1500–1750: Literary Mountebanks and Performing Quacks* (Aldershot: Ashgate, 2007).

Kelly, J., '"Drinking the waters": balneotherapeutic medicine in Ireland, 1660–1850', *Studia Hibernica*, 35 (2008), 99–146.

King, W. C., *Ambition: A History* (New Haven, CT: Yale University Press, 2013).

Kleiman-Lafon, S., and M. Louis-Courvoisier (eds), 'Les esprits animaux: 16e–21e siècles', *Épistémocritique*, 2018, p. 6, https://epistemocritique.org/category/ouvrages-en-ligne/actes-de-colloques/les-esprits-animaux/ (last consulted 13 April 2020).

Langham, M., *Buxton: A People's History* (Lancaster: Carnegie, 2001).

Laqueur, T. W., *Solitary Sex: A Cultural History of Masturbation* (New York: Zone Books, 2003).

Lefève, C., J.-C. Mino and N. Zaccaï-Reyners (eds), *Le soin: approches contemporaines* (Paris: Presses universitaires de France, 2016).

Levine, J., *Dr. Woodward's Shield: History, Science, and Satire in Augustan England* (Ithaca, NY: Cornell University Press, 1977).

Lewis, C. M. B., *Ladies and Gentlemen on Display: Planter Society at the Virginia Springs, 1790–1860* (Charlottesville, VA: University of Virginia Press, 2001).

Linn, T., *The Health Resorts of Europe* (London: H. Kimpton, 1894).

Long, K. P., *Gender and Scientific Discourse in Early Modern Culture* (New York: Routledge, 2016).

Lowndes, W., *The Royal Crescent in Bath: A Fragment of English Life* (Bristol: Redcliffe Press, 1981).

Mankin, R., 'La maladie comme triomphe de la nature? *My Own Life* de David Hume', in S. Vasset and A. Wenger (eds), 'Raconter la maladie au dix-huitième siècle', *Dix-Huitième Siècle*, 47 (2015), 181–96.

Mansel, P., 'Courts in exile: Bourbons, Bonapartes and Orléans in London, from George III to Edward VII', in D. Kelly and M. Cornick (eds), *A History of the French in London* (London: University of London Press, 2013), pp. 99–128.

March, F., 'La Mise en scène du mariage dans la comédie de la Restauration: vide rituel et anti-rites', *Revue de la Société d'études Anglo-Américaines des XVIIe et XVIIIe siècles*, 62 (2006), 51–66.

Marchal, H. (ed.), *Muses et Ptérodactyles: la poésie de la science de Chénier à Rimbaud* (Paris: Seuil, 2013).

Marshall, A., *The Practice of Satire in England, 1658–1770* (Baltimore, MD: Johns Hopkins University Press, 2013).

Mason, A., 'The "Political Knight Errant" at Bath: Charles Lucas's attack on the spa medical establishment in *An Essay on Waters* (1756)', *Journal for Eighteenth-Century Studies*, 36:1 (2013), 67–83.

McCarthy, W., *Anna Letitia Barbauld: Voice of the Enlightenment* (Baltimore, MD: Johns Hopkins University Press, 2008).

McCormack, R. A., '"An assembly of disorders": exploring illness as a motive for female spa-visiting at Bath and Tunbridge Wells throughout the long eighteenth century', *Journal for Eighteenth-Century Studies*, 40:4 (2017), 555–69.

Mcintyre, S., 'The mineral water trade in the eighteenth century', *Journal of Transport History*, 1 (1973), 1–19.

McKellar, E., 'Peripheral visions: alternative aspects and rural presences in mid-eighteenth-century London', *Art History*, 22:4 (1999), 495–513.

McMenemey, W. H., 'The water doctors of Malvern, with special mention to the years 1842 to 1872', *Proceedings of the Royal Society of Medicine*, 46:1 (1953), 5–12.

McNeil, P., 'Macaroni masculinities', *Fashion Theory*, 4:4 (2000), 373–403.

Mctague, J., 'Anti-Catholicism, incorrigibility and credulity in the warming-pan scandal of 1688–9', *Journal for Eighteenth-Century Studies*, 36:3 (2013), 433–48.

Meyer Spacks, P., *Gossip* (New York: Knopf, 1985).

Mitchell, P. D. (ed.), *Sanitation, Latrines and Intestinal Parasites in Past Populations* (Farnham: Ashgate, 2015).

Molinier, P., S. Laugier and P. Paperman (eds), *Qu'est-ce que le care? Souci des autres, sensibilité, responsabilité* (Paris: Payot, 2009).

Mullaney, S., 'Charles Lucas and medical legislation in eighteenth century Ireland', *Irish Journal of Medical Science*, 184:3 (2015), 555–6.

Murphy, S., 'Charles Lucas, Catholicism and Nationalism', *Eighteenth-Century Ireland / Iris an Dá Chultúr*, 8 (1993), 83–102.

Newman, W. R. and L. M. Principe, 'Alchemy vs. chemistry: the etymological origins of a historiographic mistake', *Early Science and Medicine*, 3:1 (1998), 32–65.

Nicoud, M., 'Les médecins italiens et le bain thermal à la fin du Moyen Âge', *Médiévales*, 21:43 (2002), 13–40.

O'Connell, A., 'Fashionable discourse of disease at the watering-places of literature, 1770–1820', *Journal for Eighteenth-Century Studies*, 40:4 (2017), 571–86.

O'Connell, A., and C. Lawlor, 'Fashioning illness in the long eighteenth century', *Journal for Eighteenth-Century Studies*, 40:4 (2017), 491–501.

Oliver, R. C. B., 'Diederick Wessel Linden, M.D.', *National Library of Wales Journal*, 18 (1974), 241–67.

Oren-Magidor, D., *Infertility in Early Modern England* (Basingstoke: Palgrave Macmillan, 2017).

Osborne, B., and C. Weaver, *Aquae Britannia: Rediscovering 17th Century Springs and Spas: In the Footsteps of Celia Fiennes* (Malvern: Cora Weaver, 1996).

Pelling, M., with F. White, *Medical Conflicts in Early Modern London: Patronage, Physicians, and Irregular Practitioners, 1550–1640* (Oxford: Clarendon Press, 2003).

Pomata, G., 'Sharing cases: the *Observationes* in early modern medicine', *Early Science and Medicine*, 15:3 (2010), 193–236.

Porter, R., 'Introduction: the medical history of waters and spas', *Medical History Supplement*, (1990).

Porter, R., *Quacks: Fakers and Charlatans in English Medicine* (Stroud: Tempus, 2000).

Porter, R., and G. S. Rousseau, *Gout: The Patrician Malady* (New Haven, CT: Yale University Press, 1998).

Principe, L. M., 'Reflections on Newton's alchemy in light of the new historiography of alchemy', in J. E. Force and S. Hutton (eds), *Newton and Newtonianism: New Studies* (Dordrecht: Springer Netherlands, 2004), pp. 205–19.

Rauser, A., 'Hair, authenticity, and the self-made macaroni', *Eighteenth-Century Studies*, 38:1 (2004), 101–17.

Rediker, M., 'Liberty beneath the Jolly Roger', in M. Creighton and L. Norling (eds), *Iron Men, Wooden Women: Gender and Seafaring in the Atlantic World, 1700–1920* (Baltimore, MD: Johns Hopkins University Press, 1996), pp. 1–33.

Riley, J. C., and S. Smala, *The Eighteenth-Century Campaign to Avoid Disease* (London: Springer, 1987).

Rousseau, G. S., 'Matt Bramble and the Sulphur Controversy in the XVIIIth century: medical background of *Humphry Clinker*', *Journal of the History of Ideas*, 28:4 (1967), 577–89.

Rousseau, G. S., *Nervous Acts: Essays on Literature, Culture, and Sensibility* (Basingstoke: Palgrave Macmillan, 2004).

Sabor, P., and T. Keymer (eds), *The Pamela Controversy: Criticisms and Adaptations of Samuel Richardson's Pamela, 1740–1750* (London: Pickering & Chatto, 2001).

Sahai, A., J. Abbaraju, B. Challacombe, I. Dickinson and S. Sriprasad, 'Urine therapy: from the ancient remedy of Shivambu Kalpa to modern times', *BJU International*, 103 (2009), 52.

Sanchez, J.-C., 'Eaux d'arquebusades et médecine thermale militaire dans les Pyrénées centrales (XVIe–XVIIIe siècles)', *Revue de Comminges* (2017), 257–85.

Savani, G., 'The lure of the past: ancient balneology at the turn of the eighteenth century', *Journal for Eighteenth-Century Studies*, 43:4 (2020), 433–45.

Scheid, J., et al. (eds), *Le thermalisme: approches historiques et archéologiques d'un phénomène culturel et médical* (Paris: CNRS Éditions, 2019).

Schwartz, D. G., *Roll the Bones: The History of Gambling* (London: Gotham Books, 2006).

Scribner, R. W., 'The Reformation, popular magic, and the "disenchantment of the world"', in *Religion and Culture in Germany (1400–1800)* (Leiden: Brill, 2001), pp. 346–65.

Scribner, V., '"The happy effects of these waters": colonial American mineral spas and the British civilizing mission', *Early American Studies: An Interdisciplinary Journal*, 14:3 (2016), 409–49.

Shapin, S., *Leviathan and the Air-Pump: Hobbes, Boyle, and the Experimental Life* (Princeton, NJ: Princeton University Press, 1985).

Shaw, J., *Miracles in Enlightenment England* (New Haven, CT: Yale University Press, 2006).

Smith, L., 'A gentleman's mad-doctor in Georgian England: Edward Long Fox and Brislington House', *History of Psychiatry*, 19:2 (2008), 163–84.

Sonnet, A., *Des villes en quête de capacité politique: permanences et recompositions du gouvernement municipal du thermalisme: une analyse comparée Dax (Nouvelle-Aquitaine) – Bagnoles de l'Orne (Normandie)* (PhD Thesis, Bordeaux, 2020).

Sonnet, A., L. Lestrelin and M. Honta, 'La fabrique des territoires du "bien vieillir": recompositions du thermalisme et gouvernement municipal en France', *Lien social et Politiques*, 79 (2017), 53–72.

Southgate, B. C., '"The power of imagination": psychological explanations in mid-seventeenth-century England', *History of Science*, 30:3 (1992), 281–94.

Stobart, J., 'In search of a leisure hierarchy: English spa towns and their place in the eighteenth-century urban system', in P. Borsay, G. Hirschfelder and R. E. Mohrmann (eds), *New Directions in Urban History: Aspects of European Art, Health Tourism and Leisure since the Enlightenment* (Munich: Waxmann, 2000), pp. 19–40.

Strange, C. H., 'The history of Tunbridge Wells', in J. C. M. Given (ed.), *Royal Tunbridge Wells: Past and Present* (Tunbridge Wells: Courier, 1946), pp. 36–71.

Suarez, M. F., 'The production and consumption of the eighteenth-century poetic miscellany', in I. Rivers (ed.), *Books and Their Readers in Eighteenth-Century England: New Essays* (Leicester: Leicester University Press, 2001), pp. 217–51.

Sunderland, S., *Old London's Spas, Baths, and Wells* (London: Bales, 1915).

Tadié, A. and A.-L. Rey, 'Disputes et territoires épistémiques', *Revue de Synthèse*, 4:137 (2016), 223–6.

Tadié, A. and R. Scholar, *Fiction and the Frontiers of Knowledge in Europe, 1500–1800* (Farnham: Ashgate, 2010).

Totelin, L., 'The pharmakon: concept figure, image of transgression, poetic practice', *Bulletin of the History of Medicine*, 93:3 (2019), 453–4.

Toulalan, S., '"If Slendernesse Be the Cause of Unfruitfulnesse; You Must Nourish and Fatten the body": thin bodies and infertility in early modern England', in T. Loughran and G. Davis (eds), *Infertility in History, Science and Culture* (Basingstoke: Palgrave Handbooks, 2017), pp. 171–97.

Tregear, V., 'From Stilton to Vimto: using food history to re-think typical products in rural development', *Sociologia Ruralis*, 43:2 (2003), 91–107.

Turner, D. M., *Disability in Eighteenth-Century England: Imagining Physical Impairment* (New York: Routledge, 2012).

Vasset, S., *Décrire, prescrire, guérir: médecine et fiction dans la Grande-Bretagne du XVIIIe siècle* (Paris: Hermann, 2013).

Vasset, S., 'Female impotence or obstruction of the womb? French doctors picturing female sterility in the 1820s', in G. Davis and T. Loughran (eds), *The Palgrave Handbook of Infertility in History* (London: Palgrave Macmillan, 2017), pp. 311–33.

Vasset, S., 'Medical laughter and medical polemics: the Woodward–Mead quarrel and medical satire', *Revue de la Société d'études Anglo-Américaines des XVIIe et XVIIIe Siècles*, 70 (2013), 109–33.

Vasset, S., *The Physics of Language in* Roderick Random (Paris: Presses universitaires de France, 2009).

Vigarello, G., *Concepts of Cleanliness* (Cambridge: Cambridge University Press, 1988).

Vigarello, G., *Le Propre et le Sale* (Paris: Seuil, 1985).

Vigarello, G., J.-J. Courtine and A. Corbin, *Histoire du corps: volume 1, de la renaissance aux lumières* (Paris: Éditions du Seuil, 2005).

Walsham, A., 'Reforming the waters: holy wells and healing springs in Protestant England', *Studies in Church History Subsidia*, 12 (1999), 227–55.

Watson, C., *Miscellanies, Poetry, and Authorship, 1680–1800* (Basingstoke: Palgrave Macmillan, 2021).

Weingrod, S. L., *Spa Drama from Shadwell to Sheridan* (PhD Thesis, Brandeis University, 1990).

Weisz, G., 'Le thermalisme en France au XXe siècle', *Médecine/Sciences*, 18:1 (2002), 101–8.

Wenger, A., 'Lire l'onanisme: le discours médical sur la masturbation et la lecture féminines au XVIIIe siècle', *Clio: Femmes, Genre, Histoire*, 22 (2005), 227–43.

Whaley, L., *Women and the Practice of Medical Care in Early Modern Europe, 1400–1800* (Basingstoke: Palgrave Macmillan, 2011).

Whitaker, H. A., C. U. M. Smith and S. Finger (eds), *Brain, Mind and Medicine: Essays in Eighteenth-Century Neuroscience* (New York: Springer, 2007).

Willson, A. B., 'Alexander Pope's grotto in Twickenham', *Garden History*, 26:1 (1998), 31–59.

Wilson, P. K., '"Out of sight, out of mind?" The Daniel Turner–James Blondel dispute over the power of the maternal imagination', *Annals of Science* 49 (1992), 63–85.

Zanetti, F., 'Les thérapies alternatives de John Wesley', in M. Cottret (ed.), *Normes et déviances* (Paris: Les Éditions de Paris, 2007), pp. 160–76.

Index

accessibility 58
Acheron (river) 60–1
acid 106
Acqui Terme, Italy 21
Adair, James Makittrick (1728–1802) 101
Adam, Robert (1728–92) 227
Addison, William 24
adultery 122, 135–47, 173
Agricola, Giorgius (1494–1555)
    De Re Metallica 15
air 11, 21, 26, 50, 55–6, 62, 74, 106, 107–8, 138
alchemy 17, 203
Allen, Benjamin (1663–1738) 15, 18, 53, 71
aluminium 18, 19
Amelia Princess of Great Britain (1711–86) 131
Andrew, Donna T. 214, 221
Andrews, John (1736–1809) 8, 187
anecdotes 85, 172–3, 218–21
Anglicanism 195–6, 198–9, 202
animal spirits 55, 77n.6, 120
Anne, Queen of Great Britain (1665–1714) 58, 60, 67, 138
Anstey, Christopher (1724–1805) 27, 90, 177
    The New Bath Guide 27, 138
Anthropocene 31

Antiquity 20–1, 42n.76, 42n.77, 85, 171
apothecary 18, 47, 53, 110, 224
architecture 3, 4, 12, 29, 136, 227
Arnall, William [pseud. Walsingham] (d. 1736) 179
artificial mineral waters 19, 80n.93
assembly rooms 27, 130, 142, 153–4, 169, 174–5, 206n.45
attractivity 4, 57
Augusta Sophia, Princess of the United Kingdom (1768–1840) 180
Augustus 85, 113n.7
Austen, Jane (1775–1817) 3, 54, 90, 123, 158n.8
    Northanger Abbey 27, 48, 59
    Persuasion 27, 49, 59, 165
    Sanditon 27, 108–9, 227–9, 250

Bachelard, Gaston 31
Baden-Baden 3, 251
Baker, Thomas (b. 1680/81, active 1700–9) 160n.51
    Tunbridge Walks 137, 151, 166, 168, 240
Balaruc 1
Ballston Spa, NY 188
Ballyspellan, Ireland 67, 187, 215, 254

Barbauld, Anna Laetitia (1743–1825) 229, 234–5, 237–8
Barèges, France 80n.93
Barker, John (1730–?) 89
Barnet 71, 225–6
barrenness 63, 66–9, 78n55, 80n.88, 143, 161n.72, 165
Bath 2–4, 5, 11, 20, 27, 29, 34n.6, 36n.7, 42n.76, 47, 48, 51, 59, 60, 68, 87, 102, 107, 109, 121, 123, 127, 149, 163, 178, 181–4, 217, 248
corporation 88, 126, 174, 182, 232
General Infirmary 3, 30, 232, 248
Bath, Virginia 14
bathing 19, 21, 22, 33n.1, 42n.75, 57, 60–1, 84–5, 87–8
bath women 125, 126
bathing costumes 127
bathing machines 124, 134
Batt, Jennifer 25
Beau Monde 30, 90, 178, 235
Benedict, Barbara 11, 38n.24, 150
Bickham, George, the Younger (1706–71) 131
Blackman, Cally 154
blindness 59, 200
blood
bleeding 85, 93
circulation 72, 87, 93, 139, 215
bluestockings 186–7
bog 104–5
see also marshes
Boileau, Nicolas (1636–1711) 110
bones 97–8
Bonny, Anne (1697–1721) 152, 162n.100
boredom 26, 74, 172, 216
Borsay, Anne 30, 54, 232
Borsay, Peter 7, 29, 37n.18, 147, 223, 226, 255
Boswell, James (1740–95) 73
bottled water 14, 19, 193, 253

Bourbon-l'Archambault, France 174
bowels 62, 82, 90, 103, 106, 110, 114n33, 188
Braddock, Fanny (?–1731) 221–2
Brighthelstome *see* Brighton
Brighton 6, 11, 134, 185–6
Bristol Hotwells 3, 5, 11, 27, 50, 51, 75n16, 102–3, 107, 155, 224
Bristol, Pennsylvania 107–8
Buchan, William (1729–1805) 14, 18, 23–4, 84, 112n.3, 120
Burnby, John (active 1772–85) 141, 150, 180
Burney, Frances (1752–1840) 27, 54
Evelina 27, 50, 154–6
Buxton 5, 10, 20, 37n.19, 42n.76, 47, 59, 60, 67, 68, 179, 232, 233
Byrde, Penelope 126

Cadogan, William (1711–97) 59–60
calcareous waters 9, 18, 19, 20, 105
care 2, 28, 34n.5, 49–50, 54, 56–7, 61, 64, 75n.14, 89, 125, 165–6, 186, 233, 249
carnivalesque 26, 28, 146, 150
Caroline, Princess of Great Britain (1757–13) 131
case histories 17, 20, 24, 63–4, 68, 70, 85, 95–6, 195
Casey King, William 226
casinos 215, 243n.40
Castle, Terry 151
categories (of spas) 4–6
Catherine of Braganza (1638–1705) 68
Catholicism 14, 94, 163, 182, 191, 193–204, 225, 233, 248
Causey, Bell (?–1734) 168–70
caution 18, 21, 23, 82
see also prevention

Cavendish Bentinck, Margaret,
    Duchess of Portland (1715–
    85) 55
Chalus, Elaine 30
chalybeate 18, 19, 51, 59, 61,
    63–4, 71, 87, 127, 234
    see also saline chalybeate
Chambers, Thomas 188
charity 30, 54, 230–3
Charles II (1660–49) 214
Charlotte Augusta Matilda
    (1766–1828) 180
Cheltenham 1, 5, 11, 18, 37n.20,
    88, 103, 138–9, 174, 177,
    179, 180, 231, 250
chemistry 14–20, 23, 24, 25, 67,
    95
    chemical analysis 17, 19, 23,
    24, 41n.62, 41n.65, 54, 60,
    67, 71, 91, 94–5, 194–5,
    230
chronic diseases 49, 58–71, 72–3
climate 51, 55–6
    see also air; rural environment
clinical observation 20, 54, 96–7
Cohen, Jeffrey Jerome 31
cold water 6, 24, 83, 85–6, 144
Coley, Noel 17, 29, 59
Colley, Linda 184
collieries *see* mining
Colman, George (1732–94) 85–6
    The Spleen or Islington Spa 12,
    26, 90, 136, 139–42, 156–7
colonialism 196, 252
colonies 14, 188–9, 228
Commedia dell'Arte 93
commercial interest 4, 53–5, 70,
    102, 195, 197, 212–41,
    217–18, 224–9, 230
common water 15, 93–5
comparative studies (of spas) 15,
    24, 29, 35n.3, 40n.58, 53,
    69
competition 3, 7, 29, 38n.29,
    53–4, 57, 108–9, 147, 150,
    159n.35, 166–7, 226

Conan 197–8
confectionary 31, 186
consumption 107, 137, 185, 235
contagion 119n.100, 146, 167
contamination 21, 147
controversy 17–19, 39n.42,
    41n.62, 53, 81n.99, 89, 111,
    114, 187, 194, 224–5, 250
conversation 108, 121, 131,
    154–5, 164–73, 177, 180,
    186–7, 219–20
Cooley, Ronald 140, 147–8, 179
copper 18
Corbin, Alain 31
corporations 34n.1, 110, 127,
    232, 237
cosmopolitanism 184, 251–3
Cossic, Annick 29, 58, 112n4
costiveness 71
Cotswolds 11
Cottom, Daniel 30, 53, 90, 106–7,
    126, 198
countryside 11–12, 38n.34, 105,
    120, 135–6, 184
courtship 26, 127–9, 144
Creigh, Hannah 178, 250
cross-dressing 151, 152, 240
cuckolds 140–1
cure 56, 97–9, 100, 233
Curl, James Stevens 39n.41

damps 85, 107
Dancer, Thomas (1750–1811) 189
dancing 100, 121, 122, 168, 216
danger 21, 31, 83–92, 93, 121,
    164, 213–23
    see also risk
Davies, Myles (1662–1716?)
    200–1
debauchery 121–2, 139, 157
debt 137, 213, 221, 224, 250
Defoe, Daniel (1660–1731) 218,
    225, 232
Derbyshire 9, 10
Derrick, Samuel (1724–69) 175,
    206n.41

desire 69, 120–63, 216
diarrhoea 189
    see also bowels; digestion
Dickinson, Richard (1669–1739)
    174–5, 206n35
digestion 60, 62, 71, 90, 106–7,
    144
diplomacy 171, 182, 185
disability 58, 174–5, 206n.35
'dishabille' 32, 122, 130–2,
    159n.36
doctors 142–3
    water doctors 22–3, 53, 94
Donnellan, Anne (1700–62) 55
dress 28, 130, 147, 149, 150, 152,
    167
drinking (water) 19, 22, 51, 109,
    140, 142, 144–5, 166, 180
drug 47, 57, 63, 64
    see also Materia Medica
Drummond, John, 1st Earl of
    Melfort (1650–1715)
    182
drying properties 20, 63, 71
Duckert, Lowell 31
Dulwich 5, 67, 230
Durie, Alistair 14, 187

economy 57, 88, 137, 230
Edinburgh oily well 103
efficiency 56, 95
effluvia 61, 108, 117n82
Égalité, Philippe, Duke of Orleans
    (1747–93) 185
Eglin, John 29, 172, 182, 217,
    222, 250
elite 34n.4, 35, 70, 89, 102, 107,
    178, 188
Ellis, Markman 169–70
enslaved people 20
environment 11, 55–6, 83
Epsom 5, 7, 11, 71, 111, 144,
    179, 230
evacuation 20, 89, 91
Evans, Jennifer 69
excess 89, 91, 102, 121–2, 180

exercise 51, 56, 120, 140, 152,
    214
experiments 18, 42n.75, 96
expertise 23, 91, 174

faking 54, 236
fashion 4, 28–9, 57, 141, 149,
    164, 180
    fashionable diseases 28–9,
        100–2, 117n.74
fertility 60, 66, 69, 76n.41
    see also barrenness
fibres 20, 60, 61–2
Fielding, Henry (1707–54) 215,
    218
Fiennes, Celia (1762–41) 26, 103,
    127, 159n.22
filth 103–12, 236
fixed air 17, 41n.62
Fleetwood, William (1656–1723)
    201–2
Floyer, John (1649–1734) 24,
    84–5, 126, 127
fluids 20
fluor albus or 'the whites' 62, 64,
    66
food 72, 91, 184, 185, 213, 214,
    236, 239
fops 147, 166
    see also macaronies
foreigners 185
fortune-hunters 137, 122,
    239–40
Foucault, Michel (1926–84) 28,
    157
friendship 65, 98, 140, 186

Galen 120
Gallagher, Noelle 63, 147
gambling 33, 123, 172, 171,
    213–23, 228, 235, 240,
    241n.3, 241n.9, 250
gaming 29, 123, 213–23, 234
gardens 2, 5, 12, 140, 191–2
gas 9, 17, 19, 31, 103
    see also volatility

gender 30, 42n.80, 62, 137–8,
   155, 162n106, 166–7
   gender crossings 148, 150, 151,
      152, 154, 156, 240
   gender fluidity 147–57
   gender-bending 150–2
genre 21, 24–5, 54, 97, 129, 136
geology 9, 11
George III, King of Great Britain
   (1738–1820) 6, 37n.20, 180
Germany 21, 61
Gilthwaite 70
Glastonbury 194–5, 232–3
Glauber salts 64, 65
Gloucester 11
Gloucestershire 9
Glover, Katharine 4, 14, 226–7,
   238
Goldsmith, Oliver (1728–74)
   171–3, 214, 217–18,
   219–21, 222
Gomersall, Ann (1750–1835) 100
gonorrhoea 63, 64
gossip 147, 164–78
gout 48–9, 51, 59–61, 87, 100,
   165
   internal gout 60, 85
Granville, Augustus 253
grotesque 58, 135, 148
Guerrini, Anita 53
guidebooks 5, 24, 26, 69, 200
Guidott, Thomas (1638?–1706)
   191–3

Hamlin, Christopher 17, 24, 29,
   197
Hampstead 72, 146, 174, 225
Harley, David 21, 83
Harrogate 1, 5, 9, 37n.20, 51, 60,
   107, 127, 150–1, 179, 239
   Tewit/Tuewhet Well 104–6,
      118n.86
Harrogate, Pennsylvania 14, 188
Hembry, Phyllis 3, 4, 9, 29,
   37n.16, 43n.92, 52–4, 93,
   180, 194, 212, 226, 233, 250

Herbert, Amanda 30, 47n.112, 54,
   109, 126–7, 139, 147, 186,
   252
heritage 36n.8
Hermaphrodite 148, 152
heterotopia 28, 157
Hippocrates 11, 83, 120
Hoffmann, Friedrich (1660–1742)
   95
Holt 71
holy wells 14, 39n.42, 163,
   191–204
Honwick Wells 126, 127
hot water 86–7, 128–9
hubris 27
Hume, David (1711–76) 47, 74
humoral medicine 20, 167
Hurley, Alison 140, 147, 187
Hygeia 131
hypocausts 20
hypochondria 62, 100, 165

identity 101, 121, 146, 157, 188,
   239
imagination 92, 94, 115n.49, 147,
   177–8, 187, 196–7
impotence 145
industrial environment 105
inoculation 82, 112n.1
invalids 49, 50, 58, 127
inventory 34n.3, 37n.16
investment (in spas) 1–2, 222–9,
   250
invisibility 17
Ireland 14, 187, 195–7
iron 15, 18, 19, 40n.57, 72,
   104–5, 111
Islington 7, 11, 26, 90, 111,
   130–1, 139–41, 142, 144–6,
   191–2, 225
Italy 21, 54

Jacobitism 36n.8, 163, 181–4,
   195
Jamaica 14, 189
Jennings, Eric T. 33, 189, 252

Johnson Rachael 29, 47n.110, 124, 131, 169, 250
Jonson, Samuel (1709–84) 73

Kent 11, 45n.110, 137, 141, 180
Kerhervé, Alain 37n.18, 56

lampoons 25, 152, 169
Langham, Michael 232
Lawlor, Clark 100, 117n4
Le Person, Xavier 182
Lechmere, Elizabeth Howard, Baronnes (1701–39) 222, 242n.37
Lefève, Céline 73
Leicestershire 9
leisure 32, 35n.4, 43n.92, 44n.97, 48, 121, 234
  commercialisation of 2, 57, 249–50
leprosy 98, 200
Lesage, Alain-René (1668–1747) 93
'A Letter from *Tunbridge* to a friend in *London*' 68, 89, 148, 167, 201, 215–16, 236, 238
Lewis, Charlene 14
limestone 18, 19, 105
Linden, Diederick Wessel (active 1745–68) 18, 52, 53, 62, 64, 67, 71, 78n.61, 87, 189, 203, 211n.144, 230, 247
Linn, Thomas 73
Llandrindod Wells, Wales 5, 67, 101, 211, 237
Lockman, John (1698–1771) 130, 131
lodgings 34, 50, 58, 72, 143, 165, 232, 235–7
London 11, 12, 14, 53, 83, 179, 190–2, 214
London area 9, 14, 121, 144
London Spa 110, 144
Louis-Courvoisier, Micheline 62
lower classes 5

Lucas, Charles (1713–71) 53, 71, 81n.99, 224–5
Lynch, John (1697–1760) 233–4
Lyncomb 64

macaronies 123, 147, 149, 150–1, 164
  see also fops; gender; masculinity
Madan, Patrick (dates unknown) 83
magnesia 18
male gaze 127–9, 131–5, 149, 152
Malvern 5, 11, 17, 93–9, 103
March, Florence 137
Margate 6, 30, 85–6, 124–7, 131, 141–2
Marivaux, Pierre Carlet de Chamblain de (1688–1763) 178
marriage market 122, 123, 135–47, 240
marshes 108, 109
  see also bog
Mary of Modena (1658–1718) 68, 181–4
masculinity 134–5, 149, 164, 173
Mason, Adam 225
master of ceremonies 4, 5, 29, 120, 168–78, 217–18
Materia Medica 64, 65, 71, 73, 79n76, 87, 91, 249
Matlock 5, 10
Maupassant, Guy de (1850–93) 251
Mavor, William Fordyce (1758–1837) 138–9, 177
McCormack, Rose 29, 54–5, 66, 147
Mcintyre, Sylvia 253
McKellar, Elizabeth 12
Mead, Richard (1673–1754) 111
mechanism 17, 20
medicalisation 2, 100, 197–8, 247–9
medieval medicine 20, 21, 45n.107

melancholy 51, 138–9
menstruation 63–4, 65, 66
Meyer-Spacks, Patricia 165
miasma 119n.100
microscope 15
minerals 9, 14–20, 24, 31, 87, 94, 127
mining 9, 10, 15, 105–7
miracle 20, 24, 95, 96, 98–9, 117n.70, 182, 190, 194, 196, 199, 203–4, 211n.133, 211n.142, 225, 248
miscellanies 25, 43n.90, 150, 180
resort-based miscellanies 25
Moffat 4, 14, 30, 60, 66, 187, 226–27
Moira waters 10
Monro, Donald (1728–1802) 14, 53
Mont Pallas, Ireland 62
Montagu, Elizabeth Robinson (1718–1800) 55–6, 76n.34, 76n.41, 184, 187, 222
Montagu, Mary Wortley, Lady (1689–1762) 73, 82, 242n.38
Montaigne, Michel de (1533–92) 70–1, 81n.96
Moreau, Simeon (?–1810) 174, 177, 206n.45, 231
mud 50, 102–3, 105, 107

Nash, Beau (1674–1761) 4, 29, 121, 171–4, 217–18
nation 179–80
nationalism 184–5
Native Americans 188
nature 11–12, 38n.34, 56, 60, 74, 104–5, 106, 188, 224
neoclassical poetry 25, 127–9
nerves 62, 87
nervous diseases 61–3, 100, 102
Nevill-Holt 65
Newman, William 17
Newton, Isaac (1743–27) 17
Nicoud, Marylin 21, 248

Nisbet, William (1759–1822) 64
nitre 18, 19, 26, 71, 111, 128, 130
Northen Ireland 191
nostalgia 36n.8, 145, 149, 189
Notting Hill House 6
Nottington Well 6
nourishment 20
nudity 121, 123–35
number (of spas in Britain) 2

O'Connell, Anita 29, 100
O'Keeffe, John (1747–1833)
The Irish Mimic; Or Blunders at Brighton 134, 240
oak galls 15, 40n.57
obstruction 71, 91
Oliver, William (1658–1716) 36n.7, 81n.99
Oliver, William (1695–1764) 3, 36n.7, 87–8, 89
Oren-Magidor, Daphne 68, 198

pain 56, 60, 61, 72
Pannanich, Scotland 14
pastoral 25, 139, 144, 177, 227
patient experience 58, 61, 72, 101
patronage 5, 29, 180, 250
peat 103, 106
Pelling, Margaret 53
Pennant, Thomas (1726–98) 202
performance 26
periodicals 27
permeability 17
Peterhead, Scotland 14, 187
petrifying wells 9
pharmakon 82, 83–92, 112n.6
Pierce, Robert (1622–1710) 24
Piozzi, Hester Lynch (Hester Thrale, 1741–1821) 57
Pitkeathly, Scotland 14
placebo 92, 94
Plombières, France 1
plotting 182, 193, 209n.106
poetry 25
poison 83, 222

politeness 107, 122–35, 175, 177, 218, 219–20, 227
Pomata, Giana 95
poor 30, 54, 180, 229–41
Pope, Alexander 73
    grotto 15
Poretta 21
porosity 20, 21
Porter, Roy 29, 36n.8, 52–4, 59, 60
preparation 85, 88, 89
prescription 21, 22, 23, 72, 84
    self-prescription 89–91
pretext 55
prevention 21, 24, 82, 91, 163, 210, 216, 220–1
prices 228, 229, 236, 244n.77
Principle, Lawrence 17
Pringle, John (1707–82) 47
private space 30, 50, 165, 230
proliferation (of spas) 4
promiscuity 122, 131, 147, 238, 246n.110, 246n.112
promotion 4, 17, 23, 38n.24, 52–4, 76n.24, 95, 96, 101
prostitution 122, 137, 142–6, 171, 226, 240
public space 28, 30, 170
Pulteney, William (1707–42) 179
pump rooms 27, 33n.1
pumping 180
purge 85, 88, 89–90, 91, 102
purging waters 19, 62, 64, 71, 88, 196
Pyrmont, Germany 19

quackery 24, 25, 52, 67, 70, 83, 92–102, 143, 225

rake 68, 121–2, 138, 142, 155, 213
Ramsgate 6
Rawlins, Thomas (1620?–70)
    Tunbridge Wells 142–4
Read, Mary (c. 1680–1721) 152, 162n.100

Reformation 11, 191, 193, 247
regulation 88, 121, 141–2, 163, 170–3, 206n.29, 215, 218, 230, 233
relief 2, 48, 60, 98, 101, 249
reputation 4–5, 11, 53, 64, 68, 72, 93, 94, 102, 101, 108, 169, 222, 227
Restoration comedies 26, 123, 136, 142, 161n.87
rheumatic complaints 59–61, 167, 238
    see also gout
Richardson, John (1668/9–1747) 196
Richardson, Samuel (1689–1761)
    Pamela 170
Richmond 144
riding-habit 152–4
risk 23, 82, 83–92, 108, 223–41
    see also danger
Rochester, John Wilmot, Earl of (1647–80) 64
Roman baths 2, 20, 42
Rowlandson, Thomas (1756–1827) 123–7
Rowzee, Lodwick (1586–1632?) 63
rural environment 9, 11, 91, 112n5, 118n89, 139, 177, 228, 236–7
    see also countryside
Rush, Benjamin (1746–1813) 14, 188–9
Russel, Richard (1687–1759) 6, 11
rustic environment 12, 83
Rutty, John (1698–1775) 8, 18, 34n.3, 53, 62, 65–6, 67, 69–70, 71, 81n99, 95, 187, 224–5, 248

sacred spaces 195
Sadler's Wells 12, 136, 191–3
Saint-Gervais-les-Bains 1
saline waters 18, 19, 20, 64, 71
    saline chalybeate 67, 88
    see also purging waters

Salmacis 147
salts 14–20, 109
salubriousness 83, 103, 107, 108
Sanders, Robert (1727–83) 187–8
Sarratoga Springs, NY 188
satire 7, 25, 26, 27, 61, 62, 89–90, 94, 100, 102–3, 109, 138, 155, 164, 167
  visual 58, 122
Sawbridge, John (1732–95) 180
scandal 28, 137, 140, 165–72
Scarborough 3, 5, 9, 30, 51–2, 61, 68–9, 128, 131–4, 174, 179, 222, 237
  St Quintin 68–9
Scarron, Paul (1610–60) 174–5
scatological humour 7, 90, 110–11, 114n.35
schedule 120, 136, 140–1
Scotland 14
  Scottish doctors 14
Scribner, Vaughn 14, 107–8, 188
sea water 6, 19, 51, 83, 85–6, 124–7, 134, 187, 253
seaside resort 27, 29, 108–9, 124–7, 131, 187, 227–9, 252
seasons 5, 6, 25, 28, 73, 85, 121, 163, 169, 174, 178, 207n.52, 250
secret 65
Seltzer 19
sewers 103
(over-)sexualisation 124, 130, 142, 170, 122, 222
sexuality 69, 120–63, 217
Shadwell Spa 52, 189–90, 230
Shadwell, Thomas (1642–92)
  Epsom Wells 121
sharpers 139, 213, 217, 219–21, 238, 240
Shaw, Jane 248
Shaw, Peter (1694–1763) 18, 115n.56
Sheridan, Richard Brinsley (1751–1816)

A Trip to Scarborough 136, 164
Short, Thomas (1690?–1772) 8, 9, 15, 18, 34n.3, 42n.75, 47, 66, 69–70, 71, 91, 95, 104–5, 107, 187, 188, 247
shower 22
skin diseases 20, 60, 69–70, 95, 97, 98
smallpox 73, 82, 111, 112, 176, 200
Smith, Adam (1723–90) 47, 74
Smith, Joseph (?–ca 1798) 89, 103, 230
Smollett, Tobias (1721–71) 27, 54, 90, 94–5
  An Essay on the External Use of Water 51, 88, 94, 109, 114n.30, 115n.51, 197
  Humphry Clinker 51, 59, 60–1, 84, 122, 134, 136, 238–9
sociability 2, 5, 26, 27, 28, 29, 30, 56–7, 86, 107, 120–1, 136, 140, 165–7, 179, 186, 205n.10, 227, 249–50
sodium 18
solitude 49, 56
solvent 20, 60, 95, 147
Somerset region 9, 11
Somersham 226, 230–1
songs 25
Southampton 11
Spa (in Belgium) 3, 18
spa comedies 26, 123, 135–47, 160n.49, 240
springs 33n.1
St Chad 11
St Govor's Well 6
St Justinian 187
St Mungo's Well 3, 5
St Patrick's Well 196
St Thomas, Jamaica 189
St Winifred, Wales 163, 168, 187, 200–4, 210n.132, 211n.133, 230
status 55

steam baths 21, 22, 23
Steele, Richard (1672–1729) 25
Steele, Richard *The Guardian*
25
Stobart, Jon 38n.26, 234
stone 14–20, 103, 104–5, 234,
245n.91
stone and gravel 70–1, 81n.97,
226
stone juice 15, 67
Stoney Middleton 1
Stretham 232
Struve, Friedrich (1781–1840) 19
Suarez, Michael 25
suffering 29, 61
see also pain
suicide 218–19, 221–2
sulphur 18, 20, 41n.62, 61, 111,
127
sulphurous waters 18, 19, 59, 71,
91, 104–6
Sussex 11
Swanlinbar 187
sweating 20, 22, 60
swimming 124, 125

tables 15
tea 3, 108, 137, 121, 140, 166,
169–70, 213, 216, 235
temperature 20, 83, 94
see also cold; hot
Templeogue 187
tepidarium 20
thaumaturgic waters 14, 163, 191
theatre 121, 136, 150–7
theatricality 122, 136, 151, 192
thermal medicine 33n.2
Thorp-Arch 107
time 73–4, 88, 163, 253
see also bathing; seasons
Tissot, Samuel-Auguste (1728–97)
112n.3
tourism 11, 57, 93, 236–7
transparency 103, 105
travel 47, 50, 141
travel literature 25, 26

treatment 1, 57, 64
last chance therapy 64, 97
violence of 60, 62, 83, 87
Tunbridge Wells 1, 5, 7, 11, 18,
29, 30, 55, 56, 60, 63–4, 68,
72, 107, 111, 127, 144–5,
147, 168–74, 178, 179, 184,
198, 219–20, 226, 230,
233–4, 250
pantiles or walks 138, 173–4,
234–5
Turkish Baths 1
types of water 18–19, 71
see also calcareous; chalybeate;
saline; sulphurous; purging

ulcers 70
underground 103–4, 106
urban environment 11, 12, 29,
36n.10, 56, 57, 103, 112n.5,
120, 135–6, 147–8, 185,
227

vapours 100
venereal disease 63, 65–70, 122,
165
Vichy, France 1, 3, 251
Vigarello, George 21
Virginia 14
vitriol 18, 104–5
volatility 17, 62, 85, 94, 143, 230
vomit 91
vulnerability 29, 50

Wales 14, 187
Walker, Anthony (bap. 1622–92)
198–9
Walker, Elizabeth (1623–90) 198,
210n.126
Wall, John (1708–76) 17, 43n.85,
93–9, 115n.45
Walpole, Robert (1676–1745) 179
Walsham, Alexandra 39n.42, 57,
195, 198–9, 202
warming pan scandal 181–4
water poets 25, 43n.92, 69

water women 22, 34
watering place 33n.1
wealth 229–41
wells 33n.1
Werth, Tiffany 15
Wesley, John (1703–91) 60
West, Jane (1758–1852) 185, 252
Westwood 70
wetlands 11
Weymouth 6
White Sulphur, Virginia 188
Wigglesworth 91, 106, 107
Wilkes, John (1725–97) 180
wit 137, 144, 149, 155–6, 164, 168

women 29–30, 147, 155–7, 165, 168, 221–2, 227, 242
  correspondence 29, 187
  networks 49, 140, 147, 186
  see also gender
Wood, John (1704–54) 3
Woodward, John (1665–28) 111, 119n.110
Wyndham, Henry Penruddocke (1736–1819) 202–3

yaws 189–90
Yorkshire 9, 11, 70, 91, 101, 104–6, 107

Ingram Content Group UK Ltd.
Milton Keynes UK
UKHW051304190723
425431UK00010B/65